Working with Vulnerable Populations

Susana Castaños-Cervantes
Angélica Ojeda García
Cristina L. Reitz-Krueger
Editors

Working with Vulnerable Populations

A Multicultural Perspective

Springer

Editors
Susana Castaños-Cervantes
Escuela de Psicología, Facultad de Ciencias de la Salud
Universidad Panamericana
Ciudad de México, Mexico

Angélica Ojeda García
Universidad Iberoamericana
Ciudad de México, Mexico

Cristina L. Reitz-Krueger
Department of Psychology
Warren Wilson College
Asheville, NC, USA

ISBN 978-3-031-67709-0 ISBN 978-3-031-67710-6 (eBook)
https://doi.org/10.1007/978-3-031-67710-6

This Springer imprint is published by the registered company Springer Nature Switzerland AG
The registered company address is: Gewerbestrasse 11, 6330 Cham, Switzerland

Foreword

Humanitarian action and cooperation programs in the 1970s, derived from natural disasters (droughts, hurricanes, and earthquakes) and the recovery problems of the affected populations, mark the origins of the concept of social vulnerability. Nevertheless, in the social sciences, the concept of vulnerability was introduced in the 1980s with studies on social inequality and poverty.

Vulnerable people are those who, for different reasons, cannot prevent, resist, and overcome an impact and, therefore, are at risk (Araujo-González, 2015). In this same sense, Villa (2001) considers that "vulnerability is understood as the risk or probability that an individual, a home or a community may be injured or damaged as a result of changes in the conditions of the context in which it is located or by their own limitations". That is why studying the concept of vulnerability becomes a fundamental tool for designing and guiding public development policies and humanitarian action interventions.

The vulnerability has been associated not only with the conditions of the individual but, increasingly, with the conditions of the social environment in which their lives develop, giving rise to the need to incorporate *multicultural* perspectives in understanding this concept. Hence, vulnerable populations are often referred to as those groups of people affected by their physical and mental health. Due to the environmental conditions in which they live, they are in a situation of greater susceptibility to being harmed.

Hence, the term "vulnerability" contains considerable complexity. It refers to the possibility of harm, the finitude, and the mortal condition of the human being. The literature on this term is extensive, and there are many ways to understand the concept of vulnerability. According to the Royal Spanish Academy, the word vulnerability derives from the Latin *vulnerabilis*. It is composed of *vulnus*, which means "wound, blow, stab, and also misfortune or affliction," hence also the words *vulnero*, which means "hurt, injure," or *vulneratio*, which means "wound, injury," and by the suffix *-abilis* (-able), which indicates "possibility"; therefore, etymologically, vulnerability indicates the probability of being injured or damaged. Everything points to an external threat. These meanings of the term consider the risks and threats linked to the experience of fragility, precariousness, defenselessness, or uncertainty.

Situations that all living beings share make us susceptible to being harmed. Hence, it is crucial to delve into the term vulnerability and who and how they are affected by the vulnerability that they suffer intrinsically or extrinsically to examine different aspects of human reality: social, environmental, public health, economic, and physical, among others.

The study of vulnerability requires the collaboration of many disciplines to have a broader vision based on a holistic understanding of reality and the perspective it engenders and an understanding of people in the different vulnerability dimensions. This book integrates the work of international researchers from the social and health sciences with original chapters in the form of empirical, theoretical/conceptual studies and case studies that provide universal ideas and new perspectives on physical, psychological and social vulnerability.

The interdisciplinary approach presented in this book is crucial for studying vulnerability, as it opens up a new research and comprehensive perspective. This book is organized into three major sections referring to the physical, psychological, and social dimensions of vulnerability, with 20 chapters divided as follows:

Part I: Physical Vulnerability contains a collection of six chapters that address diverse circumstances and vulnerable groups associated with the physical dimension of vulnerability, as would be employment opportunities for individuals with disabilities; a pathogen responsible for intrahospital epidemics; a helpful assessment index in diabetic foot patients; guidelines used to improved doctor-patient communication in patients discharged from surgery for ovarian carcinoma; physical activity with vulnerable children; and the effects of the internet and social media in chronic illnesses.

Part II: Psychological Vulnerability is a selection of six chapters that focuses on the psychological dimension of vulnerability by addressing issues such as psychosocial predictors of suicide risk in Mexican medical students; Art Therapy Intervention that promotes a sense of community in a sample of women living in a Mexican community undergoing extreme poverty; a chapter that provides a general overview of treatments for autism spectrum disorders, their efficiency and empirical evidence; multicultural and narrative therapy in a woman with severe mental illness; the role of self-efficacy as a mediator of the impact of traumatic events in Palestinian refugee children; and psychosocial characteristics of Mexican girls at risk of homelessness.

Part III: Social Vulnerability incorporates a collection of eight detailed chapters that focus on the social dimension of vulnerability by addressing cognitive abilities associated with learning in children placed in residential care; ethnic identity, conflict, and discrimination between the ancient Nahuatl-speaking people; the role of higher education in incarcerated individuals; sexual assault among women who conceive in rape, homeless females, and male college students; the genesis and evolution of feminist theology; a systematic typology of femicide; training of psychologists in child care and protection; and pedagogical approaches to address vulnerability in contemporary societies.

Therefore, the book highlights that there are at least two types of human vulnerability: an anthropological vulnerability, understood as a condition of inherent and intrinsic fragility of the human being due to its biological and psychic nature; and a socio-cultural vulnerability, understood as that derived from belonging to a group, gender, locality, environment, socioeconomic condition, culture, or environment that makes individuals vulnerable. Hence, human beings are vulnerable and fragile due to their bodily and mortal condition. On the other hand, the vulnerability that refers to the biological dimension is due to the damage derived from the relationship with the environment and others, which is social vulnerability.

Director of the Business Science PhD,
Faculty of Economics and Business,
Universidad Panamericana
Ciudad de México, Mexico

Connie Atristain Suárez

Ethics Approval and Statement of Competing Interests

We, the editors of this manuscript, assert that, to the best of our knowledge, any chapter presented herein reflects research that was conducted using practices outlined in such documents as *The Declaration of Helsinki, The Belmont Report,* and the American Psychological Association's code of ethics, including obtaining informed consent from all participants. We further assert that we are unaware of any potential competing interests held on the part of the individual authors, and that we ourselves do not have any competing interests of a financial or non-financial nature.

Aprobación ética y declaración de intereses en conflicto

Nosotros, los editores de este manuscrito, afirmamos que, según nuestro leal saber y entender, cualquier capítulo presentado en este documento refleja una investigación que se llevó a cabo siguiendo las prácticas descritas en documentos como la Declaración de Helsinki, el Informe Belmont y el código de ética de la Asociación Americana de Psicología, incluida la obtención del consentimiento informado de todos los participantes. Además, afirmamos que no tenemos conocimiento de ningún posible conflicto de intereses por parte de los autores individuales, y que nosotros mismos no tenemos ningún conflicto de intereses de naturaleza financiera o no financiera.

Preface

According to the World Health Organization, vulnerability is determined by historical, political, cultural, institutional, and natural resource processes that shape people's lives and lifestyles, which may produce a range of underlying drivers of vulnerability. Societies are becoming more polarized and immersed with exponential social problems such as lack of resources, climate change, migration, racism, terrorism, and violence that have increased the susceptibility of an individual, a community, assets, or systems to the impacts of diverse processes affecting lives and lifestyles. As such, individuals, groups, communities, and societies suffer from multiple, aggravated, compounded, or intersecting forms of discrimination, marginalization, and exclusion based on grounds such as age, sex, language, religion, political or other opinion, social origin, property, disability, birth, ethnic, sexual orientation, or other status. These disadvantages are higher in emerging or developing countries that need adequate, efficient, and sustainable protection systems using a rights-based framework, leading to adverse lifelong conditions. Thus, this book, which is specifically tailored to address vulnerability in these countries, is crucial in encouraging the design and implementation of effective and sustainable culturally competent interventions and assessment measures to address these hazardous conditions, diminish their negative impact, and improve well-being and quality of life of those affected. With this book, policymakers can develop and conduct measures for collective well-being that benefit vulnerable people and the general population.

Structured into three distinct sections—Physical, Psychological, and Social Vulnerability—this meticulously curated collection delves into vulnerability in its myriad forms and among diverse populations. By offering concrete examples and in-depth analyses, it serves as a guide for those working with groups with unique vulnerabilities. Moreover, it is a pioneering research tool, paving the way for culturally competent intervention programs and informing policymakers.

Physical Vulnerability (Part I), as used in this book, alludes to internal and external conditions that increase the susceptibility of an individual, group, or community to be affected or to diminish their capacity to cope and adapt to them. Internal factors associated with a predisposition or propensity to be physically adversely affected mainly refer to aging, chronic diseases, and malnutrition. At the same time, external circumstances include environmental hazards or artificial disasters. Such situations impact the capacity to anticipate, cope with, resist, and recover from hazardous effects, which cause people to be more fragile, require more assistance and special equipment, and face more restrictions and challenges, thus being physically vulnerable. The conditions that lead to being physically vulnerable aggravate when internal (e.g., immune system, genetics, sleep hygiene, healthy eating, physical activity, healthy lifestyle) and external resources (e.g., social network, income, household, healthy lifestyle, insurance, social security, support of family) are inadequate, insufficient, and lacking. Compared with developed countries, low- and middle-income countries (LMICs) currently face numerous challenges that increase the predisposition of individuals and communities to be physically adversely affected. Furthermore, in these emerging and developing countries, resources are seldom available to help societies cope and adapt to such physical vulnerabilities, leading to multifaceted and complex problems that, in turn, pave the way for exponential growth of vulnerable conditions. Therefore, it is imperative to carry out studies addressing physical vulnerabilities, particularly in LMICs, to provide research-based interventions to tackle the problem effectively.

The book's first section comprises six chapters focused on several types of physical vulnerabilities among different vulnerable groups, emphasizing emerging and developing countries. Chapter 1 addresses the topic of disabilities and employment. Chapters 2 and 3 delve into patients with diabetes. Chapter 4 explores communication issues among doctors and patients with cancer. Chapter 5 examines physical activity in vulnerable children. Lastly, Chap. 6 studies the effects of the internet, particularly social media, on chronic illnesses.

Our aspiration is that this section of the book will not only shed light on physical vulnerability but also lay the groundwork for future research, particularly among physically vulnerable groups in LMICs. The insights gleaned from this research are invaluable, as they equip us with the tools and interventions necessary to address physical vulnerabilities across diverse settings and populations. By understanding and tackling physical vulnerability, we can significantly enhance the health and well-being of vulnerable populations, especially in LMICs.

The book's second section (Part II) addresses *Psychological Vulnerability*, which is associated with some strategies to cope with the decrease in psychological and cognitive resources because of the attention focused on some external stimulus or stressor that generates emotional instability. To recover or increase psychological resources, everything that involves thinking adequately to make a good decision-making process about the behavior to respond most appropriately to the said condition must be told or stimulated. Hence, risk situations occur that prevent such recovery, for example, the Psychosocial Predictors of Suicide Risk in Medical Students, a study that identifies specific factors in the medical student population that may contribute to increased vulnerability to suicide. These factors include academic stress, social isolation, and lack of coping mechanisms. This study is relevant as it highlights a specific context where psychological vulnerability can be observed and studied. Other examples include a lack of Sense of Community, an essential condition for growing in unity, accompanying those who suffer from Autism

Syndrome Spectrum or Children who remain in Refugee Camps in Palestine. These examples allow us to visualize that in the most extreme condition of psychological vulnerability that seems there is a possibility to emotionally accompany or teach those who suffer from it to observe themselves and change their perception of things as a point of self-support for maintaining emotional sanity and with it, the optimal functioning required according to the circumstances of adversity.

In this sense, it would be necessary to delve deep into what psychological vulnerability truly means. Wilches-Chaux (1993) stated that the term "vulnerability" is a complex concept, associated not only with the conditions of the individual but also with those of the environment (environmental, social, or other types). This complexity is further underscored by the role of external aspects from the social, economic, and cultural environment, which constitute the determinants of all situational and circumstantial conditions in people, interactive, and relational groups. Its last name, "psychological," is the result of the level of impact on the person, individually or as a member of that group, since it depends on using their personal resources and responding to the demands of the environment. The level of response, adequate, optimal, or functional, would be what we would call the "degree of psychological vulnerability." Understanding this concept is not just crucial; it is intellectually stimulating, as it forms the basis of our research and interventions, offering new perspectives and insights into the complex nature of vulnerability.

To better understand and ground the concept, unlike the other types of existing vulnerability, psychological vulnerability crosses all of them transversally since it is defined as the level of affectation and response to the latter, this being the one that goes hand in hand with all of them. It is its continuity because it exacerbates or limits it, enhancing the condition of individual and group vulnerability. Therefore, depending on the conditions of vulnerability that occur—far from the dynamics of the groups involved—they have an indirect impact, positioning these people and groups in a condition of psychological vulnerability in their integrity, dignity, autonomy in response, and sociocultural vulnerability, among others. The exciting thing is that regardless of the relational continuity that is built or accumulated as a condition of vulnerability, there is the natural condition that people have innate aspirations toward the actualization of their potential, the acquisition and search for knowledge, and the exploration of the environment, as the three elements that produce a virtuous cycle to generate the capacity for constant self-observation that allows self-regulation, whether by learning new ways of responding and reacting or improving existing ones, is that it can be addressed to reduce any condition of vulnerability. According to the Self-Determination Theory (SDT) by Deci and Ryan (1985, 2000), this potential for change and improvement is a beacon of hope in the face of psychological vulnerability.

This section comprises six chapters addressing psychological vulnerability. Chapter 7 presents a study on how suicide occurs in Mexico, proposing characteristics and details that prevention strategies in this regard should contain. The suicide risk path model analysis showed that in Mexican medical personnel, interventions should include techniques to suppress the emotional deregulation strategy. Chapter 8 focused on building a "sense of community" in promoting the social welfare of families using techniques borrowed from art therapy. A sense of community is a factor in a unit family's well-being if it happens in a community. In Chap. 9, autism spectrum disorder (ASD) is addressed as a symptom cluster of neuro-developmental origin that affects individuals at different magnitudes. It exposes different intervention approaches from the literature review focusing on the onset of childhood in early interventions, such as an extensive spectrum of possibilities in this condition. Chapter 10 alludes to the implementation of narrative therapy and critical multiculturalism with inclusive mental health paradigms to endorse vulnerable identities that intersect in this type of population. Chapter 11 depicts a particular case: Palestinian refugee children as a population suffer from a higher prevalence of psychological, cognitive, and behavioral problems, as well as unhealthy relationships and trauma. Findings reveal that traumatic experiences were related to increased academic, social, and emotional self-efficacy, suggesting resilience. However, gender, household size, and grade affected self-efficacy. Lastly, Chap. 12 examines differences in several psychosocial factors associated with violence among a group of Mexican homeless females. Findings indicate that intervention strategies must focus on psychosocial factors linked to specific forms of violence.

We trust that this book section, which delves into the complex realm of Psychological Vulnerability, will provide valuable insights and pave the way for culturally competent, research-based interventions. These interventions could potentially lead to future public policy actions, making this research a crucial step toward understanding and addressing psychological vulnerability.

Significantly, the book's third section (Part III) is a dedicated exploration of the pivotal topic of *Social Vulnerability*, which occurs when the disadvantage conveyed by poor social conditions determines the degree to which one's life and livelihood are at risk from a particular and identifiable event in health, nature, or society. Regardless of field, social vulnerability research strives to understand the social environment not just as a descriptor but as a predictor of vulnerability relative to changes in the environment, social circumstances, disasters, or health status (Mah et al., 2023). In our rapidly globalizing, technologically advancing, and socio-politically complex world, the concept of social vulnerability has emerged as a vital lens. It not only helps us comprehend and tackle the disparities and challenges that individuals and communities face but also provides a unique perspective on the complex web of interconnected factors. These factors, including economic, environmental, political, and cultural aspects, make certain groups more susceptible to adversity, crises, and systemic injustices than others. The populations discussed in this section may indeed face physical and psychological challenges, but the emphasis here is on the social environment that places these individuals at higher risk. Factors such as gender, ethnicity, and age are considered in the context of culture and religion. Residential circumstances such as incarceration and foster care provide a backdrop to consider educational challenges. This section, comprising eight chapters, invites us to consider the intersectionality of personal traits and the societies into which individuals find themselves born. Intersectionality, a term coined by legal scholar Kimberlé Crenshaw, refers to the interconnected nature of social categorizations such as race, class, and gender as they apply to a given individual or group, regarded as creating overlapping and interdependent systems of discrimination or disadvantage. It aims to tailor our problem-solving and collaboration to fit in a multicultural world. Chapter 13 presents strategies for fostering cognitive abilities in children placed in residential care. Chapter 14 delves into characteristics of ancient Nahuatl-speaking peoples, while Chaps. 15 and 16 address understudied populations in prison settings and the sexual assault literature, respectively. Chapter 17 studies women's vulnerability from a religious and theological lens. Chapter 18 provides compelling data on femicide in Brazil. Chapter 19 alludes to how to train psychologists in childcare and protection. Lastly, Chap. 20 provides pedagogical guidelines for vulnerability.

Our aspiration is that this section will not only deepen your understanding of social vulnerability but also inspire the development of interventions. These interventions, based on intersectionality and interculturality, which refers to the interaction and exchange of different cultures, hold immense potential. They can significantly diminish vulnerability conditions, paving the way for creating societies that are genuinely based on justice, equity, diversity, and inclusion.

Finally, after thoroughly analyzing the complete edited collection, the book concludes (Chap. 21). Consequently, we hope this book provides valuable insight, tools, and intervention strategies when working with vulnerable populations across multicultural contexts and groups.

Ciudad de México, México — Susana Castaños-Cervantes
Angélica Ojeda García
Asheville, NC, USA — Cristina L. Reitz-Krueger

Contents

Contributors

Ferdoos Abed-Rabo Al Issa, Ph.D. Doha Institute for Graduate Studies, Doha, Qatar

María C. Almario-Zgheib, Ph.D. Counseling Psychology Program, Department of Educational, School, & Counseling Psychology, College of Education, University of Kentucky, Lexington, KY, USA

Mira Amer, M.A. Department of Physical and Occupational Therapy, Faculty of Nursing and Health Science, Bethlehem University, Bethlehem, Palestine

Department of Physiotherapy and Rehabilitation, Faculty of Health Science, Istanbul University-Cerrahpasa, Istanbul, Turkiye

Nilay Arman, Ph.D. Department of Physiotherapy and Rehabilitation, Faculty of Health Science, Istanbul University-Cerrahpasa, Istanbul, Turkiye

Laura S. Bogardus, Ph.D., SHRM-SCP Center for Addiction and Mental Health Research, Department of Psychology, Clemson University, Clemson, SC, USA

Susana Castaños-Cervantes, Ph.D. Escuela de Psicología, Facultad de Ciencias de la Salud, Universidad Panamericana, Ciudad de México, Mexico

Estrella Cervantes-García, Ph.D. Faculty of Medicine, National Autonomous University of Mexico, Mexico City, Mexico

José de Jesús Alcalá-Anguiano, Ph.D. Universidad Popular Autónoma del Estado de Puebla, Puebla, Mexico

Alejandro Daniel Domínguez-González, Ph.D. Faculty of Medicine, La Salle University, Mexico City, Mexico

Jaime Echeverría-García, Ph.D. Humanities and Social Sciences Department, La Salle University Mexico, Mexico City, Mexico

Jacqueline Espinosa-Bautista, B.S. Universidad Nacional Autónoma de México (UNAM), Mexico City, Mexico

Jackeline Aparecida Ferreira Romio, Ph.D. State University of Campinas – UNICAMP, São Paulo, Brazil

Angélica Ojeda García, Ph.D. Universidad Iberoamericana, Ciudad de México, Mexico

Ximena Andrea González-Grandón, Ph.D. Universidad Iberoamericana (IBERO), Mexico City, Mexico

Gabriela A. González Ruíz, Ph.D. Universidad Iberoamericana, Puebla, Mexico

Lucy A. Guarnera, Ph.D. Institute of Law, Psychiatry, and Public Policy, University of Virginia, Charlottesville, VA, USA

Niceta W. Ireri, Ph.D. Africa International University, Nairobi, Kenya

Morgan McConnell, B.A. Warren Wilson College, Asheville, NC, USA

José Aníbal Ojeda-Núñez, B.S. Universidad Iberoamericana (IBERO), Mexico City, México

Michael Duncan Overton, Ph.D. Warren Wilson College, Asheville, NC, USA

Hilda Paredes-Dávila, M.Sc. Faculty of Psychology, National Autonomous University of Mexico, Mexico City, Mexico

Cristina L. Reitz-Krueger, Ph.D. Department of Psychology, Warren Wilson College, Asheville, NC, USA

Ricardo Alberto Rodríguez-Villanueva, M.Sc. UMG-Universidad Marista de Guadalajara, Guadalajara, Jalisco, Mexico

Ali Ruíz-Coronel, Ph.D. Institute for Social Research, National Autonomous University of Mexico, Mexico City, Mexico

Rosa Angélica Salcedo-Hernández, Ph.D. National Cancer Institute of Mexico (INCan), Mexico City, Mexico

Gerardo Sierra-Martínez, Ph.D. Linguistic Engineering Laboratory, National Autonomous University of Mexico, Mexico City, Mexico

Nicole M. Vélez-Agosto, Ph.D. University of Texas Rio Grande Valley, Edinburg, TX, USA

Julie Wilson, Ph.D. Warren Wilson College, Asheville, NC, USA

Katherine Wilson, B.A. Warren Wilson College, Asheville, NC, USA

About the Editors

Susana Castaños-Cervantes, PhD, as the coordinator of Social Service at the School of Psychology of the Faculty of Health Sciences at Universidad Panamericana, oversees the implementation of social service programs. In the role of coordinator of Psychology of the Mexican Panamerican Welfare Society, Dr. Castaños-Cervantes is responsible for coordinating and supervising the psychological services provided by the society. She is a cognitive-behavioral therapist, play therapist, and art therapist, specializing in mental health prevention and social and emotional learning programs for vulnerable groups. Dr. Castaños-Cervantes holds undergraduate and graduate degrees in Health and Social Psychology from the Faculty of Psychology of the Universidad Nacional Autonoma de Mexico and a postdoctoral degree in Intervention Programs for Vulnerable Groups from the Psychology Doctoral Research Program of the Psychology Department at Universidad Iberoamericana of Mexico City. She is a specialist in vulnerable populations, particularly children and adolescents placed in residential care. She has collaborated in designing Holistic Intervention Models for vulnerable children, youth, and adults, including older people. Her research includes designing Social and Emotional Intervention Models for vulnerable children, youth, and adults. Dr. Castaños-Cervantes has participated as an oral speaker at various international conferences worldwide, including the USA, France, Germany, and Spain, and has published several research studies in scientific journals indexed in SCImago, Scopus, and journal citation reports (JCR). She has taught in several undergraduate and graduate psychology and pedagogy programs. She has conducted more than 20 workshops for vulnerable groups, families of vulnerable groups, and employees working at institutions that serve vulnerable populations as their primary function.

Angélica Ojeda García, PhD, is a professor and researcher at the Universidad Iberoamericana, Mexico City. She has a degree in Psychology, and a master's degree and a PhD in Social Psychology. She is a Gestalt and Art Therapist. She has a Specialization in Brief Therapy and Psychological First Aid for populations in conditions of vulnerability. She was a member of the National System of Researchers in the National Council for Science and Technology from 2005 to 2020. She made two sabbatical collaborations: the first, from 2012 to 2013 at Loyola Marymount

University, Los Angeles, California (within the Marital and Family Art Therapy Clinic), and the second, from 2018 to 2019 at the University of California Berkeley (in the Health Initiative of the Americas [HIA] at the School of Public Health). Her line of research focuses on the work of emotional health in groups with vulnerable conditions, in order to improve their adaptation process, active coping styles, family unity, and sense of community, through use of Transdiagnostic Model and Art Therapy techniques. She has published four books and diverse national and international articles about these lines of work.

Cristina L. Reitz-Krueger, PhD, earned her master's and doctorate in Community and Developmental Psychology from the University of Virginia. She is currently an Associate Professor and the Director of Undergraduate Research at Warren Wilson College in North Carolina, United States. Her research runs the gamut from teen dating violence among high-risk adolescents, to sexual health, risk, and assault among college students. She is particularly interested in the way adolescent development intersects with risk and the legal system, and which social environments serve as protective factors for those risky behaviors. She has published and presented her research in numerous psychology and interdisciplinary outlets, and also enjoys translating scientific research for general audiences. Additionally, her work with incarcerated women over the past six years has led to an enthusiasm for and interest in higher education in prison settings.

Part I
Physical Vulnerability

Campus Recruitment Participation Among Students with Disabilities: Campus Staff and Employer Opinions

Laura S. Bogardus

Introduction

Employment of people with disabilities in typical community-based settings has been a consistent goal of disability advocates, policymakers, education leaders, and elected officials for decades (Riesen & Morgan, 2018). Among other provisions, legislations including the Vocational Rehabilitation Act of 1973, the Americans with Disabilities Act of 1991, and the Workforce Inclusion and Opportunity Act of 2014 support opportunity and outcomes for employment among people with disabilities (Ju et al., 2013; US Department of Labor [USDOL], n.d.). Most states now have "employment-first" initiatives that prioritize employment of people with disabilities in typical work settings (Winsor et al., 2019). According to research, community-based employment environments that include people with disabilities generally yield benefits for both employers and employees while normalizing an integrated workplace. Studies show that employees with disabilities generally exhibit better retention, less turnover, and similar absence rates and productivity when compared to employees with no known disabilities (Chan et al., 2010; Ju et al., 2013). Research also supports the idea that a diverse workforce including people with disabilities yields a more innovative and resourceful workforce with real financial gains for stakeholders (Accenture, 2018; Houghton, 2017). Hernandez and McDonald (2010) found that including employees with disabilities helped diversify work settings and led to positive overall work environments. Additionally, Siperstein et al. (2006) found that customers rated companies that employ people with disabilities more favorably than companies that do not visibly include people with disabilities.

L. S. Bogardus (✉)
Center for Addiction and Mental Health Research, Department of Psychology, Clemson University, Clemson, SC, USA
e-mail: lbogard@clemson.edu

S. Castaños-Cervantes et al. (eds.), *Working with Vulnerable Populations*,
https://doi.org/10.1007/978-3-031-67710-6_1

Research on employment of people with disabilities has not only explored benefits but has also examined the costs of accommodating people in the workplace. Job accommodations studies have shown that costs associated with accommodations are generally minimal (Hernandez & McDonald, 2010). According to the Job Accommodation Network (JAN) (2019), 59% of accommodations cost nothing and 36% of accommodations had a one-time median cost of $500. Accommodations with ongoing annual costs amounted to only 3%.

Yet, persistent disparities in employment participation by disability status continue (Riesen & Morgan, 2018). People with disabilities experience double the unemployment rate of that experienced by people without disabilities. The labor participation rate of people with disabilities consistently lags behind that of people without disabilities. In 2018, the labor participation rate among people with disabilities ages 16–64 was only 30.4% compared to 74% among people without disabilities (US Bureau of Labor Statistics [USBLS], 2018).

Many factors are likely at play when seeking to reconcile the disconnect between research findings that outline the benefits of employing people with disabilities and the lower statistical rates of their employment participation. Some factors, such as lack of worksite accessibility, unaccommodating public transport, and inaccessible recruitment software, may be structurally defined in terms of physical or technical barriers experienced by people with disabilities when seeking to attain or retain employment (Partnership on Employment & Accessible Technology [PEAT], 2015). Other factors may be attitudinally based among employers (Houtenville & Kalargyrou, 2011; Kaye et al., 2011; Lengnick-Hall et al., 2008; Society for Human Resource Management [SHRM], 2019). Hernandez et al. (2008) found persistent manager bias against employees with disabilities, including "… fears that supervisory time would increase, productivity would suffer, and frequent absences would incur." Misunderstandings regarding accommodation costs persist, with managers reporting concern over the perceived costs of accommodations (Baker et al., 2018). In a 2019 study, SHRM found that over 70% of human resource professionals believe the cost of accommodations poses a recruiting, hiring, or promotion challenge.

Notwithstanding the fact that people with disabilities experience less involvement in employment than those without disabilities, college attendance among students with disabilities has risen (Barnar-Brak et al., 2010; Postsecondary National Policy Institute [PNPI], 2018). The National Center for Education Statistics (NCES) (2019) reported that 19% of undergraduates in 2015–16 reported having a disability. Despite high rates of attendance and graduation, Feldman (2019) found that students and graduates with mental disabilities often struggle to secure employment. Securing employment that is appropriate to their education level may also be a challenge. People with disabilities are overrepresented in entry-level roles of employment within lower wage sectors such as manufacturing, service, and hospitality. They are underrepresented in the business and technical sectors and hold fewer professional and managerial roles (USBLS, 2018).

Because on-campus recruitment of university students remains a common tool used by corporations to secure professionally and technically qualified new hires, this study sought to understand how the practices of select university staff and corporate recruitment staff might affect levels of on-campus recruitment participation by students with disabilities, which could ultimately impact employment attainment. The following overarching questions guided this research:

1. Which employer characteristics are most important to university students in general, and more specifically, to university students with disabilities?
2. How might participation in employer outreach and recruiting activities differ between university students with disabilities and students in general?
3. What actions can universities take to facilitate the recruitment process between employers and students with disabilities?
4. What actions can employers take to improve recruitment and retention of university students with disabilities?

Method

Three standardized open-ended focus groups (Hennink et al., 2011) were conducted on July 18, 2017, during an event held specifically for the purpose of gathering feedback from select university staff and corporate recruitment staff. The event was hosted by a large multinational corporation and co-facilitated by a local disability inclusion advocacy organization, both of which were located in the southeastern United States. Both organizations secured internal approval for this study. As the researcher was an independent contractor and not university-affiliated, no IRB was sought. The corporate event was attended by 36 individuals comprised of the host's employees from its recruitment and diversity departments, and representatives from 12 regional area university partners' student accessibility/disability services, career services, and diversity offices. The event also included representatives from local governmental organizations and other corporations' recruitment and diversity offices.

The researcher developed a focus group protocol and interview discussion guide based on four overarching open-ended research questions, which were asked of each focus group. Facilitators and note-takers, comprised of employees of the host company and the disability inclusion advocacy organization, were trained in advance to elicit rich conversation on focus group topics. The advanced training provided an opportunity for volunteers to review the protocol and interview discussion guide, and ask questions about the process.

After a welcoming session, attendees were divided into three focus groups comprised of eight or nine individuals each, grouped by (1) university accessibility/disability services and university diversity representatives; (2) university career services representatives; and (3) corporate and government representatives. Within each focus group, multiple universities or employers were represented.

Focus group participants were informed that the purpose of this study was to learn more about connecting university students with disabilities to campus recruiting activities, with a goal of engaging more students with disabilities in internships and employment. Participants were guaranteed personal anonymity about responses and organizational affiliations. Participants were told that focus groups would last 1 h. Participants were asked to describe their professional experiences in response to questions (Bruner, 1991). No individual was required to answer any question, and anyone could leave at any time without reprisal.

Transcriptions and notes from the focus group sessions were analyzed using grounded theory to identify patterns across institutions and focus group type for each question. Single comments are not utilized except as examples that support themes.

Results

Demographic Information

A total of 25 individuals participated in the focus groups representing a diverse group ranging in age, gender, race, and length of employment with their organizations. The focus group consisting of university accessibility/disability service and diversity office staff included nine participants. The focus group consisting of university career services staff included eight participants. The focus group consisting of company and government employees also included eight participants. Due to the descriptive data collection parameters established within the corporate setting, participants' individual-level demographic data such as age, race, ethnicity, and gender were not collected.

Important Employer Characteristics

Company Reputation, Size, and Compensation

Participants generally felt that today's students, especially those who participate in internships or co-ops, are savvy in evaluating employment options against their career goals. Participants reported that students overall and regardless of disability status expressed interest in learning about the reputation and size of companies that recruit on-campus. A generally positive reputation was considered desirable by students across the board. There was consensus that an employer's mission and purpose are important motivators for students regardless of disability status.

Participants reported that many students prefer large company size where they may have greater choice of role, greater upward mobility, or greater opportunity to transfer to other geographic locations. It was also noted that some students prefer smaller company environments because of the greater perceived ability to contribute to a company immediately and in meaningful ways.

Regarding compensation, participants reported that the rate of pay is a primary motivator. However, students may not fully consider the value of benefits or other company perks offered when making employment decisions. Participants in one focus group agreed that health insurance is an important employment benefit to students with disabilities; however, this theme did not surface in other focus group discussions.

Culture of Community

Focus group participants reported that a sense of community in an employer's culture is important to students regardless of disability status. According to participants, students seek internships where they will be able to receive direction, mentoring, and an opportunity to contribute rather than simply do "busy work," while also working in a fun environment. Some participants reported that students with internship experience at larger companies often feel their internships did not offer the opportunity to be "seen and heard," and therefore sought future work opportunities in smaller organizations.

Established Internship Programs

Focus group participants discussed that students, especially those at universities with well-developed for-credit internship programs, may rely on the internship options developed by their university rather than searching for internships on their own. Participants noted that due to this predefined system, students participating in established internships may not necessarily identify their ideal employer characteristics prior to participation. No distinguishing factors between students with disabilities and students in general were noted in relation to established internship programs.

Geography

Participants stated that geography represented an important factor for all students when considering internship or employment options. They noted that some students want to be employed closer to home, while some seek to leave the geographical area with which they are most familiar. Participants perceived that students from the southern United States appeared less willing to leave their geographical area when compared to students from other areas of the country. Participants reported that geography may be more of an issue for students with disabilities as they seek to stay closer to known support systems such as medical professionals, relatives, or other organizations that provide important support. However, they indicated that the desire to stay locally may vary based on the type of disability. For example, one participant noted that while a student with an anxiety disorder or a physical disability may want to stay closer to their support system, a student with a learning disability may choose to "strike out on their own."

Willingness to Hire People with Disabilities

Participants reported that students with disabilities often inquired about employers' willingness to hire people with disabilities. Some reported being asked about the level of accommodations provided by employers and their openness to "... hiring someone like me." Participants felt that companies should openly communicate their interest in hiring students with disabilities. One participant offered this advice for employers:

> Let students with disabilities know positively that you want them. I think that can really be helpful. Most of our students would go for an internship regardless of whether they have a disability or not but there might be some who would be reluctant to go for something because they think, 'I'm not sure I can do that.' But if you say yes, we want folks with disabilities, then they are going to say, 'These folks are serious and they want people like me.' And so I think that that could be a real game changer for some of our students.

Employer-Sponsored Affinity Groups

Some participants in the employer and government focus group shared that their companies had formed employee affinity groups, and that such groups are inclusive of all employees that want to participate. Employer-sponsored affinity groups often serve as corporate diversity forums to promote a corporate culture of inclusion and can range in focus from women's empowerment to healthy living forums to young professional groups. Participants reported that their disability inclusion affinity groups tend to attract employees with disabilities as well as employees who have family members with disabilities. Such groups are apt to discuss topics of concern to people with disabilities and their support systems. Focus group participants agreed that the operation of disability inclusion affinity groups contributes to overall corporate inclusion goals.

University Staff Concerns

Student Nondisclosure

Participants in university-based focus groups reported that many students with disabilities do not disclose their disabilities through university mechanisms. Participants shared that some students appear not to want disability assistance at the start of their university career but may suffer in terms of university performance later due to lack of receipt of assistance. Participants perceived that students who are connected to university accessibility/disability services seem to have positive experiences, considering it a "home away from home."

Privacy

Participants in university-based focus groups expressed concerns about student privacy issues related to sharing information about students with disabilities between university offices and with potential employers. Participants noted they are not at liberty to release disability-related information about students.

University-Sponsored Affinity Groups

While employer-sponsored affinity groups were generally perceived by study participants to contribute to inclusive corporate cultures, participants of focus groups populated by university staff did not feel that the concept would be successful in a university environment. They felt that establishing such a group on campus, whether focused on career development or other shared topics, would essentially disclose students' private health information. They noted that grass-roots student affinity group formation may be possible but would need to be initiated, developed, and managed by students.

Students with Disabilities Reported Concerns

Disability Disclosure and Stigma of Disability

Focus group participants perceived students with disabilities to be reticent about disclosing their disabilities to employers due to fear of rejection. They reported that students with disabilities often experienced confusion regarding if and when a disability should be disclosed during the hiring process. Participants voiced concern that there is a general lack of awareness and understanding about people with disabilities. They felt that despite education and advocacy efforts, stigmatized narratives persist that persons with disabilities frequently cannot perform at competitive levels or do not possess the requisite work ethic. The process of finding employment, which is intimidating to most students in general, was thus perceived to be even more daunting for students with disabilities. In turn, participants felt that students' levels of comfort in communication with employers could be negatively affected by disability disclosure.

Due to perceptions of employer-based stigma, participants relayed that some students felt employers doubt their job performance abilities, which affected their interaction with employers. One participant stated that students "… kind of stay in the background, and then the employer is not the issue … it's just they don't want to divulge it." Participants felt that students who display a lack of confidence regarding disclosure and perceptions of stigma may self-sabotage connections with employers during on-campus outreach and recruiting activities. According to some participants, this can reinforce students' self-doubts about their own abilities.

University Facilitators of Employment

Normalizing Disability

Focus group participants discussed the importance of disability awareness and pride by focusing on ability instead of disability. Some participants in the accessibility/disability and diversity focus group reported helping students discover and develop their strengths, while others suggested holding awareness days or events to normalize disability status and reduce stigma on campus. They felt that students with disabilities could benefit from hearing success stories featuring other students with disabilities' positive experiences in internships and employment.

Intra-University Collaboration

Focus groups with university representatives generally agreed that collaboration between accessibility/disability services and career services would help facilitate connections between students with disabilities and career-related assistance, including on-campus recruitment. These participants generally acknowledged that more could be done to share information and resources between offices. One participant reported, "… we can put more effort into it and our career office working together with our disability office, and just kind of better prepare them." Another career service participant stated, "One thing I may have dropped the ball on is getting communications out to our student disability services department."

Co-location and Workshops

Some university-based participants shared that their career services offices and accessibility/disability offices were located within the same building, which helped facilitate working together as partners. University-based participants reported that career services offices provide student workshops on job searching, resume writing, and interviewing to students in general. Some participants suggested jointly promoting these general workshops to encourage participation by students with disabilities, while some suggested workshops tailored more specifically to the job search needs of students with disabilities.

Sharing Employment Information

Some university-based participants shared that employers may forward their internship and job opening notices to specific academic departments rather than to career services or other student services offices. Corporate recruiters seem to prefer a single point of contact per university since recruiting activities take place at multiple universities and can pose communication challenges. Participants suggested that greater sharing of internship and employment opportunities should occur between student services offices and academic departments.

University Barriers to Employment

Limited Self-Advocacy

University-based focus group participants reported that some students with disabilities are not adept at communicating their disabilities. Parental involvement in the campus lives of students with disabilities was discussed as both helpful and potentially hurtful when the involvement overshadows students' abilities. Over-involvement by parents was said to impede student growth, including development of personal advocacy skills. According to one participant,

> Often, we get students who a lot has been done for them. I really, you ask them to describe their disabilities and how it affects them. They cannot always tell you. We are trying to really work on that because we are very conscious of the fact that we are the last stop before they go on to employment or to grad school. They need to be able to do that. They need to be articulate to the workforce.

University-based participants noted that students must be self-sufficient, and that university personnel can provide training and resources but cannot interview for them. According to one participant, "My goal is to make sure by the time they're ready for the interview and that kind of thing they are ready. We have job preparation classes at our office that we can offer to help them feel more comfortable to be able to do that."

Complexity of Disability

Participants reported struggling to prepare students with disabilities for employment opportunities. The diversity of disability type was noted as complex, with the reminder that each student has individualized strengths and needs. One participant shared the following:

> I don't know how to help this student. He is [a] super smart student but he doesn't have the social skills to present well to the employers. How can we work with employers to better help students through this process? I think this is something that can be a great outcome.

Employer Facilitators of Employment

Welcoming Tone

Employers can reassure students that they are accepting of applicants with disabilities throughout the recruiting process. During the job search process, university students typically review websites of potential employers to learn of a company's purpose, culture, and job opportunities. Focus group participants suggested that employers put forth a welcoming and inclusive tone in the language used on company websites and career information webpages. University-based participants reported that students with disabilities occasionally request information about companies willing to hire "people like them," referring to their disabilities. Participants reported not knowing how to locate disability-friendly companies, with one suggesting that a Google search may be "the best option." Several participants mentioned a local retail distribution center that is widely known as disability-friendly because it publicly announced that 30% of their workforce consists of people with disabilities doing the same jobs and those without disabilities. One participant noted that this action "kind of took the stigma away … because [students] said, 'I know I can go there. If I have a disability, then I have a fair shot." Another participant noted that a local hospital system's vice president and CEO have made an impact on reducing stigma by implementing an internship program for high school students with disabilities. This program has made an impact by publicly promoting inclusive practices.

On-Campus Presence

University-based focus group participants suggested that companies allow and encourage their employees to participate in disability awareness activities held on campuses in order to reduce stigma and increase organizational familiarity with disability. They also suggested that employers conduct on-campus recruiting workshops that are open to all students but are held in locations that students with disabilities consider comfortable and familiar, such as a student disability/accessibility office. Employers can also highlight their inclusive practices during recruiting workshops. Employers may volunteer to conduct on-campus mock interviews in collaboration with disability/accessibility offices to better prepare students with disabilities while simultaneously gaining recruitment experience with this population.

They also suggested that employers share detailed information about job requirements when recruiting on campus, so that students can match those job requirements to their skill sets. One participant supported this comment by saying, "It is really again not about the disabilities but what they are able to do, and what is the job, and do they mesh? That would be for anybody."

Actions at Employer Sites

Focus group participants discussed the merits of inclusiveness training as a way for companies to build welcoming cultures among current staff. Some suggested that companies employ ADA coordinators to oversee accommodations and accessibility issues. ADA coordinators should be well known among staff for their role. For interns and new recruits with disabilities, employers can provide regular feedback so that students with disabilities know if they are doing the job correctly, and so that they can course-correct early on if there are performance problems. According to one participant,

> You know you are not treating them any differently than anybody else but just letting them know especially in the beginning of a job that they are doing it right, contributing to the company, they are a good employee and that kind of thing, so it's important they know that.

Participants suggested that employers arrange for mentors. One participant noted that, "Whether disabled or abled, everyone can benefit from having a mentor when they are new to a position."

Discussion and Implications

Research Question 1: Which employer characteristics are most important to university students in general, and more specifically, to university students with disabilities?

In addition to rates of pay, university students consider factors such as company reputation and purpose when evaluating internship and employment opportunities. Company size and geographical location are factors students weigh against their career and personal interests in the effort to make a good job match. In terms of community, university students want to develop a sense of meaning from their internships and employment. They want mentoring relationships and a chance to make a difference. Students who feel unsure of their career priorities can hone in on their preferences through participation in established internship programs.

For university students with disabilities, geography may play a larger role. They may seek employment opportunities near existing support systems, or they may take the opposite approach to distance themselves from those with knowledge of their disabilities. The provision of health insurance may be of greater importance to students with disabilities when compared with students in general, though this topic was not explored by all focus groups. The most sought-after employer characteristic appears to be openness to hiring people with disabilities. Students with disabilities look for indications from university staff, corporate recruiters, and public information sites for clues on company inclusiveness.

Research Question 2: How might participation in employer outreach and recruiting activities differ between university students with disabilities and students in general?

Students with disabilities are concerned about stigma on-campus and among employers. They worry that employers will consider them to be less capable or less suitable for work due to their disabilities. They are unsure about when and how to disclose their disabilities and ask for accommodations without inviting stigma. The stigma may lend itself to insecurity about one's own abilities. These concerns seem to result in reticence about participation in on-campus recruiting activities, thus distancing students with disabilities from resulting corporate employment opportunities supported through on-campus recruiting activities.

Research Question 3: What actions can universities take to facilitate the recruitment process between employers and students with disabilities?

University staff can improve intra-university collaboration while still enforcing privacy provisions. Those with co-located office space benefit from physical proximity in terms of developing connections between staff. Additionally, relationship development between career services, disability/accessibility, and diversity offices can be augmented for better sharing of internship, career, and recruiting information. Workshops and recruiting activities can be held in locations of familiarity to students with disabilities to encourage their attendance alongside students in general. University staff can work to share employer information between departments, including academic departments, to include greater exposure to students with disabilities.

University career services staff may be unfamiliar with how to assist students with certain types of disabilities during their job search, while other university staff lack specific knowledge on job search techniques. University staff training on understanding disability could be of benefit to staff as they assist students with disabilities in their internship and job searches. Trained staff could also provide guidance to corporate recruiters when interacting with students with disabilities.

Some students with disabilities may have limited self-advocacy skills, which affect their ability to promote themselves for career opportunities. This may be influenced by over-involvement of parents in instances when students have not been afforded the chance to speak for themselves on personal or career matters. University staff can attempt to build life skills such as self-advocacy among students with disabilities through coaching and training activities, which may ultimately affect employment success.

Research Question 4: What actions can employers take to improve recruitment and retention of university students with disabilities?

Employers can use simple techniques that illustrate their desire to hire people with disabilities, such as featuring welcoming and inclusive language and imagery on recruitment websites. They can publicly communicate their culture of inclusivity while developing existing employees' knowledge through inclusiveness, equity, and diversity (IED) training. Companies can launch affinity groups focused on disability inclusion to widen staff knowledge and comfort with disability-related topics. When preparing and promoting internship and job notices, corporate recruiters can ensure specific job and work environment details are listed, such as accommodations availability, which can help facilitate better internship and job matches between companies and students with disabilities.

Companies can orchestrate a visibly supportive on-campus presence by encouraging employees to participate in university-supported disability awareness student activities. On-campus recruiting activities such as workshops, information sessions, and mock interviews can take place in locations familiar to students with disabilities. Together, these steps communicate to students with disabilities that they are welcomed and encouraged to apply for jobs and would be valued as employees.

Limitations

This study is limited by the number of respondents and is not generalizable to the larger population. Additionally, perceptions of students' motivation regarding on-campus recruitment participation were reported by select university staff as well as corporate and government staff as opposed to university students with lived experience and expertise in these issues. Despite the obvious lack of student participation, insights from this study help illustrate university staff and employer perceptions concerning students with disabilities. It also serves as a valuable starting point for direct conversations with students with disabilities about on-campus recruitment participation. Additionally, this study provides helpful suggestions for reducing disability stigma on-campus and at job sites as well as increasing awareness of career-related information among students with disabilities.

Conclusion

Students with disabilities represent a relatively large and dynamic portion of university student bodies. Despite completion of university degree requirements, lags in employment participation persist for university graduates with disabilities when compared to university graduates in general. Explanations for the lag in employment participation by disability status, whether between college graduates or the general population, often center around structural and attitudinal barriers.

This chapter explored the opinions of university employees from career services offices, disability/accessibility service offices, and diversity offices as well as employees from corporate recruitment departments using semi-structured, open-ended focus group discussions. Participants discussed facilitators of and barriers to connections between university students with disabilities and companies that recruit students on-campus. Consistent with the literature on barriers impacting the employment of people with disabilities, this study found that lack of disability awareness as well as perceived stigma toward people with disabilities served as primary barriers to on-campus recruitment participation among students with disabilities (Baker et al., 2018; Chan et al., 2010; Hernandez, 2000; Hernandez & McDonald, 2010; Hernandez et al., 2008; Houtenville & Kalargyrou, 2011; Ju et al., 2013; Kaye et al., 2011; Lengnick-Hall et al., 2008; Riesen & Morgan, 2018). Creative ways to encourage participation among students with disabilities in on-campus recruiting activities were brought to light in group discussions. Universities and employers can work to reduce stigma about disability while offering greater exposure to internship and job opportunities offered through on-campus recruitment programs. They can promote welcoming environments both on-campus and at job sites to encourage students with disabilities to engage in competitive employment.

Future research should engage directly with students with disabilities to explore their perceptions regarding facilitators and barriers of on-campus recruitment participation. Research using validated assessment tools such as Popovich et al.'s (2003) Assessment of Attitudes Toward Individuals with Disabilities in the Workplace and Pruit and Chan's (2006) Disability Attitude Implicit Association Test can further explore attitudinal barriers among employers, university staff, and students to identify target areas for inclusiveness, equity, and diversity training.

References

Accenture. (2018). *Getting to equal 2018: The disability inclusion advantage*. AAPD & Disability: IN. https://www.accenture.com/t20181108T081959Z__w__/us-en/_acnmedia/PDF-89/Accenture-Disability-Inclusion-Research-Report.pdf#zoom=50

Baker, P. M. A., Linden, M. A., LaForce, S. S., Rutledge, J., & Goughnour, K. P. (2018). Barriers to employment participation of individuals with disabilities: Addressing the impact of employer (mis)perception and policy. *American Behavioral Scientist, 62*(5), 657–675. https://doi.org/10.1177/0002764218768868

Barnar-Brak, L., Lectenberger, D., & Lan, W. Y. (2010). Accommodation strategies of college students with disabilities. *The Qualitative Report, 15*(2), 411–429. https://nsuworks.nova.edu/tqr/vol15/iss2/10

Bruner, J. S. (1991). The narrative construction of reality. *Critical Inquiry, 18*, 1–21.

Chan, F., Strauser, D., Maher, P., Lee, E., Jones, R., & Johnson, E. (2010). Demand-side factors related to employment of people with disabilities: A survey of employers in the Midwest region of the United States. *Journal of Occupational Rehabilitation, 20*, 412–419. https://doi.org/10.1007/s10926-010-9252-6

Feldman, J. (2019). Career development for college students with mental health disabilities. *National Center for College Students with Disabilities Research Brief, 2*(4). http://www.NCCSDclearinghouse.org

Hennink, M., Hutter, I., & Bailey, A. (2011). *Qualitative research methods*. Sage.

Hernandez, B. (2000). Employer attitudes toward workers with disabilities and their ADA employment rights: A literature review. *Journal of Rehabilitation, 66*(4), 4–16.

Hernandez, B., & McDonald, K. (2010). Exploring the costs and benefits of workers with disabilities. *Journal of Rehabilitation, 76*(3), 15–23.

Hernandez, B., McDonald, K., Divilbiss, M., Horin, E., Velcoff, J., & Donoso, O. (2008). Reflections from employers on the disabled workforce: Focus groups with healthcare, hospitality and retail administrators. *Employee Responsibilities & Rights Journal, 20*, 157–164.

Houghton, J. (2017). *Driving innovation through disability inclusion*. Partnership on Employment & Accessible Technology. https://www.peatworks.org/blog/2017/aug/driving-innovation-through-disability-inclusion

Houtenville, A., & Kalargyrou, V. (2011). People with disabilities: Employers' perspectives on recruitment practices, strategies, and challenges in leisure and hospitality. *Cornell Hospitality Quarterly, 53*(1), 40–52. https://doi.org/10.1177/1938965511424151

Job Accommodation Network. (2019). *Accommodation and compliance: Low cost, high impact*. https://askjan.org/topics/costs.cfm?csSearch=2538611_1

Ju, S., Roberts, E., & Zhang, D. (2013). Employer attitudes toward workers with disabilities: A review of research in the past decade. *Journal of Vocational Rehabilitation, 38*(2), 113–123.

Kaye, H. S., Jans, L. H., & Jones, E. C. (2011). Why don't employers hire and retain workers with disabilities? *Journal of Occupational Rehabilitation, 21*(4), 526–536. https://doi.org/10.1007/s10926-011-9302-8

Lengnick-Hall, M. L., Gaunt, P. M., & Kulkarni, M. (2008). Overlooked and underutilized: People with disabilities are an untapped human resource. *Human Resource Management, 47*(2), 255–273. https://doi.org/10.1002/hrm.20211

Partnership on Employment & Accessible Technology (PEAT). (2015). *Is HR tech hurting your bottom line? A report on PEAT's 2015 eRecruiting research findings*. https://www.peatworks.org/talentworks/resources/survey-report

Popovich, P. M., Scherbaum, C. A., Scherbaum, K. L., & Polinko, N. (2003). The assessment of attitudes toward individuals with disabilities in the workplace. *The Journal of Psychology, 137*(2), 163–177. https://doi.org/10.1080/00223980309600606

Postsecondary National Policy Institute (PNPI). (2018). *Factsheets: Students with disabilities in higher education*. https://pnpi.org/students-with-disabilities-in-higher-education/

Pruett, S. R., & Chan, F. (2006). The development and psychometric validation of the Disability Attitude Implicit Association Test. *Rehabilitation Psychology, 51*(3), 202–213. https://doi.org/10.1037/0090-5550.51.3.202

Riesen, T., & Morgan, R. L. (2018). Employer views of customized employment: A focus group analysis. *Journal of Vocational Rehabilitation, 49*(1), 33–44.

Siperstein, G. N., Romano, N., Mohler, A., & Parker, R. (2006). A national survey of consumer attitudes towards companies that hire people with disabilities. *Journal of Vocational Rehabilitation, 24*(1), 3–9.

Society for Human Resource Management (SHRM). (2019). *Employing abilities @work: 2019 research report*. https://employingabilities.org/2019_EAW_research_report.pdf

U.S. Bureau of Labor Statistics (USBLS). (2018). *Persons with a disability: Labor force characteristics summary*. https://www.bls.gov/news.release/disabl.nr0.htm

U.S. Department of Education, National Center for Education Statistics. (2019). *Fast facts: Students with disabilities*. https://nces.ed.gov/fastfacts/display.asp?id=60

U.S. Department of Labor, Employment and Training Administration (USDOL). (n.d.). *Workforce Opportunity and Innovation Act: WIOA overview*. https://www.doleta.gov/wioa/about/overview/

Winsor, J. E., Gritz-Swift, S., Pearce, J., Darm, D., & Murray, M. (2019). Using the high-performing states model to facilitate Employment First in Florida. *Journal of Vocational Rehabilitation, 50*(3), 339–346. https://content.iospress.com/articles/journal-of-vocational-rehabilitation/jvr191016

Serratia marcescens Outbreak in Mexico City

Estrella Cervantes-García

Introduction

Serratia marcescens is well known worldwide as a nosocomial and opportunistic pathogen that has been responsible for frequent outbreaks, primarily affecting critically ill neonates, patients in neonatal intensive care units (NICU) (Arslan et al., 2010; Mahlen, 2011; Samonis et al., 2011), immunocompromised patients, and patients who have received prolonged antimicrobial treatment. *S. marcescens* can survive in different environments and reservoirs, such as drinking water, hospital disinfectants, soaps, and medical instrumentations (Samonis et al., 2011). It can colonize NICUs where the gastrointestinal tract and skin can be reservoirs for cross-contamination. It colonizes hospitalized adults' respiratory and urinary tracts, especially if foreign bodies such as catheters and endotracheal tubes are present. A person may also transmit it to personal contact. Moreover, *S. marcescens* strains from hospitals are multidrug-resistant and are reported to cause more invasive infections and tend to spread rapidly in nosocomial environments (Alonso et al., 1993; Grimont et al., 1979; Samonis et al., 2017).

Traditional methods for the typing of *S. marcescens* are often based on phenotypic characteristics such as biotyping, serotyping (Cervantes-García et al., 2014; Hamilton & Brown, 1972; Shi et al., 1997), antibiogram analysis, bacteriocin typing (Cervantes-García et al., 2014), phage typing (Chetoui et al., 1995), and plasmid typing. Most of these techniques are not sufficiently sensitive to distinguish different strains or are affected by physiological factors. To distinguish different strains, one can use other methods based on molecular biology, such as isolation of outer membrane proteins (Steppberger et al., 2002), whole cell protein fingerprinting, multilocus, and pulsed-field gel electrophoresis (PFGE) (Bayramoglu et al., 2011;

E. Cervantes-García (✉)
Faculty of Medicine, National Autonomous University of Mexico, Mexico City, Mexico
e-mail: estrellacervantes@yahoo.com

S. Castaños-Cervantes et al. (eds.), *Working with Vulnerable Populations*,
https://doi.org/10.1007/978-3-031-67710-6_2

Maragakis et al., 2008; Merkier et al., 2013; Morrillo et al., 2016). In recent reports, ribotyping (Sifuentes-Osornio et al., 1986) and PCR have been used for typing *S. marcescens* and have shown a high degree of discriminatory potential and reproducibility. However, most studies fail to identify the *S. marcescens* reservoirs and the correlation between the strains isolated from patients and those isolated from the environments.

In this study, we investigated the characteristics of an *S. marcescens* outbreak in the Instituto Nacional de Pediatría (INP) in Mexico City.

The project was evaluated by the Ethics Committee of the Facultad de Medicina of the Universidad Nacional Autónoma de México (UNAM).

Methods

The Instituto Nacional de Pediatría (INP) in Mexico City opened in 1992. It has a 235-bed tertiary care center and a NICU with 20 beds for critically ill neonates. When they no longer require intensive care, they are transferred to the Department of Infants on the same floor.

Bacterial Isolates Twenty-seven strains of *S. marcescens* were isolated during the outbreak in the INP. The isolates came from the following units: Neonatal Intensive Care Unit (NICU) (11), pneumology (9), neonatology (5), and infectology (2). *All clinical samples were inoculated in trypticase soy broths at 37 °C and 30 °C for 24 h and then conserved at −70 °C for future use in experiments. Afterward, all samples were subcultured in trypticase soy agar.* VITEK (Bio-Merieux, Hazelwood, Mo.) identified the clinical isolates as *S. marcescens, and the* biochemical profiles were determined.

Susceptibility Testing The bacteria were prepared by suspending the freshly grown bacteria in a standard sterile saline solution adjusted to a 0.5 McFarland tube. Then, antimicrobial susceptibility testing was performed by using the Kirby–Bauer disc-diffusion method on Müeller–Hinton agar (Merkier et al., 2013) according to CLSI guidelines (Bayramoglu et al., 2011). Antimicrobial susceptibility was determined for ampicillin, amoxicillin/clavulanic acid, cefotaxime, ceftazidime, ceftriaxone, cefepime, gentamicin, amikacin, ciprofloxacin, imipenem, chloramphenicol, and trimethoprim/sulfamethoxazole.

Biotypes and Biogroups The strains were classified in biotypes and biogroups according to the method of Grimont and Grimont (1978) of single carbon sources (m-erythritol, trigonelline, quinate, 3-hydroxybenzoate, 4-hydroxybenzoate, benzoic acid, DL-carnitine, D-ramona, lactose, adonitol, I-arabinose, d-sorbitol, lactose), as well as tetrathionate reduction.

Hemolytic Activity We also evaluated the effects of temperature on hemolytic activity. To assess the influence of temperature on the hemolytic activity of *S. marcescens*, we cultured the samples at 30 °C and 37 °C for 24 h and then harvested at log phase prior to assay for hemolysis. Then, isolated colonies of *S. marcescens* were cultured in blood agar at 30 °C and 37 °C for 24 h.

Production of Prodigiosin For the test of prodigiosin and to enhance the production of prodigiosin, the samples were cultured in glycerol-peptone agar at 30 °C and 37 °C for 24 h.

PFGE Genomic DNA was prepared as described in Goluszko and Nowacki (1989). The bacterial suspension was prepared by harvesting the colonies from trypticase soy agar plates after overnight incubation at 37 °C. An isolated colony of each sample was inoculated into 5 mL of trypticase soy broth and incubated overnight at 37 °C. The culture was adjusted to 1×10^9 CFU/ml and centrifuged. The supernatant was removed, and the pellet was resuspended in 2 mL of the buffer (10 mM Tris–HCl, 50 mM EDTA, pH 7.5). The bacterial suspension was then mixed with an equal volume of 2% low-melting agarose (Bio-Rad, Mexico) and solidified in a 100-μl plug mold at 4 °C for 45 min. The DNA block was incubated for 2 h at 37 °C in 1 ml of lysis buffer (10 mM Tris–HCl, 100 mM EDTA, 100 mM NaCl, 0.5% Brij 58, 0.2% sodium deoxycholate, 0.5% sodium lauroyl sarcosine, lysozyme [0.5 mg/ml]). Following this step, the lysis buffer was replaced with 1 ml of proteolysis buffer (1% sodium lauroyl sarcosine, 0.5 M EDTA, pH 9.5, proteinase K 500 μg/mL), and this solution was incubated at 50 °C overnight. To eliminate the lysed bacterial material and inactivate proteinase K activity, we rinsed the DNA blocks four times at room temperature in 10 mL of Tris–EDTA buffer (10 mM Tris–HCl pH 7.5, 1 mM EDTA). A slice of each plug was cut and incubated with SpeI (Roche, Mexico). PFGE separated restriction fragments of DNA with a CHEF-DRII system (Bio-Rad Laboratories) through 5–60 pulsed over to 20 h at 200 V. The gels were stained for 20 min with ethidium bromide dec, colorized in distilled water for 20 min, and photographed with filtered ultraviolet light. If the patterns were identical, the isolates had the same strain as their PFGE. The isolate was considered a closely related strain if the PFGE pattern differed from the outbreak pattern by two or three bands.

The statistical analysis was performed using R 2.15.3 (R-project, http://www.r--project.org). Medians and interquartile ranges (Q1 and Q3) were calculated for all sampling times when data were not normally distributed. Means and 95% confidence interval (95% CI) were used for normally distributed data. Kruskal–Wallis test for non-normal data was used to evaluate the differences between sampling times. Fisher's exact test was used to compare proportions. In all cases, P values of <0.05 were considered significant.

Results

All 27 patients admitted to the NICU were identified as infected by *S. marcescens*. Table 1 shows the clinical and demographic data of the infants. All the infants required anti-biotherapy, and the preterm infants remained for a longer time (45 days) at the NICU compared with the normal-term ones. In particular, prematurity of birth is associated with infections due to low weight and a not well-developed immune system.

Table 2 shows the isolated sites of the outbreak related to *S. marcescens*. The biochemical profiles were identified using the Vitek system, and no differences were observed. The results of biotyping using the method of Grimont and Grimont (1978) did not correlate with those by PFGE. The former results indicated that all the strains corresponded to biogroup A8 and that the total number of strains was biotype A5. On the other hand, all the strains had the same PFGE patterns (type A).

Table 3 shows the pattern of susceptibility of all isolates. All the *S. marcescens* outbreak isolates were resistant to ampicillin, amoxicillin/clavulanic, cefoxitin, cefepime, and ciprofloxacin. Third-generation cephalosporins (ceftazidime and cefotaxime), ceftriaxone, and piperalizina/tazobactam also exhibited high resistance rates. Imipenem exhibited high antimicrobial activity rates in our study against *S. marcescens* strains. In addition, macrolides and the combination of trimethoprim with sulfonamides were found to be highly active against *S. marcescens*.

Table 1 Clinic and demographic data of the infants ($N = 27$)

Gestational age	
Preterm	4 (15%)
Normal term delivery	23 (85%)
Gender	
Male	10 (37%)
Female	17 (63%)
Delivery mode	
Vaginal	15 (56%)
Cesarean section	12 (44%)
Birth weight	2.000–2.700 kg
Antibiotherapy	
Yes	27
No	0
Bronchopulmonary dysplasia	
Yes	6 (22%)
No	21 (78%)
Parenteral nutrition (days)	10
Enteral nutrition (days)	45
Preterm infants NICU (days)	45
Average hospital (days)	68

Table 2 *S. marcescens* isolates ($N = 27$)

Unit	Cases	Type of simple
NICU	11 (40.8%)	Blood
Pneumology	9 (33.3%)	Bronchial aspiratc
Infectology	2 (7.4%)	Catheter
Neonatology	3 (11.1%)	Peritoneal fluid
	2 (7.4%)	Cerebrospinal fluid
Total	27	

Table 3 Antimicrobial susceptibility

Antibiotic	% of susceptible cases
Ampicillin	0
Amoxicillin/clavulanic	0
Cefoxitin	0
Cefepime	0
Ciprofloxacin	0
Cefotaxime	25
Ceftazidime	25
Ceftriaxone	28
Piperalizina/tazobactam	30
Amikacin	70
Gentamicin	75
Trimethoprim/sulfamethoxazole	75
Imipenem	96

Another virulence factor is hemolysin. We observed hemolysis around the colony when cultured in blood agar at 30 °C. On the other hand, when cultured in blood agar at 37 °C, there was no hemolysis. We observed the same result with prodigiosin when *S. marcescens* strains were cultured in glycerol-peptone agar at 30 °C and 37 °C. They developed the red pigment (prodigiosin) at 30 °C, and the strains were white colonies at 37 °C (Fig. 1).

Discussion

S. marcescens is an opportunistic, Gram-negative, and well-recognized nosocomial pathogen. It causes severe illnesses commonly seen in immunocompromised patients. In newborns, these organisms can be responsible for sepsis and meningitis, which have a high fatality rate (Dessi et al., 2009; Grimont & Grimont, 1978; Sifuentes-Osornio & Groschel, 1987; Tenover et al., 1995). However, the source of *S. marcescens* outbreaks remains unknown (Merkier et al., 2013; Sifuentes-Osornio & Groschel, 1987). This can partially be explained by the prevalence and resistance of the microorganism since it can survive for long periods on inanimate surfaces

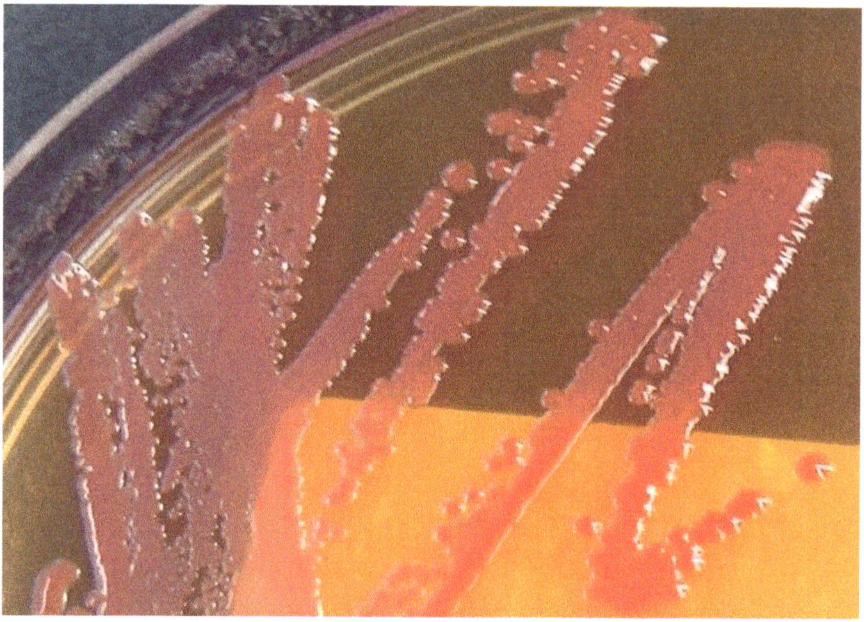

Fig. 1 *Serratia marcescens* prodigiosin. (Source: Author's research)

such as medical devices, soap, breast pumps, antiseptic solutions, catheters, and endotracheal tubes (Dessi et al., 2009; Goluszko & Nowacki, 1989; Grimont & Grimont, 1978; Ligozzi et al., 2010; Poole & Braun, 1988; Tenover et al., 1995). Also, *S. marcescens* colonizes symptomatic and asymptomatic hosts' respiratory and/or gastrointestinal tract (Carbonell et al., 2003; Sifuentes-Osornio et al., 1986; Steppberger et al., 2002).

In newborns, the main risk factors for the acquisition of an *S. marcescens* infection are the following: immaturity of the immune system and low birth weight (<1.500 kg) in preterm newborns (Cervantes-García et al., 2014), length of stay (Martineau et al., 2018), and the use of antibiotics, especially if they are broad-spectrum and administered empirically (Villari et al., 2001). In our study, the infants initially received empirical antibiotic therapy because it was not known which pathogen was causing the symptomatology, and this may have contributed to developing the multi-resistance of the pathogen. Afterward, our study revealed that *S. marcescens* was responsible for the outbreak and determined that antibiotic effectively eradicated the infection. In this regard, a study by Villari et al. suggested that empirical antibiotic therapy with ampicillin associated with an aminoglycoside (gentamicin or netilmicin) was a predisposing factor for the acquisition of *S. marcescens* in newborns involved in an epidemic event (Perotti et al., 2007).

Due to its diverse antibiotic resistance, infections caused by *S. marcescens* may be challenging to treat. This species displays intrinsic resistance to several classes of antibiotics, including some b-lactams and tetracyclines (Maragakis et al., 2008;

Merkier et al., 2013; Steppberger et al., 2002). In our study, the *S. marcescens* strains were resistant to ampicillin, amoxicillin/clavulanic, cefoxitin, cefepime, and ciprofloxacin. They also exhibited high resistance rates to third-generation cephalosporins (ceftazidime and cefotaxime), ceftriaxone, and piperalizina/tazobactam. These are all b-lactams. Tetracyclines were not administered because they can damage the teeth, delay the development of the skeleton and bones, and, in some cases, cause kidney damage in children less than 8 years old.

S. marcescens is intrinsically susceptible to other classes of antimicrobials, including quinolones and aminoglycosides, though chromosomal or plasmid-mediated resistance to some of these has been reported (Maragakis et al., 2008; Merkier et al., 2013; Steppberger et al., 2002). Our study found that *S. marcescens* is highly susceptible to imipenem and macrolides (amikacin and gentamicin) and the combination of trimethoprim/sulfamethoxazole. This is consistent with the results of other works (Ligozzi et al., 2010; Poole & Braun, 1988).

Our results indicate that all the strains belonged to biogroup A8 and biotype A5, which agrees with other works (Carbonell et al., 2003; Carbonell et al., 2000; Goluszko & Nowacki, 1989). Phenotypic approaches based on metabolic or biological characteristics such as the ones used in our study (biotyping with the Grimont and Grimont method and tetrathionate reduction and antibiograms) (Jang et al., 2001; Shi et al., 1997) can be carried out rapidly, and their results can be used as epidemiological markers. Nevertheless, they only provide presumptive evidence of infection by *S. marcescens* because their applicability has been limited due to insufficient discrimination between closely related organisms. On the other hand, molecular genotyping methods such as PFGE (Abrahantes-Pérez et al., 2013; Gulani et al., 2012; Lapenda et al., 2015) have gained popularity due to their sensitivity. In our study, the PGFE method showed an identical clone in all the samples, confirming that cross-infection occurred. In addition, *S. marcescens* was the only pathogen responsible for the outbreak. It is possible that other pathogens were being horizontally transmitted simultaneously, but they were not detected and, thus, were not investigated. These outbreaks seldom have one cause or source, and several factors are more likely (El-Bialy & Abou El-Nour, 2015).

We also found that the hemolytic activity in *S. marcescens* was related to the temperature at which the strains were grown. We noted that strains cultured at 30 °C presented hemolysis around the colonies and that this was not observed when the strains were cultured at 37 °C. This agrees with other works (Cristina et al., 2019; Martineau et al., 2018; Prasad et al., 2001). This result is significant because several experiments in vitro show that the hemolysin of *S. marcescens* stimulates the release of inflammatory mediators such as histamine and leukotrienes, suggesting its role as a pathogenic factor.

On the other hand, we obtained that the strains produced prodigisin, a nondiffusible red pigment, when cultured at 30 °C and that this did not happen when incubated at 37 °C. This result also agrees with other works. Some species and biotypes of *Serratia* produce prodigiosin. These are mostly recovered from a natural environment, whereas the nonpigmented biotypes are prevalent in hospitals. Nonpigmented strains of *S. marcescens* are more resistant to antibiotics than pigmented strains because they often carry resistance plasmids. Infections caused by the organism may be difficult to treat because of its resistance to various antibiotics, as shown in the results of our study. Characterizing at which temperature *S. marcescens* produces prodigiosin is vital because it has been observed that it is antibacterial and antimalarial, kills some fungi, and has been used against cancer (Perotti et al., 2007; Palacio-Castañeda et al., 2019; Villari et al., 2001).

This work had limitations. We did not take samples from the staff members, environment, incubators, humidifiers, suction jars, antiseptics, soap, irrigation fluids, distilled water, inhalation therapy equipment, intravenous solutions, sinks, and stethoscopes.

Conclusions

We identified the outbreak in the hospital using phenotypic and genotypic methods. Phenotypic characterization of the isolates helps study the relatedness of microbial pathogens. Relatedness of one clinical isolate to another during an outbreak is essential in motivating the search for a common source or mode of transmission. Phenotypic methods have some limitations, and using genotypic methods such as PFGE typing is a gold-helpful standard for studying outbreaks of *S. marcescens*. This facilitated the implementation of effective preventive measures and an effective antibiotic treatment. During the outbreak, several control measures were introduced. Strict hand washing by personnel during their handling of patients was stressed. Nurses were encouraged to wear gloves when suctioning and during any catheter manipulation of the patients. To prevent outbreaks, it is necessary to pay attention to healthcare workers, mothers, neonates, and general risk factors. In neonatal intensive care units, colonized or infected newborns are the primary potential source of *S. marcescens*, particularly in the respiratory apparatus and gastrointestinal tract.

References

Abrahantes-Pérez, M. C., Reyes-González, J., Véliz-Ríos, G., Bequet-Romero, M., Gómez-Riera, R., Anas-Gasmury, C., Huerta, V., González, L., Canino, C., García, J., Váldez, J., Reyes, B., Váldes, R., & Martínez, E. (2013). Cytotoxic proteina combined with prodigiosin obtained from *Serratia marcescens* have both broad and selective cytotoxic activity on tumor cells. *Journal of Chemotherapy, 18*(2), 172–181. https://doi.org/10.1179/joc.2006.18.2.172

Alonso, R., Aucken, H. M., Perez-Diaz, J. C., Cookson, B. D., Baquero, F., & Pitt, T. L. (1993). Comparison of serotype, biotype, and bacteriocin type with rDNA RFLP patterns for the type identification of *Serratia marcescens*. *Epidemiology and Infection, 111*(1), 99–107. https://doi.org/10.1017/s0950268800056727

Arslan, U., Erayman, I., Kirdar, S., Yuksekkaya, S., Cimen, O., Tuncer, I., & Bozdogan, B. (2010). *Serratia marcescens* sepsis outbreak in a neonatal intensive care unit. *Pediatrics International, 52*(2), 208–212. https://doi.org/10.1111/j.1442-200X.2009.02934.x

Bayramoglu, G., Buruk, K., Dinc, U., Mutlu, M., Yilmaz, G., & Aslan, Y. (2011). Investigation of an outbreak of *Serratia marcescens* in a neonatal intensive care unit. *Journal of Microbiology, Immunology, and Infection = Wei mian yu gan ran za zhi, 44*(2), 111–115. https://doi.org/10.1016/j.jmii.2010.02.002

Carbonell, G. V., Della Colleta, H. H., Yano, T., Darini, A. L., Levy, C. E., & Fonseca, B. A. (2000). Clinical relevance and virulence factors of pigmented Serratia marcescens. *FEMS Immunology and Medical Microbiology, 28*(2), 143–149. https://doi.org/10.1111/j.1574-695X.2000.tb01469.x

Carbonell, G. V., Amorim, C. R., Furumura, M. T., Darini, A. L., Fonseca, B. A., & Yano, T. (2003). Biological activity of *Serratia marcescens* cytotoxin. *Brazilian Journal of Medical and Biological Research = Revista brasileira de pesquisas medicas e biologicas, 36*(3), 351–359. https://doi.org/10.1590/s0100-879x2003000300010

Cervantes-García, E., García-Gonzalez, R., & Salazar-Schettino, P. M. (2014). Proteínas de Membrana externa de *Serratia marcescens*. *Revista Latinoamericana de Patologia Clinica y Medicina de Laboratorio, 61*(4), 224–228.

Chetoui, H., Delhalle, E., Osterrieth, P., & Rousseaux, D. (1995). Ribotyping for use in studying molecular epidemiology of *Serratia marcescens*: Comparison with biotyping. *Journal of Clinical Microbiology, 33*(10), 2637–2642. https://doi.org/10.1128/jcm.33.10.2637-2642.1995

Cristina, M. L., Sartini, M., & Spagnolo, A. M. (2019). *Serratia marcescens* infections in Neonatal Intensive Care Units (NICUs). *International Journal of Environmental Research and Public Health, 16*(4), 610. https://doi.org/10.3390/ijerph16040610

Dessì, A., Puddu, M., Testa, M., Marcialis, M. A., Pintus, M. C., & Fanos, V. (2009). *Serratia marcescens* infections and outbreaks in neonatal intensive care units. *Journal of Chemotherapy (Florence, Italy), 21*(5), 493–499. https://doi.org/10.1179/joc.2009.21.5.493

El-Bialy, H. A., & Abou El-Nour, S. A. (2015). Physical and chemical stress on *Serratia marcescens* and studies on prodigiosin pigment production. *Annales de Microbiologie, 65*, 59–68. https://doi.org/10.1007/s13213-014-0837-8

Goluszko, P., & Nowacki, M. R. (1989). Extracellular haemolytic activity of *Serratia marcescens*. *FEMS Microbiology Letters, 52*(1–2), 207–211. https://doi.org/10.1016/0378-1097(89)90198-5

Grimont, P. A., & Grimont, F. (1978). Biotyping of *Serratia marcescens* and its use in epidemiological studies. *Journal of Clinical Microbiology, 8*(1), 73–83. https://doi.org/10.1128/jcm.8.1.73-83.1978

Grimont, P. A., Grimont, F., Le Minor, S., Davis, B., & Pigache, F. (1979). Compatible results obtained from biotyping and serotyping in *Serratia marcescens*. *Journal of Clinical Microbiology, 10*(4), 425–432. https://doi.org/10.1128/jcm.10.4.425-432.1979

Gulani, C., Bhattacharya, S., & Das, A. (2012). Assessment of process parameters influencing the enhanced production of prodigiosin from *Serratia marcescens* and evaluation of its antimicrobial, antioxidant, and dyeing potentials. *Malaysian Journal of Microbiology, 8*(2), 116–122.

Hamilton, R. L., & Brown, W. J. (1972). Bacteriophage typing of clinically isolated *Serratia marcescens*. *Applied Microbiology, 24*(6), 899–906. https://doi.org/10.1128/am.24.6.899-906.1972

Jang, T. N., Fung, C. P., Yang, T. L., Shen, S. H., Huang, C. S., & Lee, S. H. (2001). Use of pulsed-field gel electrophoresis to investigate an outbreak of *Serratia marcescens* infection in a neonatal intensive care unit. *The Journal of Hospital Infection, 48*(1), 13–19. https://doi.org/10.1053/jhin.2001.0947

Lapenda, J. C., Silva, P. A., Vicalvi, M. C., Sena, K. X., & Nascimento, S. C. (2015). Antimicrobial activity of prodigiosin isolated from Serratia marcescens UFPEDA 398. *World Journal of Microbiology & Biotechnology, 31*(2), 399–406. https://doi.org/10.1007/s11274-014-1793-y

Ligozzi, M., Fontana, R., Aldegheri, M., Scalet, G., & Lo Cascio, G. (2010). Comparative evaluation of an automated repetitive-sequence-based PCR instrument versus pulsed-field gel electrophoresis in the setting of a *Serratia marcescens* nosocomial infection outbreak. *Journal of Clinical Microbiology, 48*(5), 1690–1695. https://doi.org/10.1128/JCM.01528-09

Mahlen, S. D. (2011). *Serratia infections*: From military experiments to current practice. *Clinical Microbiology Reviews, 24*(4), 755–791. https://doi.org/10.1128/CMR.00017-11

Maragakis, L. L., Winkler, A., Tucker, M. G., Cosgrove, S. E., Ross, T., Lawson, E., Carroll, K. C., & Perl, T. M. (2008). Outbreak of multidrug-resistant *Serratia marcescens* infection in a neonatal intensive care unit. *Infection Control and Hospital Epidemiology, 29*(5), 418–423. https://doi.org/10.1086/587969

Martineau, C., Li, X., Lalancette, C., Perreault, T., Fournier, E., Tremblay, J., Gonzales, M., Yergeau, É., & Quach, C. (2018). *Serratia marcescens* outbreak in a Neonatal Intensive Care Unit: New insights from next-generation sequencing applications. *Journal of Clinical Microbiology, 56*(9), e00235–e00218. https://doi.org/10.1128/JCM.00235-18

Merkier, A. K., Rodríguez, M. C., Togneri, A., Brengi, S., Osuna, C., Pichel, M., Cassini, M. H., Serratia marcescens Argentinean Collaborative Group, & Centrón, D. (2013). Outbreak of a cluster with epidemic behavior due to *Serratia marcescens* after colistin administration in a hospital setting. *Journal of Clinical Microbiology, 51*(7), 2295–2302. https://doi.org/10.1128/JCM.03280-12

Morrillo, A., González, V., Aguayo, J., Carreño, C., Torres, M., Jarana, D., Artacho, M., Jiménez, F., Conde, M., & Aznar, J. (2016). A six-month *Serratia marcescens* outbreak in a Neonatal Intensive Care Unit. *Enfermedades Infecciosas y Microbiología Clínica, 34*(10), 645–651. https://doi.org/10.1016/j.eimc.2016.01.006

Palacio-Castañeda, V., Pérez-Hoyos, A., Carrascal-Correa, D., & Osorio-Echeverri, V. (2019). Antibacterial pigment production by *Serratia marcescens* using different casein types obtained from milk. *Revista Colombiana de Biotecnología, 21*(1), 82–90. https://doi.org/10.15446/rev.colomb.biote.v21n1.62435

Perotti, G., Bernardo, M. E., Spalla, M., Matti, C., Stronati, M., & Pagani, L. (2007). Rapid control of two outbreaks of *Serratia marcescens* in a Northern Italian neonatal intensive care unit. *Journal of Chemotherapy (Florence, Italy), 19*(Suppl 2), 56–60. https://doi.org/10.1080/1120009x.2007.11782448

Poole, K., & Braun, V. (1988). Influence of growth temperature and lipopolysaccharide on hemolytic activity of *Serratia marcescens*. *Journal of Bacteriology, 170*(11), 5146–5152. https://doi.org/10.1128/jb.170.11.5146-5152.1988

Prasad, G. A., Jones, P. G., Michaels, J., Garland, J. S., & Shivpuri, C. R. (2001). Outbreak of *Serratia marcescens* infection in a neonatal intensive care unit. *Infection Control and Hospital Epidemiology, 22*(5), 303–305. https://doi.org/10.1086/501906

Samonis, G., Vouloumanou, E. K., Christofaki, M., Dimopoulou, D., Maraki, S., Triantafyllou, E., Kofteridis, D. P., & Falagas, M. E. (2011). *Serratia* infections in a general hospital: Characteristics and outcomes. *European Journal of Clinical Microbiology & Infectious Diseases, 30*(5), 653–660. https://doi.org/10.1007/s10096-010-1135-4

Samonis, G., Vardakas, K., Marki, S., Stamouli, P., Mavromanolaki, E., Kofteridis, D., & Falagas, M. (2017). Resistance phenotypes and susceptibility of contemporary *Serratia* isolates in the university hospital of Crete, Greece. *Infectious Diseases, 49*(11–12), 847–853. https://doi.org/10.1080/23744235.2017.1361546

Shi, Z. Y., Liu, P. Y., Lau, Y. J., Lin, Y. H., & HU, B. S. (1997). Use of pulsed-field gel electrophoresis to investigate an outbreak of *Serratia marcescens*. *Journal of Clinical Microbiology, 35*(1), 325–327. https://doi.org/10.1128/jcm.35.1.325-327.1997

Sifuentes-Osornio, J., & Gröschel, D. H. (1987). Modification of Grimont biotyping system for epidemiologic studies with nosocomial *Serratia marcescens* isolates. *Journal of Clinical Microbiology, 25*(3), 567–568. https://doi.org/10.1128/jcm.25.3.567-568.1987

Sifuentes-Osornio, J., Ruiz-Palacios, G. M., & Gröschel, D. H. (1986). Analysis of epidemiologic markers of nosocomial *Serratia marcescens* isolates with special reference to the Grimont biotyping system. *Journal of Clinical Microbiology, 23*(2), 230–234. https://doi.org/10.1128/jcm.23.2.230-234.1986

Steppberger, K., Walter, S., Claros, M. C., Spencker, F. B., Kiess, W., Rodloff, A. C., & Vogtmann, C. (2002). Nosocomial neonatal outbreak of *Serratia marcescens*--analysis of pathogens by pulsed field gel electrophoresis and polymerase chain reaction. *Infection, 30*(5), 277–281. https://doi.org/10.1007/s15010-002-2141-y

Tenover, F. C., Arbeit, R. D., Goering, R. V., Mickelsen, P. A., Murray, B. E., Persing, D. H., & Swaminathan, B. (1995). Interpreting chromosomal DNA restriction patterns produced by pulsed-field gel electrophoresis: Criteria for bacterial strain typing. *Journal of Clinical Microbiology, 33*(9), 2233–2239. https://doi.org/10.1128/jcm.33.9.2233-2239.1995

Villari, P., Crispino, M., Salvadori, A., & Scarcella, A. (2001). Molecular epidemiology of an outbreak of *Serratia marcescens* in a neonatal intensive care unit. *Infection Control and Hospital Epidemiology, 22*(10), 630–634. https://doi.org/10.1086/501834

Utility of the Ankle-Brachial Pressure Index in Detecting Peripheral Arterial Disease in Diabetic Foot Patients

Estrella Cervantes-García

Introduction

Diabetes mellitus type 2 (t2DM) is a chronic disease due to a maintained hyperglycemia. The high demand for medical care for this pathology leads to an increase in costs for both the healthcare system and the patient's family (Cervantes-García & Salazar-Schettino, 2017; Nussbaum et al., 2018; Zhang et al., 2010). Among the complications of t2DM, diabetic foot (DF) is one of the most frequent and devastating problems (Boulton, 2015).

DF ulcers develop due to numerous interacting factors, such as peripheral neuropathy and peripheral arterial disease (PAD). The latter has a considerable impact since up to 50% of t2DM patients have circulation problems (Armstrong et al., 1998). Usually, PAD is a silent, asymptomatic disease whose diagnosis is often made when it is in an advanced state. In addition, there is a strong link between PAD and cardiovascular diseases, and the latter can lead to more severe complications and even death (Wacher, 2009).

Vascular alterations can be diagnosed quickly and easily using the ankle-brachial pressure index (ABI), a low-cost test that has a sensitivity of 95% and a specificity of 99% (Ferreira & Macedo, 2010; Julio & Galleguillos, 2009). The ABI has an ideal predictive value for an early diagnosis to help prevent vascular morbi-mortality (Medina et al., 2010; Norgren et al., 2007). Nevertheless, the use of the ABI is limited in DF patients with medial arterial calcification due to a high prevalence of false negative values (Rac-Albu et al., 2014; Reardon et al., 2020).

The objectives of this study were twofold: to show the usefulness of the ABI in the regular physical examination of DF patients and to determine how accurately the ABI identifies vascular complications in DF patients. It is crucial to be able to

E. Cervantes-García (✉)
Faculty of Medicine, National Autonomous University of Mexico, Mexico City, Mexico
e-mail: estrellacervantes@yahoo.com

S. Castaños-Cervantes et al. (eds.), *Working with Vulnerable Populations*,
https://doi.org/10.1007/978-3-031-67710-6_3

make inferences on vascular complications in diabetic foot patients using the ABI so PAD can be attended timely and a better, more efficient treatment can be provided.

The study research was approved by the Facultad de Medicina Ethics Committee, Universidad Nacional Autonoma de México (UNAM), and by the Hospital General de Mexico committee.

Materials and Methods

A prospective, descriptive, and correlational study was conducted from June 2015 to September 2016. During this study, 248 patients (163 males and 85 females) with t2DM and infected diabetic foot ulcers were attended at the emergency department of the Hospital General de Mexico, a tertiary care hospital in Mexico City. They were all given a questionnaire to collect data and informed consent. Afterward, all the patients had a clinical examination, and only 30 (24 males and 6 females) were accepted for the study. Inclusion criteria were patients with ambulatory management and age greater than or equal to 18 years who were diagnosed with t2DM and infected DF ulcers of grades II–IV according to Wagner's scale (Wagner, 1981). The exclusion criteria were the following: patients diagnosed with infected DF ulcers of grade V according to Wagner's classification; patients who had suffered a significant amputation; patients who had been hospitalized for five or more days; patients with cancer, endocrine disease, neurological disorders, or collagenopathies; users of monoamine oxidase inhibitors; and patients who did not want to participate in the study.

The first examination found that the 30 patients presented foot ulcers that had not healed in at least 5 months and that they had received empiric antibiotic treatment before the study. The posterior pedal and tibial pulses were detected and registered. The first one is laterally located in the dorsal area of the foot in the space between the first and second metatarsal. In contrast, the second is located immediately behind the tibial malleolus. The examination was completed by measuring the ABI (also called Yao's index) (Yao et al., 1969) using a sphygmomanometer and a portable vascular Doppler model EdanSD3V. In order to do this, patients were asked to take a supine decubitus position with the legs at the same level as the heart. First, their brachial systolic blood pressures from both arms were registered. Then, the sphygmomanometer handle was placed above each ankle's articulation. Afterward, each leg pulse's posterior tibial and dorsal pedal arteries were located, and the portable vascular Doppler equipment was placed over them. Finally, the value obtained from each ankle was divided by the value obtained from the corresponding arm. We always chose the highest value, and the result was compared with the reference values (Table 1).

PAD is a disorder that affects the blood vessels (arteries) that carry blood to the legs, arms, and stomach. PAD was mild to moderate if the ABI was between 0.5 and 0.9. An ABI of less than 0.5 was graded as severe PAD. Severe PAD is the hardening of arteries caused by deposits of fat, cholesterol, and other substances within the

Table 1 Yao's classification (1969)

Value	Meaning
>1.2	Incompressible artery, possible calcification
0.9–1.1	Normal
0.7–0.89	Mild condition
0.4–0.69	Moderate condition
<0.4	Severe condition

blood vessels. It is diagnosed by observing a restriction in the blood supply to the legs, which causes pain and cramps and limits the ability to walk (intermittent claudication). It can be diagnosed with the ABI using a Doppler.

ABI values above 1.4 suggest a noncompressible calcified vessel. In this case, the blood pressure cuff may resist the vessel's collapse, and a signal may be heard at high cuff pressures.

After the first examination, minor amputations (an amputation of one or several toes or a transmetatarsal amputation) were carried out on some patients who presented necrosis on some toes.

Afterward, using the ABI results and the state of the lesions, it was decided to revascularize the lower extremity of all 30 patients with the infected ulcer. This procedure was performed to prevent major amputations and help heal the wounds by improving blood flow.

During the study, the patients received an antimicrobial treatment using an antibiogram. The evolution of the wound's healing was assessed one day every week for 6 months at the hospital's diabetic foot clinic. During the assessment, each patient received surgical washing or, if necessary, debridement to help heal the wound. In addition, the patients received instructions on foot care (cleaning the foot and changing the bandages).

Surgical washing consisted of the following steps. First, the wounds were vigorously washed with a gauze or sterile sponge soaked with serum or physiological saline. Second, the wounds were vigorously washed with surgical soap (chlorhexidine or glycerin). Finally, the wounds were vigorously washed with a sterile gauze or sponge soaked with serum or physiological saline to remove all contaminants and soap. Finally, the foot was dried with sterile gauze and was bandaged with sterile gauze.

Debridement consisted of the following steps: first, surgical washing was performed. Second, all the border tissue, callus, hyperkeratosis, and dead or necrotic tissue were removed with a scalpel. Third, the wounds were vigorously washed with sterile gauze or a sponge soaked with serum or physiological saline. Finally, the foot was dried with sterile gauze and bandaged with sterile gauze.

In approximately 3 months, some patients required major amputations (above or below the knee).

The data was registered and analyzed using the SPSS v.22 program. We used the chi-square test and discriminant analysis.

Results

In this research, we studied 30 patients, 24 (80%) males and 6 females (20%). All patients were diagnosed with t2DM and infected diabetic foot ulcers. The patients ranged in age from 39 to 89 years old, and the average age was 57.6 years. Also, 17% of the patients reported smoking (a daily pack of 20 cigarettes), and 40% presented high blood pressure. High blood pressure was defined as a systolic blood pressure ⩾ 140 mmHg and/or a diastolic blood pressure ⩾ 90 mmHg. In addition, 13% had dyslipidemia (an increased plasma concentration of cholesterol and lipids in the blood).

The degree of the lesion in the diabetic foot was classified according to Wagner's scale. Most of the patients were grade 3 (47%), followed closely by grade 2 (40%) and then grade 4 (13%). In particular, the right (left) foot was affected in 63% (37%) of the cases (Table 2).

Table 2 Data of the study ($N = 30$)

Gender	Frequency (% of cases)
Male	24 (80%)
Female	6 (20%)
Wagner's scale	
Grade 2	12 (40%)
Grade 3	14 (47%)
Grade 4	4 (13%)
Comorbidities	
HAS	12 (40%)
Smoking	5 (17%)
Dyslipidemia	4 (13%)
Affected limb	
Right	19 (63%)
Left	11 (37%)
Antibiotherapy scheme	
Ciprofloxacin/clindamycin	8 (26.7%)
Levofloxacin/clindamycin	17 (56.7%)
Ceftriaxone/clindamycin	5 (16.7%)
Procedure carried out	
Surgical washing	7 (23%)
Fasciotomy	5 (17%)
Amputation of a toe	14 (47%)
Transmetatarsal amputation	4 (13%)

Seven patients (23%) required only surgical washing, while the rest needed a surgical procedure. Minor amputations (amputations of one or several toes) were performed in 14 patients (47%), a fasciotomy was carried out in 5 patients (17%), and a metatarsal amputation was performed in 4 patients (13%). Hospitalization lasted from 1 to 4 days, averaging 2.1 days (Tables 2 and 3).

All patients were given antibiotics according to an antibiogram. Three antibiotherapy schemes were used to treat the patients: the combination ciprofloxacin/clindamycin (8 cases, 26.7%), levofloxacin/clindamycin (17 cases, 56.7%), or ceftriaxone/clindamycin (5 cases, 16.7%) (Tables 2 and 3).

Table 3 shows the patient's blood pressure with which the ABI was calculated. In contrast, Table 4 shows the average ABI according to the type of procedure performed (surgical washing, fasciotomy, amputation of a toe, or transmetatarsal amputation). In particular, the patients who suffered a transmetatarsal amputation presented a low ABI, while the rest presented an average ABI close to 0.9. It is important to note that two patients who suffered an amputation of a toe had an ABI of 1.75. They were excluded from calculating the average ABI and the standard deviation because they were considered extreme points.

Findings obtained with chi-squared revealed a positive and statistically significant correlation between dyslipidemia and the type of surgical procedure, $X^2_{(30,3)} = 9.017$, $p = 0.029$. The effect size was moderate according to Cramer's V coefficient = 0.548, $p = 0.029$, and contingency coefficient = 0.489, $p = 0.029$. As such, when patients presented an absence of dyslipidemia, the most common types of procedures carried out were surgical washing and amputation of toes. In contrast, the presence of dyslipidemia was associated with fasciotomy and transmetatarsal amputation procedures.

Also, a discriminant analysis was performed to determine the utility of the ABI-type classification of vascular complications (Table 5). Values of canonical

Table 3 ABI and pressure measurements

Variable	Minimum	Maximum	Average	Standard deviation
Age (years)	39	89	57.6	11
Hospitalization days	1	4	2.14	1
ABI	0.5	1.75	0.99	0.28
Systolic pressure of the left leg	80	300	160.6	51.6
Systolic pressure of the left arm	100	210	149.6	30.3
Systolic pressure of the right leg	80	300	148	43.3
Systolic pressure of the right arm	80	300	154.4	41.6

Table 4 ABI, according to the procedure

Procedure	Patients	Average ABI	Standard deviation
Surgical washing	7	0.84	0.22
Fasciotomy	5	0.9	0.12
Amputation of a toe	12	0.87	0.12
Transmetatarsal amputation	4	0.55	0.1

Table 5 Discriminant analysis for types of vascular problems according to ABI ($N = 30$)

						Exact F					
Factor	Standardized coefficient of the canonical discriminant function	*Wilks' lambda*	X^2	df	*p*	Value	df1	df2	*p*	Eigenvalue	*Canonical correlation*
ABI	1	0.202	18.213	2	0.000	24.765	4	25	0.000	3.962	0.894

correlation and eigenvalue were close to 1, which implied that ABI, the discriminant factor, accurately distinguished between the types of vascular problems (normal, mild, moderate, severe, and calcification). Additionally, since Wilks' lambda value was close to 0, it can be inferred that the types of vascular problems were differentiated. Furthermore, ABI successfully classified patients according to their degree of vascular problems with 83.3% accuracy. Individuals with normal blood flow, mild vascular problems, or severe ones were classified correctly with 100% accuracy. Those with calcification were accurately classified as such in 80% of the cases (20% were classified as average blood flux). On the contrary, 25% of the patients with moderate vascular problems were classified as presenting a low vascular problem and 75% as having a severe vascular problem. Therefore, ABI seems to classify diabetic patients with moderate vascular problems wrongly.

Discussion

t2DM is increasing each year worldwide, and one of the complications causing a greater disability is diabetic foot. This becomes a public health problem due to the costs and the complications it represents, such as a diabetic foot with high morbidity and mortality (Faglia et al., 2006; Hingorani et al., 2016; Hinchlife et al., 2012; Monteiro-Soares et al., 2020; Noor et al., 2015).

In this work, we treated 30 t2DM patients (24 men and 6 women) diagnosed with infected diabetic foot ulcers that had not healed in at least 5 months. The patients ranged from 39 to 89 years old, averaging 57.6 years. The right (left) foot was affected in 63% (37%) of the cases. According to Wagner's classification, grade III ulcers were the most common ones (47%) and required an amputation of one or several toes. Also, grade II ulcers were common (40%) and most only required surgical washing. Finally, grade IV ulcers were present in 13%, and all suffered a transmetatarsal amputation. These results are similar to other studies (Bandyk, 2018; Cervantes-García et al., 2015).

Throughout the treatment, three antibiotherapy schemes were used. These included clindamycin combined with ciprofloxacin (26.7%), levofloxacin (56.7%), or ceftriaxone (16.7%). The antibiotic therapy was chosen depending on each patient's antibiogram and clinical history, considering which antibiotics the patient had received before the realization of this study.

All the patients presented nocturnal or resting pain and intermittent claudication, while some reported swelling of the legs, and others had a background of cardiovascular diseases. This indicated that all patients had some degree of PAD. Among the comorbidities, smoking (17% of the cases) is the most critical risk factor for the development of PAD and its complications since smoking increases the risk of PAD 2–6 times (Hirsch et al., 1997). This increase in risk depends on the number of cigarettes per day and the number of years with the smoking habit. Active smoking increases the risk of progression and seriousness of PAD, increases the risk of both the amputation of a lower member and the occlusion of arteries, and makes revascularization procedures difficult (Anderson et al., 2012; Pal et al., 2016). The patients abandoned the smoking habit, which progressively reduced the risk of developing PAD.

Within the physiopathology of diabetic foot are infections, neuropathy, and vasculopathy. The latter usually appears in patients with an age greater than or equal to 50 years, and it consists in the development of arteriosclerosis, vascular degeneration, endothelial damage, chronic capillary hypertension, or increase of platelet aggregation (Alexiadou & Doupis, 2012; Iraj et al., 2013; Shahbazian et al., 2013). Also, 40% of the cases presented arterial hypertension. Since this is an angiopathic factor, mainly when it is associated with smoking and with diabetic microangiopathy, almost half the patients are at significant risk of aggravating their PAD and developing arteriosclerosis. In addition, 13% of the patients presented dyslipidemia. Hence, they are at risk of aggravating their PAD, developing cardiovascular disease, and suffering an amputation (Bonafede et al., 2015; Edwards, 2004; Mahmood et al., 2014; Mendis, 2010; Mucha et al., 2006) since a high level of cholesterol in the blood decreases the flow of blood and oxygen in the arteries (Isordia-Salas et al., 2012; Pérez-Panero et al., 2021).

The ankle-brachial pressure index (ABI) was determined in each patient, and different levels of vascular affection were found. At the beginning of the study, the patients who suffered a transmetatarsal amputation presented a low ABI (average 0.55). In contrast, the rest presented an average ABI close to 0.9, excluding two patients who suffered an amputation of a toe that had an ABI of 1.75. It is essential to highlight that arterial calcification and Mönckeberg sclerosis are frequent in diabetic patients. The calcification of the middle arterial tunic avoids the occlusion of the blood vessel when compressed by the handle to more than 200 mmHg (David Smith et al., 2008). This process may be observed in 60% of diabetic patients (Lanzer et al., 2014; McCullough et al., 2008; Potier et al., 2011). In this case, the predictive value of the ABI is limited.

Several statistical tests were performed. It was found that when patients presented an absence of dyslipidemia, the most common types of procedures carried out were surgical washing and amputation of toes. In contrast, the presence of dyslipidemia was associated with fasciotomy and transmetatarsal amputation procedures. In addition, it was found that ABI accurately distinguished between the types of PAD (normal, mild, moderate, severe, and calcification) with 83.3% accuracy. In particular, individuals classified as having normal blood flow, mild vascular problems, or severe ones were classified correctly with 100% accuracy. These results concur with similar studies (Chan & Lo, 2020).

After approximately 3 months, 8 (26.7%) patients were readmitted to the hospital because they once again presented an infected foot ulcer. They were all male, and all required a major amputation. One of the leading causes of this was that the patients could not follow the instructions for managing their feet due to economic problems. Income is a factor that hinders diabetic treatment in patients with diabetic foot ulcers (Fernández-Torres et al., 2020).

Conclusion

The diabetic patient may show different degrees of the condition of the foot, such as neuropathy and silent vascular disease in which there is no manifestation of skin injury or gangrene throughout the limb according to Wagner's classification (Mavrogenis et al., 2018; Palomo-López et al., 2019; Wagner, 1981). To partially remedy this situation, the determination of the ABI should be implemented. From the results presented above, the ABI is an excellent predictor of PAD. In diabetic foot patients, it is essential to carry out an adequate physical exploration of the diabetic foot from the beginning, particularly to determine the ABI. It can detect early PAD in the asymptomatic phase and can be a cutoff parameter to consider more aggressive preventive interventions before the existing vascular damage becomes symptomatic. This test can be used to identify patients requiring extra preventive care. A limitation of our study is that we had a small number of patients.

References

Alexiadou, K., & Doupis, J. (2012). Management of diabetic foot ulcers. *Diabetes Therapy, 3*(1), 4. https://doi.org/10.1007/s13300-012-0004-9

Anderson, J. J., Boone, J., Hansen, M., Spencer, L., & Fowler, Z. (2012). A comparison of diabetic smokers and non-smokers who undergo lower extremity amputation: A retrospective review of 112 patients. *Diabetic Foot & Ankle, 3*. https://doi.org/10.3402/dfa.v3i0.19178

Armstrong, D. G., Lavery, L. A., & Harkless, L. B. (1998). Validation of a diabetic wound classification system. The contribution of depth, infection, and ischemia to risk of amputation. *Diabetes Care, 21*(5), 855–859. https://doi.org/10.2337/diacare.21.5.855

Bandyk, D. F. (2018). The diabetic foot: Pathophysiology, evaluation, and treatment. *Seminars in Vascular Surgery, 31*(2–4), 43–48. https://doi.org/10.1053/j.semvascsurg.2019.02.001

Bonafede, M. M., Johnson, B. H., Richhariya, A., & Gandra, S. R. (2015). Medical costs associated with cardiovascular events among high-risk patients with hyperlipidemia. *ClinicoEconomics and Outcomes Research: CEOR, 7*, 337–345. https://doi.org/10.2147/CEOR.S76972

Boulton, A. J. M. (2015). The diabetic foot. *Medicine J, 43*(1), 33–37. https://doi.org/10.1016/j.mpmed.2014.10.006

Cervantes-García, E., & Salazar-Schettino, P. M. (2017). Clinical and surgical characteristics of infected diabetic foot ulcers in a tertiary hospital of Mexico. *Diabetic Foot & Ankle, 8*(1), 1367210. https://doi.org/10.1080/2000625X.2017.1367210

Cervantes-García, E., García-González, R., Reséndiz-Albor, A., & Salazar-Schettino, P. M. (2015). Infections of diabetic foot ulcers with methicillin-resistant Staphylococcus aureus. *The International Journal of Lower Extremity Wounds, 14*(1), 44–49. https://doi.org/10.1177/1534734614564053

Chan, K. S., & Lo, Z. J. (2020). Wound assessment, imaging and monitoring systems in diabetic foot ulcers: A systematic review. *International Wound Journal, 17*(6), 1909–1923. https://doi.org/10.1111/iwj.13481

David Smith, C., Gavin Bilmen, J., Iqbal, S., Robey, S., & Pereira, M. (2008). Medial artery calcification as an indicator of diabetic peripheral vascular disease. *Foot & Ankle International, 29*(2), 185–190. https://doi.org/10.3113/FAI.2008.0185

Edwards, R. (2004). The problem of tobacco smoking. *BMJ (Clinical research ed.), 328*(7433), 217–219. https://doi.org/10.1136/bmj.328.7433.217

Faglia, E., Clerici, G., Caminiti, M., Quarantiello, A., Gino, M., & Morabito, A. (2006). The role of early surgical debridement and revascularization in patients with diabetes and deep foot space abscess: Retrospective review of 106 patients with diabetes. *The Journal of Foot and Ankle Surgery, 45*(4), 220–226. https://doi.org/10.1053/j.jfas.2006.04.002

Fernández-Torres, R., Ruiz-Muñoz, M., Pérez-Panero, A. J., García-Romero, J. C., & Gónzalez-Sánchez, M. (2020). Clinician assessment tools for patients with Diabetic Foot Disease: A systematic review. *Journal of Clinical Medicine, 9*(5), 1487. https://doi.org/10.3390/jcm9051487

Ferreira, A. C., & Macedo, F. Y. (2010). A review of simple, non-invasive means of assessing peripheral arterial disease and implications for medical management. *Annals of Medicine, 42*(2), 139–150. https://doi.org/10.3109/07853890903521070

Hinchliffe, R. J., Andros, G., Apelqvist, J., Bakker, K., Friederichs, S., Lammer, J., Lepantalo, M., Mills, J. L., Reekers, J., Shearman, C. P., Valk, G., Zierler, R. E., & Schaper, N. C. (2012). A systematic review of the effectiveness of revascularization of the ulcerated foot in patients with diabetes and peripheral arterial disease. *Diabetes/Metabolism Research and Reviews, 28*(Suppl 1), 179–217. https://doi.org/10.1002/dmrr.2249

Hingorani, A., LaMuraglia, G. M., Henke, P., Meissner, M. H., Loretz, L., Zinszer, K. M., Driver, V. R., Frykberg, R., Carman, T. L., Marston, W., Mills, J. L., Sr., & Murad, M. H. (2016). The management of diabetic foot: A clinical practice guideline by the Society for Vascular Surgery in collaboration with the American Podiatric Medical Association and the Society for Vascular Medicine. *Journal of Vascular Surgery, 63*(2 Suppl), 3S–21S. https://doi.org/10.1016/j.jvs.2015.10.003

Hirsch, A. T., Treat-Jacobson, D., Lando, H. A., & Hatsukami, D. K. (1997). The role of tobacco cessation, antiplatelet, and lipid-lowering therapies in the treatment of peripheral arterial disease. *Vascular medicine (London, England), 2*(3), 243–251. https://doi.org/10.1177/1358863X9700200314

Iraj, B., Khorvash, F., Ebneshahidi, A., & Askari, G. (2013). Prevention of diabetic foot ulcer. *International Journal of Preventive Medicine, 4*(3), 373–376.

Isordia-Salas, I., Santiago-Germán, D., Rodrìguez-Navarro, H., Almaráz-Delgado, M., Leaños-Miranda, A., Anaya-Gómez, F., Borrayo-Sánchez, G., & Majluf-Cruz, A. (2012). Prevalence of metabolic syndrome components in an urban Mexican sample: Comparison between two classifications. *Experimental Diabetes Research, 202540*. https://doi.org/10.1155/2012/202540

Julio, R., & Galleguillos, I. (2009). Diabetes y enfermedad vascular periférica [Diabetes and peripheral vascular disease]. *Revista Médica Clínica Las Condes, 20*, 687–697.

Lanzer, P., Boehm, M., Sorribas, V., Thiriet, M., Janzen, J., Zeller, T., St Hilaire, C., & Shanahan, C. (2014). Medial vascular calcification revisited: Review and perspectives. *European Heart Journal, 35*(23), 1515–1525. https://doi.org/10.1093/eurheartj/ehu163

Mahmood, S. S., Levy, D., Vasan, R. S., & Wang, T. J. (2014). The Framingham Heart Study and the epidemiology of cardiovascular disease: A historical perspective. *Lancet (London, England), 383*(9921), 999–1008. https://doi.org/10.1016/S0140-6736(13)61752-3

Mavrogenis, A. F., Megaloikonomos, P. D., Antoniadou, T., Igoumenou, V. G., Panagopoulos, G. N., Dimopoulos, L., Moulakakis, K. G., Sfyroeras, G. S., & Lazaris, A. (2018). Current concepts for the evaluation and management of diabetic foot ulcers. *EFORT Open Reviews, 3*(9), 513–525. https://doi.org/10.1302/2058-5241.3.180010

McCullough, P. A., Agrawal, V., Danielewicz, E., & Abela, G. S. (2008). Accelerated atherosclerotic calcification and Monckeberg's sclerosis: A continuum of advanced vascular pathology in chronic kidney disease. *Clinical Journal of the American Society of Nephrology: CJASN, 3*(6), 1585–1598. https://doi.org/10.2215/CJN.01930408

Medina, G. E., Rubio, A. F., Vargas, A. G., & Rivera, X. (2010). Insuficiencia arterial periférica en pacientes diabéticos comparada con pacientes diabéticos e hipertensos [Peripheral arterial insufficiency in diabetic patients compared to hypertensive diabetic patients]. *Medicina Interna de Mexico, 26*(6), 568–572.

Mendis, S. (2010). The contribution of the Framingham Heart Study to the prevention of cardiovascular disease: A global perspective. *Progress in Cardiovascular Diseases, 53*(1), 10–14. https://doi.org/10.1016/j.pcad.2010.01.001

Monteiro-Soares, M., Boyko, E. J., Jeffcoate, W., Mills, J. L., Russell, D., Morbach, S., & Game, F. (2020). Diabetic foot ulcer classifications: A critical review. *Diabetes/Metabolism Research and Reviews, 36*(Suppl 1), e3272. https://doi.org/10.1002/dmrr.3272

Mucha, L., Stephenson, J., Morandi, N., & Dirani, R. (2006). Meta-analysis of disease risk associated with smoking by gender and intensity of smoking. *Gender Medicine, 3*(4), 279–291. https://doi.org/10.1016/s1550-8579(06)80216-0

Noor, S., Zubair, M., & Ahmad, J. (2015). Diabetic foot ulcer--A review on pathophysiology, classification, and microbial etiology. *Diabetes & Metabolic Syndrome, 9*(3), 192–199. https://doi.org/10.1016/j.dsx.2015.04.007

Norgren, L., Hiatt, W. R., Dormandy, J. A., Nehler, M. R., Harris, K. A., Fowkes, F. G., & TASC II Working Group. (2007). Inter-Society consensus for the management of peripheral arterial disease (TASC II). *Journal of Vascular Surgery, 45*(Suppl S), S5–S67. https://doi.org/10.1016/j.jvs.2006.12.037

Nussbaum, S. R., Carter, M. J., Fife, C. E., DaVanzo, J., Haught, R., Nusgart, M., & Cartwright, D. (2018). An economic evaluation of the impact, cost, and medicare policy implications of chronic nonhealing wounds. *Value in Health: The Journal of the International Society for Pharmacoeconomics and Outcomes Research, 21*(1), 27–32. https://doi.org/10.1016/j.jval.2017.07.007

Pal, B., Raveender, N., & Sudipta, P. (2016). A study on the impact of smoking and alcoholism as determinant factors in the prognosis and outcome of diabetic foot ulcer disease. *International Journal of Research in Medical Sciences, 4*(5), 1720–1724. https://doi.org/10.18203/2320-6012.ijrms20161257

Palomo-López, P., Losa-Iglesias, M. E., Becerro-de-Bengoa-Vallejo, R., López-López, D., Rodríguez-Sanz, D., Romero-Morales, C., & Calvo-Lobo, C. (2019). Specific foot health-related quality-of-life impairment in patients with type II versus type I diabetes. *International Wound Journal, 16*(1), 47–51. https://doi.org/10.1111/iwj.12984

Pérez-Panero, A. J., Ruiz-Muñoz, M., Fernández-Torres, R., Formosa, C., Gatt, A., & Gónzalez-Sánchez, M. (2021). Diabetic foot disease: A systematic literature review of patient-reported outcome measures. *Quality of Life Research.* https://doi.org/10.1007/s11136-021-02892-4

Potier, L., Abi Khalil, C., Mohammedi, K., & Roussel, R. (2011). Use and utility of ankle-brachial index in patients with diabetes. *European Journal of Vascular and Endovascular Surgery, 41*(1), 110–116. https://doi.org/10.1016/j.ejvs.2010.09.020

Rac-Albu, M., Iliuta, L., Guberna, S. M., & Sinescu, C. (2014). The role of ankle-brachial index for predicting peripheral arterial disease. *Maedica, 9*(3), 295–302.

Reardon, R., Simring, D., Kim, B., Mortensen, J., Williams, D., & Leslie, A. (2020). The diabetic foot ulcer. *Australian Journal of General Practice, 49*(5), 250–255. https://doi.org/10.31128/AJGP-11-19-5161

Shahbazian, H., Yazdanpanah, L., & Latifi, S. M. (2013). Risk assessment of patients with diabetes for foot ulcers according to risk classification consensus of International Working Group on Diabetic Foot (IWGDF). *Pakistan Journal of Medical Sciences, 29*(3), 730–734. https://doi.org/10.12669/pjms.293.3473

Wacher, N. (2009). Epidemiologia del síndrome metabólico. *Gac Méd Méx, 145*(5), 384–391.

Wagner, F. W., Jr. (1981). The dysvascular foot: A system for diagnosis and treatment. *Foot & Ankle, 2*(2), 64–122. https://doi.org/10.1177/107110078100200202

Yao, S. T., Hobbs, J. T., & Irvine, W. T. (1969). Ankle systolic pressure measurements in arterial disease affecting the lower extremities. *The British Journal of Surgery, 56*(9), 676–679. https://doi.org/10.1002/bjs.1800560910

Zhang, P., Zhang, X., Brown, J., Vistisen, D., Sicree, R., Shaw, J., & Nichols, G. (2010). Global healthcare expenditure on diabetes for 2010 and 2030. *Diabetes Research and Clinical Practice, 87*(3), 293–301. https://doi.org/10.1016/j.diabres.2010.01.026

Poor Doctor–Patient Communication: How Social Vulnerability Turns into Physical Vulnerability

Alí Ruiz-Coronel, Rosa Angélica Salcedo-Hernández, and Gerardo Sierra-Martínez

Introduction

This study was conducted to improve patient guidelines after hospital discharge from surgery for ovarian carcinoma. The overarching hypothesis is that doctor–patient communication affects the outcomes after ovarian surgery as it impacts patient behavior once they have left the hospital. At home, the surgical outcome mainly depends on the information of the patient and her caregivers and the decisions they make regarding her care. Incorrect care could cause readmission to the hospital emergency room, another surgical intervention, or even the death of the patient. Thus, the quality of communication when giving discharge instructions is critical to determining positive patient outcomes.

A. Ruiz-Coronel (✉)
Institute for Social Research, National Autonomous University of Mexico, Mexico City, Mexico
e-mail: ali@sociales.unam.mx

R. A. Salcedo-Hernández
National Cancer Institute of Mexico (INCan), Mexico City, Mexico
e-mail: rosasalher@gmail.com

G. Sierra-Martínez
Linguistic Engineering Laboratory, National Autonomous University of Mexico, Mexico City, Mexico
e-mail: gsierram@iingen.unam.mx

S. Castaños-Cervantes et al. (eds.), *Working with Vulnerable Populations*,
https://doi.org/10.1007/978-3-031-67710-6_4

Background Information

We know that the occurrence of hospital readmission after gynecological malignancy surgery is between 12% in the next 30 days after discharge (ESGO, 2016). The principal causes are infections (45%) and gastrointestinal disturbances such as nausea, vomiting, ileus, and intestinal occlusion (19.4%) (Nakayama et al., 2015; Uppal et al., 2016). The French Gynecological Society distinguishes between three types of associated factors: those that are strictly medical, regarding treatment and/or the staff giving treatment; those that are patient characteristics, such as age, race, and socioeconomic status; and those attributable to the care received by the patient from discharge (Querleu et al., 2013). Those relating to the last set of factors include poor communication with patients, insufficient follow-up care after discharge, and inadequate postoperative care. Uppal et al. (2016) include post-discharge accommodation as a predictive variable.

Furthermore, poor health illiteracy is a component of social vulnerability that may negatively affect the communication process and even lead to misunderstandings of the doctor's care instructions by the patient or the caregiver, indirectly provoking adverse outcomes. In order to question this hypothesis, we registered and analyzed the process of communication in instruction transmission for hospital discharge after surgery for ovarian carcinoma carried out by the oncological gynecological service at the National Cancer Institute of Mexico (INCan) and what the patient and his or her primary caregiver could recall of the care instructions. This protocol was submitted as an addition to the primary investigation and approved along with the letter of informed consent, which was given to the patients on May 7, 2018, at the Sixth Ordinary Session of the Research Committee and the Sixth Ordinary Session of the Ethics on Research Committee (INCAN/CI/392/18).

Methodology

Participants

Twenty-one actual events were recorded (audio only). Each event consisted of a patient receiving medical instructions for hospital discharge and repeating (having been asked to) the instructions immediately afterwards. The events occurred at the National Cancer Institute of Mexico INCan, between May 30 and August 15, 2018. The sample was based on convenience. The inclusion criteria for the patients were that they had been operated on (as a primary, interval, or secondary surgery) for epithelial ovarian carcinoma, they were more than 18 years of age, and that they had signed informed consent. To guarantee the authenticity of the recorded events, consent to participate in the study came from the medical team on the oncological gynecology service and the tenured professors of the subspecialties as a collective, not as individuals. Though the doctors were aware of the study, they did not know which event would be recorded.

Analysis

After sessions were recorded, a linguistic analysis was carried out. Linguistic corpora constitute a model of the linguistic reality one wishes to observe (Sierra, 2017). The linguistic corpus that was analyzed in this study comprises a variety of texts that were acquired through the literal transcription of the 21 communication events:

- *The corpus object Co* is the primary source. It is a literal transcript of the instructions the attending physician gave following a written script, which was checked in advance to ensure it contained all the necessary and sufficient instructions.
- *The reference corpus M* consists of texts taken from a literal transcript of medical doctor instructions given to patients.
- *The reference corpus P* is made up of a literal transcript of the repeated instructions by the patients immediately after being given these instructions.

The analysis consists of a formal and semantic comparative study of the various linguistic corpora. In the current study, the relevance of this perspective rests on the fact that it allows for an objective measurement of the correspondence between the reference corpus *P* and the reference corpus *M*, and both reference corpora can be compared with the object corpus *Co*.

The *comparative formal analysis* involved quantifying the information in the messages by counting the number of words, disregarding their meaning. The *comparative semantic analysis* consisted of identifying the topics addressed, counting the number of instructions, and finding a hierarchy between them, meaning that some instructions are more important than others according to the impact that they may have on the patient's outcome.

In both the formal and the semantic analysis, the closer the total amount of information, topics, or instructions are to the object corpus Co, the better. More information might be distracting, and less information might be insufficient.

Results

Comparative Formal Analysis

Formal analysis is a quantitative approximation with an explicit instrumental aim of reducing communication to the quantity of information. Figure 1 shows the size of the texts in order of their word count.

Words

	M	P
CO	793	793
Case	M	P
1	145	58
2	259	39
3	846	139
4	241	200
5	1478	112
6	1237	46
7	84	32
8	392	69
9	467	60
10	89	40
11	147	26
12	167	133
13	143	64
14	276	127
15	264	44
16	1145	80
17	280	77
18	96	88
19	338	55
20	214	44
21	241	38
P	407	74.8

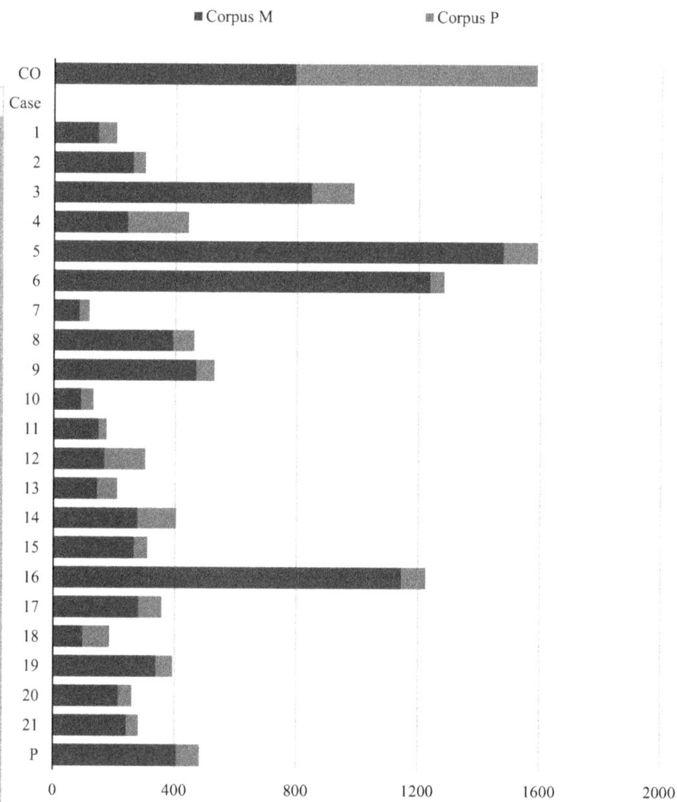

Fig. 1 Number of words. (Source: Authors' elaboration)

The line *Co* shows the number of words in the object corpus. On average, the patients' text is 70% smaller than the text from the doctor giving them the instructions. The doctors' text is only more extensive than the object corpus text in cases 5, 6, and 16, when an attending physician gave the instructions and in case 3, when a patient asked to discuss a different issue. The average number of words in the reference corpus *P* (74.8) is 18.3% of the average word count in the reference corpus *M* (407) and only 9.4% of the object corpus (793). Similarly, the average number of words in reference corpus *M* is 51.3% of the total word count in the object corpus. The componential analysis provides evidence of the constant reduction in the quantity of information as it is being transmitted from attending to resident to patient.

Comparative Semantic Analysis: Topics

Semantic analysis refers to the signified in the transmitted information; it highlights the meaning of the communication. In this research, the meaning of the object corpus and the reference corpora *P* and *M* is the same: the meaning is that patients who have been operated on for ovarian carcinoma know the instructions for their postoperative care on discharge from the hospital. Hammel (1965) described that the corpora were compared as partially identical emissaries.

The topics addressed are similar to semantic fields as they are categories "whose tokens are the points in experiential space that cluster in a particular target area; they are discrete formal entities manifested as infinite classes of actual experiences" (Chafe, 1965, p. 24). The purpose of communication determines the relevant topics. Thus, the topics that form part of the object corpus are based on the experience of the specialized medical team and to ensure patients have the necessary tools to guarantee adequate care.

The topics that refer to hospital discharge are *administrative issues*, which must be resolved to be discharged, and *warning symptoms*, which can prevent discharge or cause readmittance. Infection prevention is present in the semantic fields of *prescribed medication* and *wound care*. Gastrointestinal disturbances are tackled by two semantic fields, one regarding *diet* and the other regarding *physical activity*, which patients should participate in to avoid digestive atrophy or malfunction. One semantic field present in the object corpus but absent in the reference corpora is the reference to using the incentive *spirometer*, as shown in Fig. 2. Figure 2 shows the order of appearance of the topics in the corpora. Line *Co* shows how the topics appear in the object corpus. Line *T* shows the order of importance from 1 to 7, as assigned theoretically by the medical team, to the topics in a personal communication carried out to this aim. The following lines show the order in which the doctor and the patient addressed each unit in each event. An *N* indicates that the topic was not discussed. Line *R* is the natural hierarchy in which the units appear with the highest frequency in the reference corpora.

Administrative issues are sixth in the theoretical hierarchical order used by the medical team. However, in practice, more than half of the doctors discussed this. It is the only item in all the medical interventions considered even more critical than prescription medication, which was omitted twice. Given that gastrointestinal disturbances are associated with diet, it is interesting that doctors ignored this topic in half of the cases. In the same way, ileus, intestinal occlusion, and similar disturbances are often associated with a lack of activity. However, in 17 of the events, the medical team did not mention activity.

Logically, the topics in reference corpus *P* can only be the same or less than those of reference corpus *M* because the patient repeated the instructions received from the medical team. In the same way, the order of appearance of the topics in the reference corpora is very similar. In all the cases except 12, the number of topics included in the patient texts was fewer than those received. The maximum number of topics addressed in the reference corpus *M* was six, and only in cases 5, 6, and 16, where

	Prescribed Medication		Wound Care		Diet		Warning Symptoms		Physical Activity		Administrative Issues		Spirometer		Total	
Co	1		4		2		5		3		7		6		7	
T	1		2		3		4		5		6		7		7	
Case	M	P	M	P	M	P	M	P	M	P	M	P	M	P	M	P
1	4	1	5	N	2	N	3	2	N	N	1	N	N	N	5	2
2	1	N	4	1	3	N	5	N	N	N	2	2	N	N	5	2
3	1	N	3	1	N	2	4	N	N	N	2	N	N	N	4	2
4	2	N	3	N	5	1	N	2	N	N	1	N	N	N	4	2
5	3	1	4	N	5	3	1	2	6	4	2	N	N	N	6	4
6	2	N	1	N	5	1	4	N	6	2	3	3	N	N	6	3
7	2	2	N	N	N	N	N	N	N	N	1	1	N	N	2	2
8	1	2	4	N	N	N	5	3	3	N	2	1	N	N	5	3
9	N	N	2	1	3	2	N	N	N	N	1	3	N	N	3	3
10	2	N	N	N	N	N	3	1	N	N	1	2	N	N	3	2
11	3	N	2	N	N	N	N	1	N	N	1	N	N	N	3	1
12	3	1	4	3	N	2	2	5	N	4	1	N	N	N	4	5
13	N	N	N	N	N	N	2	1	N	N	1	N	N	N	2	1
14	3	N	4	N	N	N	2	N	N	N	1	1	N	N	4	1
15	2	N	3	N	5	N	4	N	N	N	1	1	N	N	5	1
16	4	N	2	N	6	N	3	N	5	N	1	N	N	N	6	0
17	2	1	N	N	N	N	3	2	N	N	1	N	N	N	3	2
18	3	N	3	2	N	1	2	4	N	N	1	3	N	N	4	4
19	2	1	N	N	N	N	3	2	N	N	1	N	N	N	3	2
20	3	N	N	N	4	N	2	2	N	N	1	1	N	N	4	2
21	2	2	N	N	3	N	4	N	N	N	1	1	N	N	4	2
R	2	2	4	5	5	4	3	3	6	6	1	1	0	0	4	2

Fig. 2 Topics. (Source: Authors' elaboration)

an attending physician was giving the instructions, was this number reached. The minimum was 2, *and there were administrative issues* and *prescribed medication*. In corpus P, the maximum reached was 4, and the minimum was 0. On average, the reference corpus texts *M* included four topics, while reference corpus texts *P* consisted of two on average.

Comparative Semantic Analysis: Instructions

The minimal semantic units of the corpus are the specific instructions relevant to each topic. The instructions were reduced to basic units following three rules: the rule of sequential difference in a range, the rule of different matching sequences in a range, and the rule of reciprocals within a range (Goodenough, 1956). Figure 3 summarizes the number of instructions within each topic in the object corpus and the *M* and *P* reference corpora by case. The information was gathered in a correlation matrix where all the instructions of the object corpus were listed by topic. When the instruction was present in the reference corpora, *1* was assigned, *2* if it dealt with an instruction with greater ancestry, *0* if it was absent, −*1* when it was present but erroneously, and −*2* if there was an erroneous item of greater ancestry.

Caso	Prescribed Medication		Wound Care		Diet		Warning Symptoms		Physical Activity		Administrative Issues		Spirometer		Total	
Co	4		7		34		21		11		4		3		84	84
1	8	2	5	1	-34	-34	6	2	0	0	2	0	0	0	-13	-29
2	8	0	6	2	4	1	4	0	0	0	2	2	0	0	24	5
3	8	0	4	1	0	0	2	0	0	0	2	0	0	0	16	1
4	6	0	3	0	-34	-34	0	0	0	0	3	0	0	0	-22	-31
5	5	0	7	3	31	-3	14	6	16	5	0	0	0	0	73	11
6	8	0	9	0	30	0	15	0	16	1	3	0	0	0	67	14
7	8	0	2	1	0	0	0	0	0	0	2	2	0	0	12	3
8	4	0	2	0	0	0	7	2	2	0	3	2	0	0	18	44
9	0	0	1	1	-26	-30	0	0	0	0	4	2	0	0	-21	-27
10	4	0	2	0	0	0	2	2	0	0	4	2	0	0	10	2
11	4	0	4	0	0	0	2	3	0	0	3	0	0	0	13	3
12	6	0	4	2	0	0	7	5	0	0	2	0	0	0	19	7
13	0	0	2	-8	0	-34	4	4	0	0	2	0	0	0	8	-38
14	4	0	4	0	0	0	3	0	0	0	4	-4	0	0	15	-4
15	4	0	2	1	-33	0	-18	0	2	0	4	2	0	0	-42	2
16	8	0	7	0	29	0	10	0	21	0	4	0	0	0	79	0
17	8	6	3	3	0	0	7	4	0	0	4	0	0	0	22	13
18	4	0	4	2	0	-33	-19	-22	0	0	2	-3	0	0	-9	-56
19	6	0	7	1	0	0	7	-20	0	0	2	0	0	0	22	-19
20	8	0	6	0	-34	0	6	-18	0	0	4	-1	0	0	-10	-19
21	8	0	6	0	-31	0	3	0	0	0	3	-1	0	0	-11	-1
P	5.6	0.38	4.2	0.47	-4.6	-7.9	2.9	-1.5	2.7	0.28	2.8	0.14	0	0	12.8	-5.6

Fig. 3 Instructions. (Source: Authors' elaboration)

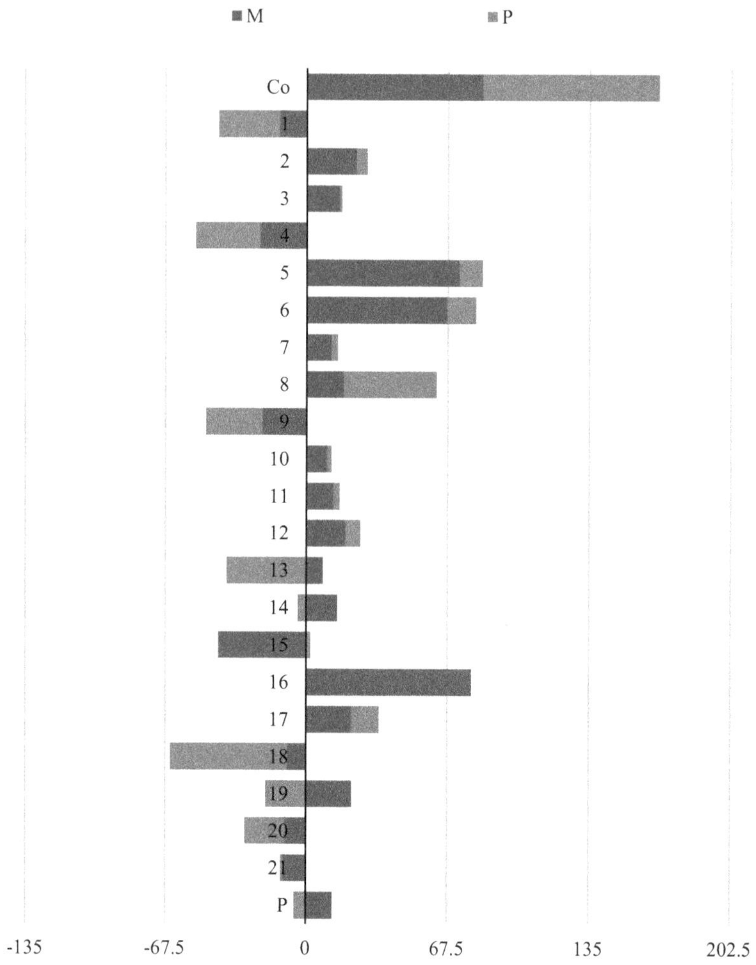

Fig. 3 (continued)

Line *Co* lists all the instructions by topic within the object corpus. The lines below list the exact data for the reference corpora case by case. Line *P* shows the averages given using all 21 cases.

There is even more significant evidence of the depth of information loss at this level of detail. The object corpus consists of 84 instructions. The average instructions found in reference corpus *M* was 12.8 and −5.6 in reference corpus *P*. This shows that the information given to patients was far smaller and incorrect. Regarding medical instructions, incorrect generalizations and ambiguous instructions could cause the patient to make adverse decisions. Examples include: "You can eat *everything*" and "Follow your *usual diet*." Due to cultural differences between doctors and patients, what is considered "normal" by each group varies greatly. If the patients were to continue with their "normal" diet, they could be risking an adverse surgical outcome by following this doctor-(mis)approved "normal" diet.

Discussion

Recommendations from the Comparative Formal Analysis

Information degrades constantly as the distance between the source and the receiver increases. In this case, the source is the doctor giving the instructions, and the receiver is the patient. Creating other sources is one way to mitigate information degradation and increase uncertainty. These could be written (leaflets, brochures), images (infographics, drawings), audio or video. Medical personnel should base their talking points on these sources to increase the amount of mutual information with the object corpus. The source should be portable and accessible to the patient so that they can consult it whenever necessary. This will reduce uncertainty around the source and the amount of intuition or other methods used that could (mis)guide aftercare. These instruments constitute a support, not a substitute for communication.

Recommendations from the Comparative Semantic Analysis of Topics

Looking at the theory and their professional experience, the medical team members identified seven topics to address with patients. In practice, the majority addressed four when giving instructions, and the majority of patients only two, at a proportion of 4:2. There is a great deal of research literature about the capacity of patients to remember medical information (Ley, 1979, 1972; Ley & Spelman, 1965, 1967; Ley et al., 1973). According to these authors, "studies of outpatients from various treatment settings indicate that patients recall approximately half of what they are told" (Ley & Spelman, 1965, p. 116). As corroborated in our data, reducing the number of topics to be addressed by the medical team upon discharge may be advisable, strengthening the interdisciplinary intervention of the health team.

Instructions for using the spirometer and wound care could be delegated to the nursing team and given during the hospital stay, emphasizing that this should be done in the same way at home. Additionally, administrative issues take up much space in reference corpus *M*. It seems more prudent for the social work team to coordinate administrative decisions based on each patient's needs and circumstances. By contrast, with their prescribing authority, the medical team should coordinate topics such as warning symptoms, medication, diet, and activity, mainly because these subjects are sometimes culturally counterintuitive, as seen in case 12.

In case 12, the patient addressed two topics the medical doctor did not include. They stated that they had been prescribed a bland diet and rest, although the doctor did not mention anything related to these. This case highlights the influence of culture in the communicative process through the patients' preconceptions. Some patients hold a cultural association that they need to rest and eat plain food to recover faster. For this particular patient, this constitutes an increased risk for their health.

Recommendations from the Comparative Semantic Analysis of Instructions

General instructions such as "you can do *everything*," "if there are *any problems*, come to the emergency room," or ambiguous instructions, such as "if you have any *abnormal symptoms*, come back in" not only increase patient uncertainty regarding correct aftercare. Instead, they could increase or even encourage harmful behaviors. This study shows that patients fill communicative spaces opened with false generalizations and ambiguities with what their cultural knowledge and intuition dictate. Due to social differences between doctors and patients, knowledge and cultural intuition could be at odds with medical advice.

Morrow et al. (1983) reported a linear relationship between the number of sentences given by the doctor and the number of sentences forgotten by the patient. Ley et al. (1973) found that the longer the medical instructions, the greater the amount of information the patient forgets. Our findings back up this assertion; therefore, we suggest following the communication strategies proposed by those researchers to achieve more efficient communication: divide the information into categories, verbally introduce each one, present information in order of importance, make declarative sentences that are short and simple, and use colloquial, jargon-free words.

Conclusions

The merit of this study does not lie in the discovery that information is lost and distorted in the communication process between doctor and patient; this is something both parties are aware of. It proposes interweaving corpus linguistics and information theory to describe and quantify this loss objectively. Thus, it is possible to link the loss of this information to an increase in the patient's uncertainty about their care and draw attention to the tendency to fill this gap with erroneous information from other sources or their intuition.

Using this method, we have identified that the first significant loss of information comes from within the medical team. The number of words in the object corpus was 793, the average number of words in the reference corpus M was 407, the number of topics integrated into the object corpus was 7, and the average number present in reference corpus *M* was 4. There were 84 instructions in the object corpus and 12.8 average instructions in *M*. Evidently, the information that reaches the patient is lesser in quantity and content. In terms of quantity, the average number of words in a patient's text is 70% less than that of the doctor who gave them the instructions. The average number of words in reference corpus *P* is 18.3% of the average number of words in reference corpus *M* and 9.4% of the object corpus. Regarding content, none of the corpus texts *P* included the seven semantic units present in the object corpus, and the majority included two. Furthermore, the instructional average was −5.6, meaning that the information transmitted to patients was much reduced and incorrect. Among the suggestions proposed is to create additional information sources that provide a unifying script on which the medical team can base their instructions. This source should be available to the patient so they can consult it whenever necessary. A further suggestion is to reduce the number of topics the medical team addresses to four and redistribute the remaining units to relevant professionals on the wider interdisciplinary care team. Finally, for greater understanding and to improve the linguistic character of communication, all false generalizations and ambiguities should be removed and replaced by simple declarative sentences. Information should be grouped by topic and order of importance, emphasizing instructions that may be culturally counterintuitive and using straightforward language without medical jargon.

References

Chafe, W. (1965). Meaning in language. *American Anthropologist, 67*(5), 23–36. https://www.jstor.org/stable/668755

European Society of Gynaecological Oncology. (2016). Advanced (StageI II-IV) ovarian cancer. *Quality Indicators*. ESCGO. https://doi.org/10.1097/IGC.0000000000000767

Goodenough, W. C. (1956). Componential analysis and the study of meaning. *Language, 32*(1), 195–216. https://www.jstor.org/stable/410665

Hammel, E. A. (Ed.). (1965). Formal semantic analysis. *American Anthropologist, 67*(5), 316. http://www.jstor.org/browse/00027294/ap020365

Ley, P. (1972). Primary, rated importance and recall of medical information. *Journal of Health and Social Behavior, 13*(3), 311–317. https://doi.org/10.2307/2136768

Ley, P. (1979). Memory for medical information. *British Journal of Social and Clinical Psychology, 18*, 245–255. https://doi.org/10.1111/j.2044-8260.1979.tb00333.x

Ley, P., & Spelman, M. S. (1965). Communications in an outpatient setting. *British Journal of Social and Clinical Psychology, 4*, 114–116. https://doi.org/10.1111/j.2044-8260.1965.tb00449.x

Ley, P., & Spelman, M. S. (1967). *Communication with the patient*. Staples Press.

Ley, P., Bradshaw, P. W., Eaves, D. E., & Walker, C. M. (1973). A method for increasing patients' recall of information presented to them. *Psychological Medicine, 3*, 217–220. https://doi.org/10.1017/s0033291700048558

Morrow, G., Alice, C., Hoagland, M. A., & Carpenter, P. J. (1983). Improving physician-patient communications in cancer treatment. *Journal of Psychosocial Oncology, 1*(2), 93–101. https://doi.org/10.1300/J077v01n02_07

Nakayama, J., Ou, J. P., Friedman, C., Smolkin, M., & Duska, L. (2015). The risk factors of read mission in post-operative gynecologic oncology patients at a single institution.

International Journal of Gynecological Cancer, 25(9), 1697–1703. https://doi.org/10.1097/IGC.0000000000000535

Querleu, D., Ray-Coquard, I., Classe, J. M., Aucouturier, J. S., Bonnet, F., Bonnier, P., Darai, E., De Vouassoux, M., Gladieff, L., Glehen, O., Haie-Meder, C., Joly, F., Lécuru, F., Lefranc, J. P., Lhommé, C., Morice, P., Salengro, A., Stoeckle, E., Taieb, S., Zeng, Z. X., & Leblanc, E. (2013). Quality indicators in ovarian cancer surgery: Report from the French Society of Gynecologic Oncology. *Annals of Oncology, 24*(11), 2732–2739. https://doi.org/10.1093/annonc/mdt237

Sierra, G. (2017). *Introducción a los corpus lingüísticos*. Universidad Nacional Autónoma de México-Instituto de Ingeniería.

Uppal, S., Penn, C., Del Carmen, M., Rauh-Hain, A., Reynolds, K., & Rice, L. (2016). Readmissions after major gynecologic oncology surgery. *Gynecologic Oncology, 141*, 287–229. https://doi.org/10.1016/j.ygyno.2016.02.031

Overcoming Obstacles and Promoting Physical Activity in Vulnerable Children Through Identified Challenges and Solutions: From a HIIT Perspective

Mira Amer and Nilay Arman

Introduction

In addressing the urgent challenges confronted by children in vulnerable areas, where constrained environments may result in maladaptive behavior and significant health issues, there is a crucial demand for effective interventions. This chapter proposes a tailored physical activity program as a solution, specifically designed to overcome time constraints in disadvantaged communities. By integrating behavior change theories into the implementation of a high-intensity interval training (HIIT) program, the goal is to enhance both the physical and mental well-being of these children, positively impacting their behavior and motivation levels.

Within developed nations, socioeconomic disparities influence the participation in physical activity, with a substantial proportion of adolescents and adults failing to meet recommended levels (Chaput et al., 2020). Children in disadvantaged areas face additional challenges, including limited parental physical activity levels, insufficient physical education classes at school, and the necessity for child labor (Carson et al., 2020; Eyre et al., 2022; Tucker et al., 2015). The cumulative effect of these factors hinders children from achieving the recommended 60 min of daily physical activity prescribed by the World Health Organization (WHO) (Chaput et al., 2020).

M. Amer (✉)
Department of Physical and Occupational Therapy, Faculty of Nursing and Health Science, Bethlehem University, Bethlehem, Palestine

Department of Physiotherapy and Rehabilitation, Faculty of Health Science, Istanbul University-Cerrahpasa, Istanbul, Turkiye

N. Arman
Department of Physiotherapy and Rehabilitation, Faculty of Health Science, Istanbul University-Cerrahpasa, Istanbul, Turkiye
e-mail: nilayarman@iuc.edu.tr

S. Castaños-Cervantes et al. (eds.), *Working with Vulnerable Populations*,
https://doi.org/10.1007/978-3-031-67710-6_5

To address these obstacles, implementing a HIIT program emerges as a viable solution due to its time efficiency and potential benefits for both advantaged and disadvantaged children (Miller, 2016). HIIT involves short bursts of vigorous activity interspersed with brief periods of rest and has demonstrated positive impacts on cardiovascular health, metabolic health, and overall physical development in children (Eddolls et al., 2017; Gibala et al., 2012). Moreover, its engaging nature can turn exercise into an enjoyable experience, fostering a positive attitude toward physical activity (Heisz et al., 2016).

Children in vulnerable populations, situated in economically disadvantaged or marginalized areas, face unique challenges that impact their development (Paul-Sen Gupta et al., 2007). Addressing these challenges is not only a moral imperative but also a strategic investment in societal well-being. By focusing on vulnerable populations, particularly in childhood, we can break the cycle of intergenerational disadvantage, ensuring better healthcare, educational opportunities, and resources (de Souza et al., 2021; Kruk et al., 2018).

Behavior change theories play a pivotal role in implementing effective physical activity programs for children in disadvantaged areas. The theory of planned behavior (TPB), social cognitive theory (SCT), self-determination theory (SDT), trans-theoretical model (TTM), and the health belief model (HBM) offer systematic frameworks to understand, predict, and influence behavior (Ajzen, 1991; Bandura, 2001; Hagger & Chatzisarantis, 2008; Jones et al., 2015; Prochaska & Velicer, 1997). Tailoring interventions based on these theories allows for a nuanced understanding of the unique challenges and motivations in disadvantaged communities, addressing specific barriers and leveraging social support networks (Bagherniya et al., 2018; Bélanger-Gravel & Godin, 2010).

In this chapter, we explore the vulnerability of children as a demographic, examining the diverse factors influencing their levels of physical activity. We discuss the challenges linked to implementing effective solutions and present an alternative framework for physical activity that shows promise for successful implementation.

Children as a Vulnerable Population, Physical Activity, and Related Factors

Childhood vulnerability, often rooted in economic disadvantage or marginalization, underscores the pressing need to understand and address the unique challenges faced by children in these populations, particularly concerning physical activity. The vulnerability of children manifests in various ways, shaping their access to resources, opportunities, and overall well-being. In the context of physical activity, these vulnerabilities contribute to disparities in engagement, limiting children's ability to meet recommended activity levels. Understanding the intricate factors influencing physical activity in children is crucial for developing targeted interventions that cater to the specific needs of vulnerable populations (Craike et al., 2018; Stevens et al., 2006; Tangcharoensathien et al., 2018).

Socioeconomic disparities, for example, play a significant role in shaping the physical activity landscape for children. Economic disadvantage often translates into limited access to safe play spaces, structured physical activities, and quality physical education (Somerset & Hoare, 2018). The challenges extend beyond the immediate environment, affecting parental engagement in physical activity and creating a cycle that hinders children from developing healthy habits. These disparities are not confined to a specific age group, with influences on physical activity observed from early childhood through adolescence (Carson et al., 2020; Ke et al., 2022). As we delve into the multifaceted factors influencing vulnerable children's physical activity, we uncover the complex interplay between socioeconomic circumstances, educational access, and environmental considerations.

Vulnerability as a factor and as a definition is a nuanced state that extends across diverse facets of well-being, encapsulating a susceptibility to harm in various dimensions. Physically vulnerable individuals or groups find themselves at an elevated risk of health-related adversities, be it from preexisting health conditions, exposure to environmental hazards, or a lack of access to essential healthcare services (Gordon, 1965; Waisel, 2013). Economic vulnerability unveils itself through a scarcity of financial resources or stability, leaving individuals or communities more exposed to the throes of poverty, financial crises, and economic shocks (Arnault et al., 2021). Simultaneously, social vulnerability involves facing discrimination, marginalization, or grappling with insufficient social support, thereby amplifying the risk of negative social outcomes (Mah et al., 2023). Emotional vulnerability delves into heightened sensitivity or fragility in emotional well-being, often influenced by past traumas, mental health struggles, or a dearth of emotional support (LoBue & Ogren, 2022). Environmental vulnerability is entwined with exposure to environmental risks and a diminished resilience when confronted with challenges such as natural disasters, climate change, or other environmental adversities (Etzel, 2020).

In children, vulnerability arises from the convergence of factors, influencing their susceptibility to adverse conditions and shaping overall well-being. Recognizing and addressing vulnerabilities is crucial for designing interventions and policies that meet specific needs. Communities can work toward creating environments fostering resilience and equal opportunities for all, regardless of their starting point (Embleton et al., 2020).

According to the WHO, children need to do 60 min of moderate-to-vigorous physical activity daily (Chaput et al., 2020) while a small percentage of children can achieve this goal, children in disadvantaged areas struggle more to achieve it.

In developed countries, engagement in physical activity and the resulting health outcomes exhibit a social distribution shaped by socioeconomic status (Melhuish, 2014). Despite the health benefits physical activity has on people of all ages, according to the WHO report on physical activity in 2022, more than 80% of adolescents do not do the required minimum levels of physical activity and 27% of adults do not as well (Chaput et al., 2020). Individuals with higher socioeconomic advantage are more prone to achieving recommended levels of physical activity, thereby lowering the risk of adverse health consequences linked to a sedentary lifestyle, in comparison to their less advantaged counterparts (Ball et al., 2015). This substantial socioeconomic gradient in physical activity engagement is consistently observed across all age groups, commencing from early childhood (Salmon et al., 2005).

Children's levels of physical activity are usually connected to their parents' levels of physical activity (Ruedl et al., 2021). Mothers in disadvantaged areas have shown lower levels of physical activity than their peers in developed countries (Morris et al., 2020). This respectively affects the children (Carson et al., 2020). Another reason is the children not doing enough physical activity at school as schools might opt to cancel physical education class to give more time and focus on other subjects. Here it isn't just the schools but some parents in disadvantaged areas believe that physical education classes could affect the child's academic performance negatively (Eyre et al., 2022; Tucker et al., 2015).

The absence of regular physical activity among vulnerable children in disadvantaged areas has its consequences. Firstly, the health implications are substantial, with inadequate physical activity contributing to heightened risks of obesity, cardiovascular diseases, and mental health challenges such as stress and anxiety (Gibala et al., 2012). Developmentally, the lack of physical activity hinders the refinement of motor skills crucial for daily functioning and may impact cognitive development, potentially influencing academic performance (Pan et al., 2019). Socially and emotionally, these children may face social isolation and emotional challenges as the communal aspects of physical activity, such as team sports, provide valuable opportunities for interaction and mood regulation (Ball et al., 2015; Tandon et al., 2021).

Implementing modifications through targeted physical activity programs that consider both the physical and the psychological aspects has shown promise in addressing maladaptive behavior (Li et al., 2022). Regular physical activity brings about improvements in self-regulation, emotional control, and enhanced coping mechanisms. Structured interventions develop social skills, foster teamwork, and instill discipline but also contribute to modifying maladaptive behavior patterns and improving well-being (Biddle & Asare, 2011).

Focusing on vulnerable populations in childhood aligns with the principles of equity. It recognizes that not all children start from the same baseline and that tailored support is necessary to ensure that every child has an equal chance to thrive (Embleton et al., 2020). Implementing physical activity programs for children in vulnerable areas faces numerous challenges and barriers. We will address these obstacles and provide potential solutions.

Challenges in Implementing Physical Activity Programs for Children in Vulnerable Areas

Children in vulnerable areas and populations face distinct challenges that significantly impact their ability to embrace and sustain physical activity programs. These challenges span socioeconomic, cultural, and environmental factors, necessitating tailored approaches in behavior change initiatives.

First, socioeconomic barriers, in economically disadvantaged areas, children confront obstacles related to restricted access to resources like sports facilities, proper equipment, and qualified trainers, hindering their engagement in structured physical activity programs. Economic disparities further contribute to financial constraints, creating barriers to participation in organized sports or fitness programs. The associated costs of enrollment, equipment, and transportation become significant hindrances, limiting the accessibility of physical activity initiatives for children in such disadvantaged circumstances (Cleland et al., 2012; Eyre et al., 2022; Larrinaga-Undabarrena et al., 2023).

In economically disadvantaged areas, an additional layer of complexity arises with the prevalence of child labor, where children are compelled to work to support their families. This compromises their health and physical activity levels, subjecting them to hazardous conditions that can lead to physical strain, injuries, malnutrition, and stunted growth. Child labor not only denies these children the essential play and exercise necessary for overall well-being but also exacerbates existing economic challenges faced by families (Ibrahim et al., 2019). According to a 2021 UNICEF report, an estimated 160 million children are in child labor worldwide (UNICEF, 2021).

Cultural perceptions of exercise play a pivotal role in shaping children's attitudes toward physical activity, influencing their views on the acceptability and importance of such programs (Mohammadi et al., 2023). The cultural context significantly informs program design, necessitating careful consideration to align with community values and preferences. Moreover, gender norms within a culture can influence the types of physical activities deemed appropriate for boys and girls, underscoring the need for culturally sensitive and inclusive programs (Mohammadi et al., 2023; Rio & Saligan, 2023).

The environment restrictions and safety concerns pose a significant challenge for children in vulnerable areas, particularly concerning the lack of secure outdoor spaces for physical activities especially during war or natural disasters. Addressing these safety issues is crucial for establishing a conducive and secure environment for effective physical activity engagement. Additionally, the limited availability of recreational spaces, such as parks or playgrounds, presents an obstacle to implementing physical activity programs, emphasizing the need for innovative solutions to make these programs accessible in resource-limited settings (Pouliou et al., 2015).

Education barriers like the lack of access to education and limited awareness and education pose significant barriers to the successful promotion of physical activity programs, especially in vulnerable areas (Ruedl et al., 2021). Research shows that children can do most of the required physical activity levels at school since it is the most awake time they spend during the day (Grao-Cruces et al., 2020). In areas torn by war, conflict, and natural disasters, many children do not go to school. A UNESCO report estimates that 250 million children are out of school (UNICEF, 2018). This, with many other factors, hinders the opportunities for those children to be physically active. The lack of understanding about the benefits of physical activity, coupled with insufficient educational resources, hampers the dissemination of information and community support. Overcoming these barriers requires robust educational initiatives that not only highlight the advantages of physical activity but also actively engage communities in the promotion of a healthier lifestyle (Pouliou et al., 2015).

Parental constraints play a pivotal role in shaping children's participation in extracurricular activities (Carson et al., 2020). In vulnerable areas, parents often encounter challenges such as time constraints and a lack of awareness regarding the significance of physical activity. The limited availability of time or understanding can hinder parents from actively supporting and encouraging their children to engage in physical activity programs (Ruedl et al., 2021). Addressing parental constraints necessitates community-focused initiatives that not only educate parents about the positive impact of physical activity on their children's well-being but also provide practical solutions to overcome time-related challenges (Nyberg et al., 2016). By involving and empowering parents, children can more readily participate and benefit from physical activity programs.

Children in vulnerable populations often contend with preexisting health disparities that significantly affect their capacity to participate in physically demanding activities. The presence of elevated health inequalities may be a barrier to engaging in strenuous exercises, requiring a nuanced and inclusive approach in program design. Tailoring interventions for diverse health conditions in these populations is crucial to create an inclusive environment for all children, irrespective of health disparities, to actively participate (Cleland et al., 2012).

Addressing health inequalities not only contributes to the inclusivity of physical activity programs but also underscores the broader goal of promoting equitable access to physical activity, ensuring that health disparities do not impede children in vulnerable populations from reaping the benefits of such interventions (Aboud & Singla, 2012).

After discussing potential challenges in implementing a physical activity program in this population, we will explore behavior change theories that can effectively address these challenges and support the successful implementation of such programs.

Behavior Change Theories/Models and Their Implementation in Physical Activity Programs

Implementing behavior change theories in the context of physical activity programs for children in disadvantaged areas is paramount for fostering positive and sustainable health outcomes (Smokowski, 1998). These theories offer a systematic framework to understand, predict, and influence behavior. In the context of vulnerable populations, including children facing socioeconomic challenges, the application of these theories could become a crucial tool. Tailoring interventions based on the key constructs of these theories—such as attitudes, subjective norms, perceived behavioral control, and observational learning—allows for a nuanced understanding of the unique challenges and motivations prevalent in disadvantaged communities.

By incorporating behavior change theories into program design, interventions can address specific barriers, enhance self-efficacy, and leverage social support networks to promote sustained engagement in physical activity among children in vulnerable areas (Bélanger-Gravel & Godin, 2010). This approach not only acknowledges the multifaceted influences on behavior but also provides a strategic and evidence-based foundation for crafting interventions that resonate with the needs and circumstances of children facing adversity (Aboud & Singla, 2012).

The SCT by Albert Bandura highlights the impact of observational learning and social factors on behavior change, recognizing individual, social, and environmental influences. Although the SCT has advantages, such as a robust framework incorporating self-efficacy and social support, limitations include a potential oversight of external environmental factors and reliance on self-report measures (Bandura et al., 1999).

The HBM delves into health-related behaviors, emphasizing factors like perceived susceptibility, severity, benefits, barriers, cues to action, and self-efficacy. While advantageous for its structured approach, HBM's limitations lie in assuming rational decision-making and potentially overlooking emotional and contextual factors. To align HBM with physical activity programs for children, addressing their beliefs and reducing barriers is crucial for successful behavior change (Ar-yuwat et al., 2013; Green et al., 2020; Rosenstock, 1977).

The SDT, crafted by Deci and Ryan, focuses on intrinsic motivation and psychological needs, promoting autonomy, competence, and relatedness. The SDT aligns with cultivating genuine interest and enjoyment in physical activity, emphasizing supportive environments. Despite cultural context variations, the SDT offers a holistic approach to sustained engagement, acknowledging intrinsic and extrinsic motivations. Implementing the SDT in physical activity programs involves creating autonomy-supportive environments, fostering skill development, and encouraging positive social interactions (Deci & Ryan, 1985; Hagger & Chatzisarantis, 2008; Ryan & Deci, 2000).

The TPB, by Ajzen, predicts behavior through attitudes, subjective norms, and perceived behavioral control. While effective in diverse health-related domains, the TPB's focus on individual factors may overlook broader social and environmental influences. Integrating the TPB into physical activity programs includes leveraging key constructs, assessing participant attitudes, creating supportive environments, and incorporating behavior change techniques (Ajzen, 1991; Armitage, 2005).

The TTM, developed by Prochaska and DiClemente, views behavior changes as a gradual process with stages. Recognizing individual readiness levels, the TTM allows tailored interventions. Despite focusing on individual-level factors, the TTM may overlook sociocultural and environmental influences. Implementing the TTM in physical activity programs entails assessing readiness, providing education, and employing processes of change to facilitate sustained behavior change (Hashemzadeh et al., 2019; Prochaska & Velicer, 1997; Sheng et al., 2023).

Influencing Factors, Possible Solutions, and Implementations

Promoting physical activity is crucial for public health, employing various strategies aimed at encouraging regular exercise and lifelong physical activity habits (Chaput et al., 2020). The effectiveness of these strategies is influenced by factors like gender, socioeconomic status, social support, and motivation (Bloemen et al., 2015). Recognizing these influences is vital for tailoring interventions and maximizing the impact of physical activity promotion strategies (Michie et al., 2018). Additionally, developing lifelong physical activity habits from early childhood to adulthood is key for sustaining a healthy lifestyle. Longitudinal studies, like Telama et al. (2005), offer valuable insights into the enduring effects of physical activity on adult exercise habits, emphasizing the importance of interventions across the developmental spectrum.

Gender significantly moderates the effectiveness of physical activity promotion strategies, with research indicating differential responses between males and females due to varying preferences, barriers, and motivations (Bloemen et al., 2015). Tailoring physical activity programs to address gender-specific needs enhances participation and adherence (Schlund et al., 2021). Socioeconomic status (SES) is another influential factor affecting strategy effectiveness, particularly for lower SES individuals facing barriers like limited access to resources (Kyan & Takakura, 2022).

Social support serves as a crucial mediator impacting the effectiveness of physical promotion strategies. Positive support from family, friends, and peers enhances motivation and adherence to exercise (Zou et al., 2023). Interventions incorporating social support mechanisms, such as group activities or buddy systems, foster a sense of belonging, promoting sustained engagement in physical activity (Lee et al., 2020).

Motivation, both intrinsic and extrinsic, plays a pivotal role in strategy effectiveness. Intrinsic motivation, driven by personal enjoyment and perceived competence, is linked to long-term physical activity adherence as well as extrinsic motivation, such as rewards (Hagger & Chatzisarantis, 2008). Aligning program design with individuals' motivational factors, including appropriate external incentives, maximizes participation and adherence, capitalizing on intrinsic motivation (Markland & Tobin, 2010).

Designing Inclusive HIIT Programs for Children in Vulnerable Populations

There is no research evidence on the benefits of a HIIT program in this population; however, there are many highlighting the importance of HIIT in increasing children's levels of physical activity and their many benefits. Crafting effective HIIT programs for children in vulnerable populations requires a meticulous and adaptable approach to address unique challenges. Considerations include program duration, intensity, progression, inclusivity, and exercise adaptation (Eddolls et al., 2017; Miller, 2016). Program duration should balance short, engaging intervals with sufficient rest, catering to children's attention spans and preventing burnout (Heisz et al., 2016). Intensity and progression involve a gradual start with low to moderate intensity, avoiding overwhelm, and incorporating progressive challenges for continual improvement (Gibala et al., 2012).

Inclusivity demands culturally relevant activities and accessible exercises to align with community preferences (Mohammadi et al., 2023). Adaptation to varying fitness levels includes tiered exercises and individualized progress plans. Fun and engagement are crucial, achieved through gamification, challenges, and playful elements (Heisz et al., 2016). A supportive environment involves community cultivation, including parents and influencers. Educational components highlight HIIT's health benefits (Lee et al., 2020; Pouliou et al., 2015; Tucker et al., 2015). Aligning HIIT program design with children's unique needs ensures impactful and sustainable interventions, promoting physical activity and well-being in vulnerable populations.

Implementation of Behavior Change Strategies in a HIIT Program

HIIT programs for children require evidence-based behavior change strategies to ensure both initial engagement and sustained participation (Al-walah et al., 2023). Drawing from behavior change theories, practitioners deploy a range of interventions. These include establishing social support through buddy systems and peer demonstrations (Zou et al., 2023), promoting accountability with goal-setting and self-monitoring tools, offering recognition systems and tangible rewards for positive reinforcement, fostering a supportive environment through family involvement and community partnerships (Karmali et al., 2020; Nyberg et al., 2016), introducing variety and enjoyment through diverse activities and interactive games, and incorporating educational components on health and nutrition (Heisz et al., 2016).

By combining these strategies, practitioners create a holistic environment that not only sparks children's interest in HIIT but also cultivates a lasting commitment to regular physical activity. This multifaceted approach recognizes the importance of addressing social, psychological, and environmental factors in shaping behavior. It acknowledges that sustained engagement goes beyond the initial attraction, requiring ongoing support, motivation, and a sense of accomplishment.

A Possible Implementation of a HIIT Framework

A HIIT program stands out as a time-effective solution to address the time limitations children might face due to environmental constraints. Its versatility makes it easily adaptable to the diverse needs of children in various settings. Offering the benefits of an hour of physical activity in just 5–20 min, it serves as a practical substitute until other options become viable (Eddolls et al., 2017; Miller, 2016). The cost-effective and tools-free nature of the program enables implementation at home or community centers if available (Albustami et al., 2023). This time-efficient approach fosters a sense of accomplishment, enjoyment, and mood improvements that could be particularly beneficial for children who might be experiencing burnout, such as those involved in child labor (Saanijoki et al., 2017).

Furthermore, integrating behavior change theories into physical activity programs is crucial to overcoming barriers hindering children from being physically active while providing effective solutions (Lubans et al., 2017). The SCT, for instance, emphasizes social norms and the importance of support from the surrounding environment, including parental and peer support (Bandura, 2001). Implementing a HIIT program in group settings that involve parents could yield better results for both children and their parents, addressing both physical and psychological aspects (Rhodes et al., 2010). Physical activity has the potential to improve maladaptive behavior in children and enhance their psychological well-being (Biddle & Asare, 2011).

The effectiveness of such an approach was investigated in a quasi-experimental research study conducted as part of an unpublished master's thesis at Istanbul University-Cerrahpasa (Amer & Arman, 2023). The study focused on the potential effectiveness of a physical activity program, incorporating four behavior change theories, in Turkish children aged 7–12. The program recommended a 25-min HIIT session, comprising a 3-min warm-up, 12 min of HIIT, and a 10-min cooling down period, conducted twice a week for 8 weeks at a community center-like venue. The SCT guided meetings, presentations, and interactive tools. The SDT empowered children through autonomy and consistent group sessions. The TPB motivational interviewing to promote equality in effort. The TTM informed personalized strategies, ensuring timely support. This holistic approach fostered a supportive environment for sustained behavior change.

Notably, the results indicated a significant increase in motivation levels, physical activity levels, and self-efficacy levels in the participants in the intervention group, underscoring the success of the integrated behavior change theories in promoting positive behavior change.

Challenges and Future Directions in Implementing HIIT Programs in Vulnerable Areas

Challenges

Implementing HIIT programs in vulnerable areas faces diverse challenges. Resource limitations in these regions impact access to essential facilities, exacerbated by economic disparities. Limited time and family responsibilities hinder children's participation in physical activity. Addressing cultural sensitivities is crucial for program acceptance, requiring alignment with local values. Safety concerns require collaboration with local authorities. Fostering community engagement is vital, demanding extensive outreach and partnerships for program success.

Future Directions

To overcome challenges, future HIIT programs must prioritize adaptability and inclusivity. Tailoring interventions to vulnerable populations, considering cultural, economic, and environmental factors, is crucial. Empowering communities through capacity-building initiatives ensures program sustainability. Leveraging technology, especially virtual platforms, enhances accessibility. Longitudinal studies are vital to assess lasting impact. A holistic health approach integrating nutrition, mental well-being, and lifestyle is key. Scalability relies on policy advocacy, collaborating with policymakers. Multisectoral collaboration between public health entities, educational institutions, NGOs, and community organizations amplifies program impact and sustainability.

In addressing these challenges and charting future directions, the goal is to cultivate sustainable, culturally sensitive HIIT interventions that positively impact the health and well-being of children in vulnerable communities.

Conclusion

In conclusion, the implementation of HIIT programs in vulnerable areas is a complex endeavor fraught with challenges but brimming with potential. The multifaceted issues, ranging from resource limitations and economic disparities to cultural sensitivities and safety concerns, demand innovative and adaptive solutions. As we look toward the future, the outlined strategies for adaptability, inclusivity, and community empowerment serve as guiding principles for the next phase of HIIT interventions. By tailoring programs to the unique needs of vulnerable populations, leveraging technology, and fostering collaborative partnerships, we can navigate the hurdles and unlock the transformative power of HIIT. This holistic approach not only addresses immediate challenges but sets the stage for sustainable, culturally sensitive interventions that have a lasting impact on the health and well-being of children in these communities. The journey ahead requires continued dedication, research, and collaborative efforts, but the promise of positive change beckons us to forge ahead on this important path of health and community empowerment.

References

Aboud, F. E., & Singla, D. R. (2012). Challenges to changing health behaviours in developing countries: A critical overview. *Social Science & Medicine, 75*(4), 589–594. https://doi.org/10.1016/J.SOCSCIMED.2012.04.009

Ajzen, I. (1991). The theory of planned behavior. *Organizational Behavior and Human Decision Processes, 50*(2), 179–211. https://doi.org/10.1016/0749-5978(91)90020-T

Albustami, M., Hartfiel, N., Charles, J. M., Powell, R., Begg, B., Birkett, S. T., Nichols, S., Ennis, S., Hee, S. W., Banerjee, P., Ingle, L., Shave, R., McGregor, G., & Edwards, R. T. (2023). Cost-effectiveness of high-intensity interval training (HIIT) versus moderate intensity steady-state (MISS) training in UK cardiac rehabilitation. *Archives of Physical Medicine and Rehabilitation*. https://doi.org/10.1016/J.APMR.2023.09.005

Al-walah, M. A., Donnelly, M., Cunningham, C., & Heron, N. (2023). Which behaviour change techniques are associated with interventions that increase physical activity in pre-school children? A systematic review. *BMC Public Health, 23*(1), 1–18. https://doi.org/10.1186/S12889-023-16885-0

Amer, M., & Arman, N. (2023). *Developing a physical activity program based on behavior change models in children and investigating of its efficiency* [Master thesis]. Istanbul University-Cerrahpasa.

Armitage, C. J. (2005). Can the theory of planned behavior predict the maintenance of physical activity? *Health Psychology, 24*(3), 235–245. https://doi.org/10.1037/0278-6133.24.3.235

Arnault, L., Jusot, F., & Renaud, T. (2021). Economic vulnerability and unmet healthcare needs among the population aged 50 + years during the COVID-19 pandemic in Europe. *European Journal of Ageing, 19*(4), 811–825. https://doi.org/10.1007/S10433-021-00645-3

Ar-yuwat, S., Clark, M. J., Hunter, A., & James, K. S. (2013). Determinants of physical activity in primary school students using the health belief model. *Journal of Multidisciplinary Healthcare, 6*, 119. https://doi.org/10.2147/JMDH.S40876

Bagherniya, M., Darani, F. M., Sharma, M., Maracy, M. R., Birgani, R. A., Ranjbar, G., Taghipour, A., Safarian, M., & Keshavarz, S. A. (2018). Assessment of the efficacy of physical activity level and lifestyle behavior interventions applying social cognitive theory for overweight and

obese girl adolescents. *Journal of Research in Health Sciences, 18*(2). https://pubmed.ncbi.nlm.nih.gov/29784890/
Ball, K., Carver, A., Downing, K., Jackson, M., & O'rourke, K. (2015). Addressing the social determinants of inequities in physical activity and sedentary behaviours. *Health Promotion International, 30*(S2). https://doi.org/10.1093/heapro/dav022
Bandura, A. (2001). Social cognitive theory: An agentic perspective. *Annual Review of Psychology, 52*, 1–26. https://doi.org/10.1146/ANNUREV.PSYCH.52.1.1
Bandura, A., Freeman, W. H., & Lightsey, R. (1999). Self-efficacy: The exercise of control. *Journal of Cognitive Psychotherapy, 13*(2), 158–166. https://doi.org/10.1891/0889-8391.13.2.158
Bélanger-Gravel, A., & Godin, G. (2010). Key beliefs for targeted interventions to increase physical activity in children: Analyzing data from an extended version of the theory of planned behaviour. *International Journal of Pediatrics, 2010*, 1–7. https://doi.org/10.1155/2010/893854
Biddle, S. J. H., & Asare, M. (2011). Physical activity and mental health in children and adolescents: A review of reviews. *British Journal of Sports Medicine, 45*(11), 886–895. https://doi.org/10.1136/BJSPORTS-2011-090185
Bloemen, M. A. T., Backx, F. J. G., Takken, T., Wittink, H., Benner, J., Mollema, J., & de Groot, J. F. (2015). Factors associated with physical activity in children and adolescents with a physical disability: A systematic review. *Developmental Medicine and Child Neurology, 57*(2), 137–148. https://doi.org/10.1111/DMCN.12624
Carson, V., Langlois, K., & Colley, R. (2020). Associations between parent and child sedentary behaviour and physical activity in early childhood. *Health Reports, 31*(2), 3–10. https://doi.org/10.25318/82-003-X202000200001-ENG
Chaput, J. P., Willumsen, J., Bull, F., Chou, R., Ekelund, U., Firth, J., Jago, R., Ortega, F. B., & Katzmarzyk, P. T. (2020). 2020 WHO guidelines on physical activity and sedentary behaviour for children and adolescents aged 5–17 years: Summary of the evidence. *International Journal of Behavioral Nutrition and Physical Activity, 17*(1), 1–9. https://doi.org/10.1186/S12966-020-01037-Z/TABLES/6
Cleland, C. L., Tully, M. A., Kee, F., & Cupples, M. E. (2012). The effectiveness of physical activity interventions in socio-economically disadvantaged communities: A systematic review. *Preventive Medicine, 54*(6), 371–380. https://doi.org/10.1016/J.YPMED.2012.04.004
Craike, M., Wiesner, G., Hilland, T. A., & Bengoechea, E. G. (2018). Interventions to improve physical activity among socioeconomically disadvantaged groups: An umbrella review. *International Journal of Behavioral Nutrition and Physical Activity, 15*(1), 1–11. https://doi.org/10.1186/S12966-018-0676-2/TABLES/1
de Souza, L. B., Aragão, F. B. A., da Cunha, J. H. S., & Fiorati, R. C. (2021). Intersectoral actions in decreasing social inequities faced by children and adolescents. *Revista Latino-Americana de Enfermagem, 29*. https://doi.org/10.1590/1518-8345.4162.3427
Deci, E. L., & Ryan, R. M. (1985). *Intrinsic motivation and self-determination in human behavior*. Springer. https://doi.org/10.1007/978-1-4899-2271-7
Eddolls, W. T. B., McNarry, M. A., Stratton, G., Winn, C. O. N., & Mackintosh, K. A. (2017). High-intensity interval training interventions in children and adolescents: A systematic review. *Sports Medicine (Auckland, N.z.), 47*(11), 2363. https://doi.org/10.1007/S40279-017-0753-8
Embleton, L., Shah, P., Gayapersad, A. A., Kiptui, R., Ayuku, D., & Braitstein, P. (2020). Identifying strategies to advance health equity through action on social determinants of health and human rights for street-connected children and youth in Kenya. *Health and Human Rights, 22*(2), 177. https://www.ncbi.nlm.nih.gov/pmc/articles/PMC7762894/.
Etzel, R. A. (2020). The special vulnerability of children. *International Journal of Hygiene and Environmental Health, 227*, 113516. https://doi.org/10.1016/J.IJHEH.2020.113516
Eyre, E. L. J., Adeyemi, L. J., Cook, K., Noon, M., Tallis, J., & Duncan, M. (2022). Barriers and facilitators to physical activity and FMS in children living in deprived areas in the UK: Qualitative study. *International Journal of Environmental Research and Public Health, 19*(3). https://doi.org/10.3390/IJERPH19031717

Gibala, M. J., Little, J. P., Macdonald, M. J., & Hawley, J. A. (2012). Physiological adaptations to low-volume, high-intensity interval training in health and disease. *The Journal of Physiology, 590*(Pt 5), 1077. https://doi.org/10.1113/JPHYSIOL.2011.224725

Gordon, E. W. (1965). Chapter I: Characteristics of socially disadvantaged children. *Review of Educational Research, 35*(5), 377–388. https://doi.org/10.3102/00346543035005377/ASSET/00346543035005377.FP.PNG_V03

Grao-Cruces, A., Velásquez-Romero, M. J., & Rodriguez-Rodríguez, F. (2020). Levels of physical activity during school hours in children and adolescents: A systematic review. *International Journal of Environmental Research and Public Health, 17*(13), 1–23. https://doi.org/10.3390/IJERPH17134773

Green, E. C., Murphy, E. M., & Gryboski, K. (2020). The health belief model. *The Wiley Encyclopedia of Health Psychology*, 211–214. https://doi.org/10.1002/9781119057840.CH68

Hagger, M., & Chatzisarantis, N. (2008). Self-determination theory and the psychology of exercise. *International Review of Sport and Exercise Psychology, 1*(1), 79–103. https://doi.org/10.1080/17509840701827437

Hashemzadeh, M., Rahimi, A., Zare-Farashbandi, F., Alavi-Naeini, A., & Daei, A. (2019). Transtheoretical model of health behavioral change: A systematic review. *Iranian Journal of Nursing and Midwifery Research, 24*(2), 83–90. https://doi.org/10.4103/IJNMR.IJNMR_94_17

Heisz, J. J., Tejada, M. G. M., Paolucci, E. M., & Muir, C. (2016). Enjoyment for high-intensity interval exercise increases during the first six weeks of training: Implications for promoting exercise adherence in sedentary adults. *PLoS One, 11*(12). https://doi.org/10.1371/JOURNAL.PONE.0168534

Ibrahim, A., Abdalla, S. M., Jafer, M., Abdelgadir, J., & De Vries, N. (2019). Child labor and health: A systematic literature review of the impacts of child labor on child's health in low- and middle-income countries. *Journal of Public Health (Oxford, England), 41*(1), 18. https://doi.org/10.1093/PUBMED/FDY018

Jones, C. L., Jensen, J. D., Scherr, C. L., Brown, N. R., Christy, K., & Weaver, J. (2015). The health belief model as an explanatory framework in communication research: Exploring parallel, serial, and moderated mediation. *Health Communication, 30*(6), 566. https://doi.org/10.1080/10410236.2013.873363

Karmali, S., Battram, D. S., Burke, S. M., Cramp, A., Johnson, A. M., Mantler, T., Morrow, D., Ng, V., Pearson, E. S., Petrella, R. J., Tucker, P., & Irwin, J. D. (2020). Perspectives and impact of a parent-child intervention on dietary intake and physical activity behaviours, parental motivation, and parental body composition: A randomized controlled trial. *International Journal of Environmental Research and Public Health, 17*(18), 1–41. https://doi.org/10.3390/IJERPH17186822

Ke, Y., Shi, L., Peng, L., Chen, S., Hong, J., & Liu, Y. (2022). Associations between socioeconomic status and physical activity: A cross-sectional analysis of Chinese children and adolescents. *Frontiers in Psychology, 13*, 904506. https://doi.org/10.3389/FPSYG.2022.904506/BIBTEX

Kruk, M. E., Gage, A. D., Arsenault, C., Jordan, K., Leslie, H. H., Roder-DeWan, S., Adeyi, O., Barker, P., Daelmans, B., Doubova, S. V., English, M., Elorrio, E. G., Guanais, F., Gureje, O., Hirschhorn, L. R., Jiang, L., Kelley, E., Lemango, E. T., Liljestrand, J., et al. (2018). High-quality health systems in the sustainable development goals era: Time for a revolution. *The Lancet. Global Health, 6*(11), e1196. https://doi.org/10.1016/S2214-109X(18)30386-3

Kyan, A., & Takakura, M. (2022). Socio-economic inequalities in physical activity among Japanese adults during the COVID-19 pandemic. *Public Health, 207*, 7–13. https://doi.org/10.1016/J.PUHE.2022.03.006

Larrinaga-Undabarrena, A., Río, X., Sáez, I., Martinez Aguirre-Betolaza, A., Albisua, N., Martínez de Lahidalga Aguirre, G., Sánchez Isla, J. R., Urbano, M., Guerra-Balic, M., Fernández, J. R., & Coca, A. (2023). Effects of socioeconomic environment on physical activity levels and sleep quality in basque schoolchildren. *Children, 10*(3), 551. https://doi.org/10.3390/CHILDREN10030551

Lee, J., Hoornbeek, J., & Oh, N. (2020). Social cognitive orientations, social support, and physical activity among at-risk urban children: Insights from a structural equation model. *International Journal of Environmental Research and Public Health, 17*(18), 1–17. https://doi.org/10.3390/IJERPH17186745

Li, J., Huang, Z., Si, W., & Shao, T. (2022). The effects of physical activity on positive emotions in children and adolescents: A systematic review and meta-analysis. *International Journal of Environmental Research and Public Health, 19*(21), 14185. https://doi.org/10.3390/IJERPH192114185/S1

LoBue, V., & Ogren, M. (2022). How the emotional environment shapes the emotional life of the child. *Policy Insights From the Behavioral and Brain Sciences, 9*(1), 137. https://doi.org/10.1177/23727322211067264

Lubans, D. R., Lonsdale, C., Cohen, K., Eather, N., Beauchamp, M. R., Morgan, P. J., Sylvester, B. D., & Smith, J. J. (2017). Framework for the design and delivery of organized physical activity sessions for children and adolescents: Rationale and description of the 'SAAFE' teaching principles. *International Journal of Behavioral Nutrition and Physical Activity, 14*(1), 1–11. https://doi.org/10.1186/S12966-017-0479-X

Mah, J. C., Penwarden, J. L., Pott, H., Theou, O., & Andrew, M. K. (2023). Social vulnerability indices: A scoping review. *BMC Public Health, 23*(1), 1–11. https://doi.org/10.1186/S12889-023-16097-6/FIGURES/3

Markland, D., & Tobin, V. J. (2010). Need support and behavioural regulations for exercise among exercise referral scheme clients: The mediating role of psychological need satisfaction. *Psychology of Sport and Exercise, 11*(2), 91–99. https://doi.org/10.1016/J.PSYCHSPORT.2009.07.001

Melhuish, E. (2014). The impact of early childhood education and care on improved wellbeing. *Faculty of Social Sciences - Papers (Archive)*. https://ro.uow.edu.au/sspapers/1642

Michie, S., Carey, R. N., Johnston, M., Rothman, A. J., De Bruin, M., Kelly, M. P., & Connell, L. E. (2018). From theory-inspired to theory-based interventions: A protocol for developing and testing a methodology for linking behaviour change techniques to theoretical mechanisms of action. *Annals of Behavioral Medicine, 52*(6), 501–512. https://doi.org/10.1007/S12160-016-9816-6

Fred, L., & Miller, I. (2016). High-intensity interval training versus traditional continuous training. *AMAA Journal, 29*(1), 8–10. https://go.gale.com/ps/i.do?p=AONE&sw=w&issn=&v=2.1&it=r&id=GALE%7CA453907241&sid=googleScholar&linkaccess=fulltext

Mohammadi, M., Elahipanah, F., & Amani-shalamzari, S. (2023). The role of the cultural environment in the development of physical literacy and physical activity of Iranian children. *BMC Pediatrics, 23*(1), 1–9. https://doi.org/10.1186/S12887-023-04297-3/TABLES/4

Morris, K. A., Arundell, L., Cleland, V., & Teychenne, M. (2020). Social ecological factors associated with physical activity and screen time amongst mothers from disadvantaged neighbourhoods over three years. *International Journal of Behavioral Nutrition and Physical Activity, 17*(1), 1–11. https://doi.org/10.1186/S12966-020-01015-5/TABLES/6

Nyberg, G., Norman, Å., Sundblom, E., Zeebari, Z., & Elinder, L. S. (2016). Effectiveness of a universal parental support programme to promote health behaviours and prevent overweight and obesity in 6-year-old children in disadvantaged areas, the Healthy School Start Study II, a cluster-randomised controlled trial. *International Journal of Behavioral Nutrition and Physical Activity, 13*(1), 1–14. https://doi.org/10.1186/S12966-016-0327-4/TABLES/5

Pan, C. Y., Tsai, C. L., Chu, C. H., Sung, M. C., Huang, C. Y., & Ma, W. Y. (2019). Effects of physical exercise intervention on motor skills and executive functions in children with ADHD: A pilot study. *Journal of Attention Disorders, 23*(4), 384–397. https://doi.org/10.1177/1087054715569282

Paul-Sen Gupta, R., De Wit, M. L., & McKeown, D. (2007). The impact of poverty on the current and future health status of children. *Paediatrics & Child Health, 12*(8), 667. https://doi.org/10.1093/PCH/12.8.667

Pouliou, T., Sera, F., Griffiths, L., Joshi, H., Geraci, M., Cortina-Borja, M., & Law, C. (2015). Environmental influences on children's physical activity. *Journal of Epidemiology and Community Health, 69*(1), 77–85. https://doi.org/10.1136/JECH-2014-204287

Prochaska, J. O., & Velicer, W. F. (1997). The transtheoretical model of health behavior change. *American Journal of Health Promotion, 12*(1), 38–48.

Rhodes, R. E., Naylor, P. J., & McKay, H. A. (2010). Pilot study of a family physical activity planning intervention among parents and their children. *Journal of Behavioral Medicine, 33*(2), 91–100. https://doi.org/10.1007/S10865-009-9237-0

Rio, C. J., & Saligan, L. N. (2023). Understanding physical activity from a cultural-contextual lens. *Frontiers in Public Health, 11*, 1223919. https://doi.org/10.3389/FPUBH.2023.1223919/BIBTEX

Rosenstock, I. M. (1977). The health belief model and preventive health behavior. *Health Education & Behavior, 2*(4), 354–386. https://doi.org/10.1177/109019817400200405/ASSET/109019817400200405.FP.PNG_V03

Ruedl, G., Niedermeier, M., Wimmer, L., Ploner, V., Pocecco, E., Cocca, A., & Greier, K. (2021). Impact of parental education and physical activity on the long-term development of the physical fitness of primary school children: An observational study. *International Journal of Environmental Research and Public Health, 18*(16). https://doi.org/10.3390/IJERPH18168736

Ryan, R. M., & Deci, E. L. (2000). Self-determination theory and the facilitation of intrinsic motivation, social development, and well-being. *The American Psychologist, 55*(1), 68–78. https://doi.org/10.1037/0003-066X.55.1.68

Saanijoki, T., Tuominen, L., Tuulari, J. J., Nummenmaa, L., Arponen, E., Kalliokoski, K., & Hirvonen, J. (2017). Opioid release after high-intensity interval training in healthy human subjects. *Neuropsychopharmacology, 43*(2), 246–254. https://doi.org/10.1038/npp.2017.148

Salmon, J., Timperio, A., Cleland, V., & Venn, A. (2005). Trends in children's physical activity and weight status in high and low socio-economic status areas of Melbourne, Victoria, 1985-2001. *Australian and New Zealand Journal of Public Health, 29*(4), 337–342. https://doi.org/10.1111/J.1467-842X.2005.TB00204.X

Schlund, A., Reimers, A. K., Bucksch, J., Brindley, C., Schulze, C., Puil, L., Coen, S. E., Phillips, S. P., Knapp, G., & Demetriou, Y. (2021). Do intervention studies to promote physical activity and reduce sedentary behavior in children and adolescents take sex/gender into account? a systematic review. *Journal of Physical Activity & Health, 18*(4), 461–468. https://doi.org/10.1123/JPAH.2020-0666

Sheng, J., Shi, P., Sun, J., & Feng, X. (2023). Predictors of physical activity behavior transitions in children and adolescents: A systematic review based on a transtheoretical model. *Journal of Healthcare Engineering, 2023*. https://doi.org/10.1155/2023/5786841

Smokowski, P. R. (1998). Prevention and intervention strategies for promoting resilience in disadvantaged children. *Social Service Review, 72*(3), 337–364. https://doi.org/10.1086/515762

Somerset, S., & Hoare, D. J. (2018). Barriers to voluntary participation in sport for children: A systematic review. *BMC Pediatrics, 18*(1), 1–19. https://doi.org/10.1186/S12887-018-1014-1/FIGURES/3

Stevens, G. D., Seid, M., Mistry, R., & Halfon, N. (2006). Disparities in primary care for vulnerable children: The influence of multiple risk factors. *Health Services Research, 41*(2), 507. https://doi.org/10.1111/J.1475-6773.2005.00498.X

Tandon, P. S., Kroshus, E., Olsen, K., Garrett, K., Qu, P., & McCleery, J. (2021). Socioeconomic inequities in youth participation in physical activity and sports. *International Journal of Environmental Research and Public Health, 18*(13). https://doi.org/10.3390/IJERPH18136946

Tangcharoensathien, V., Mills, A., Das, M. B., Patcharanarumol, W., Buntan, M., & Johns, J. (2018). Addressing the health of vulnerable populations: Social inclusion and universal health coverage. *Journal of Globalization and Health, 8*(2). https://doi.org/10.7189/JOGH.08.020304

Telama, R., Yang, X., Viikari, J., Välimäki, I., Wanne, O., & Raitakari, O. (2005). Physical activity from childhood to adulthood: A 21-year tracking study. *American Journal of Preventive Medicine, 28*(3), 267–273. https://doi.org/10.1016/J.AMEPRE.2004.12.003

Tucker, S., Trotman, D., & Martyn, M. (2015). Vulnerability: The role of schools in supporting young people exposed to challenging environments and situations. *International Journal of Educational Development, 41*, 301–306. https://doi.org/10.1016/J.IJEDUDEV.2014.09.005

UNICEF. (2018, September 18). *1 in 3 children and young people is out of school in countries affected by war or natural disasters—UNICEF*. https://www.unicef.org/press-releases/1-3-children-and-young-people-out-school-countries-affected-war-or-natural-disasters

UNICEF. (2021, June 9). *Child labour rises to 160 million—first increase in two decades*. https://www.unicef.org/press-releases/child-labour-rises-160-million-first-increase-two-decades

Waisel, D. B. (2013). Vulnerable populations in healthcare. *Current Opinion in Anaesthesiology, 26*(2), 186–192. https://doi.org/10.1097/ACO.0B013E32835E8C17

Zou, Y., Liu, S., Guo, S., Zhao, Q., & Cai, Y. (2023). Peer support and exercise adherence in adolescents: The chain-mediated effects of self-efficacy and self-regulation. *Children, 10*(2), 401. https://doi.org/10.3390/CHILDREN10020401

Chronic Illnesses and the Internet: Effects of Idolizing the Stars

Katherine Wilson, Cristina L. Reitz-Krueger, and Michael Duncan Overton

Introduction

With massive technological advancements in a short amount of time, information and people are more accessible than ever before. For chronically ill individuals, this means a longer lifespan and through the use of social media, they have a way to obtain support, educational resources, and improved disease management techniques. Almost half of the studies investigating the benefits of social media for chronically ill individuals suggest positive benefits, while 45% were neutral or undefined, and 7% suggested social media to be harmful (Patel et al., 2015). Despite these findings from Patel et al., the impact of social media heavily depends on the accessibility of technology and applications, how easily they can be navigated, and the individuals' age (2015). For chronically ill adolescents and emerging adults turning to social media, there may be a new risk to look out for: parasocial relationships. With a decreased ability to socialize with peers, the need for connection may cause strong emotional attachments that create additional distress, loneliness, and social isolation at a time when relationships are pivotal for social development.

K. Wilson · M. D. Overton
Warren Wilson College, Asheville, NC, USA
e-mail: kw.parasocially.yours@gmail.com; overton.phd@gmail.com

C. L. Reitz-Krueger (✉)
Department of Psychology, Warren Wilson College, Asheville, NC, USA
e-mail: creitz-krueger@warren-wilson.edu

S. Castaños-Cervantes et al. (eds.), *Working with Vulnerable Populations*,
https://doi.org/10.1007/978-3-031-67710-6_6

Parasocial Relationships

Parasocial relationships (PSRs) are unreciprocated relationships between an individual and a media figure, where time, emotions, and money are invested into someone unaware of their existence (Bond, 2022). PSRs are formed as safe alternatives to real-life connections as there is no chance of rejection with illusionary interactions and emotions projected onto the media figure. These connections also potentially function as components of an individual's social circle that closely mimic real-life friends during periods of media dependency and may be beneficial for emotional or coping purposes during crises that hinder social relationships (Bond, 2022; Hoffner & Bond, 2022). PSRs are not without their problems, however, as some individuals have reported genuine distress due to the emotions they have devoted to them (Murray, 2022a, b).

The phenomena of parasocial relationships were recognized as early as 1956 by Donald Horton and R. Richard Wohl. According to Horton and Wohl, the difference between having a parasocial relationship and simply being a fan is a continued association and a meaningful bond (1956). Individuals in a parasocial relationship may feel that they know the media persona and understand them on an intimate level, despite there being no reciprocation. Giles and Maltby state "they are 'parasocial' because they exist beyond the person's social network" (2006). Currently, social psychologists remain hesitant to acknowledge how parasocial relationships differ from ordinary relationships or whether they should count as relationships at all, considering they do not abide by the mechanics of a typical connection (2006).

There are three levels to how a parasocial relationship develops: entertainment-social, intense-personal, and borderline-pathological: with the relationships becoming more intense the further down an individual progresses (Giles & Maltby, 2006; Espinal, 2021). The first stage, entertainment-social, functions as a form of entertainment or a way to supplement a lack of real-life social interactions. Intense-personal progresses from a relationship purely for entertainment to the forming of an emotionally intense relationship. The last stage, borderline-pathological, results from fans overidentifying with the celebrity to the point that their illusions have become uncontrollable behaviors.

The COVID-19 pandemic created an interesting situation that compelled people to engage in social distancing protocols, increased media exposure, and transitioned social interactions to digital spaces (Bond, 2022). This created an environment in which parasocial relationships could flourish. Parasocial relationships may have also served a compensation function during this time, and increased exposure to real-life friends through social media may have further blurred the lines between social and parasocial. For example, during the beginning of the pandemic, *Mashable* published an article titled "'Emotional support K-pop boys' help fans with their mental health" that elaborates on the strong attachments K-pop fans can have toward idols that provide comfort and inspiration when it is difficult to find elsewhere. While not the only type of celebrity to inspire parasocial attachments, the K-pop industry is unique in the way it almost facilitates them.

K-pop refers to the Korean pop music industry and an "idol" is an artist working in the industry, either as a solo act or within a group. Veronica Espinal from *EnVi Media* states forming this sort of [parasocial] attachment is not unusual for the K-pop industry as entertainment companies count on fans to experience some level of connection (2021). Within the K-pop industry, Korean entertainment companies have devised a structure that creates a specific relationship between fans and the idol, without either party having met in real life (2021). "The structure: the building of exposure, the physical attraction, the task attraction (voting, streaming), and social attraction," all of which contribute to and increase the relationship (2021).

Personal moments and struggles the idols face are made public, increasing feelings of empathy and love toward them, and stimulating social interactions that the fans are looking for. Espinal asserts that "as a result [of the exposure], this special bond has led to the establishment of parasocial relationships" (2021). While the K-pop industry originally marketed groups around the mystery and intrigue their image produced, companies now use social media as a way to promote their idols differently: they capitalize heavily off of the parasocial relationship they have created. By manufacturing their K-pop idols, companies have established a sense of loyalty amongst fans for growth while ensuring constant engagement. The vast distribution of idol content such as comebacks, live streams, and subscription-based applications all factor into building the structure of the relationship.

While entertainment companies and brands capitalize off these connections, they can be detrimental when boundaries get crossed. By marketing idols as a commodity rather than a person or artist, they are not perceived as real people and the relationship becomes blurred. Even when presenting a more "human" side through personal content, they remain unobtainable in the eyes of their fans. Tumblr user fontainexpert states in a post from September 17, 2022:

> Little by little this admiration starts to feel like you know the person, even when deep down you know you don't … You start to see their life behind the screens more and more and then you know your delusion got worse when the admiration starts to taste like 'we could be good friends in real life' … then, next thing you know, they're your safe and comfort place, you start to seek for their comfort when you're sad or happy, starts to wonder how they're such an amazing person, and how unfair is that you'll never get to meet them, or be their friend. It's like watching a person behind a window.

These relationships can positively influence and improve the psychological well-being of those who take part in them, especially when they do not have support from those around them in their daily lives. However, a problem arises when the bond develops into an intense attachment built upon emotional dependency (such as a real-life unhealthy or toxic relationship). Instead of the relationship being approached as a form of enjoyment, the idol is now used as a form of escapism from current events in the individuals' lives, with more time being spent consuming content allowing the attachment to become more intense. The constant influx of content available does not allow fans to take a step back from fandom life, creating a space for them to slip into the borderline-pathological stage of the relationship. These fans, known as sasaengs (사생팬) in K-pop or stalkers in the West, are the byproduct of the inability to control intense emotions and are individuals slipping into an overly obsessive persona (Espinal, 2021). Due to the time and money invested into the idols or artists, they believe they have a right to information surrounding their private lives and resort to unlawful acts and possessive behaviors. This behavior is enabled by companies due to the marketing of the "boyfriend/girlfriend" fantasy and the enforcement of dating bans, bringing harm to fans who have found solace in these relationships and the idols who are just doing their job and fulfilling the requirements of their contract (Espinal, 2021).

While these types of relationships could be observed with Western artists such as One Direction, Justin Bieber, and older boy bands such as NSYNC and New Kids on the Block, K-pop artists stand out due to their constant presence, messaging, and approachable demeanors; all of which are carefully curated through the use of social media (Stec, 2013). With easy direct access and interactive methods of communication, fans may feel like they "know" celebrities and experience increased intimacy and a stronger parasocial relationship (Kim & Song, 2016). A vast majority of fans regularly post on social media sites such as Instagram and Twitter, and celebrities have mastered the art of using this social engagement to remain relevant. This relevancy allows them to establish familiarity by posting updates about their schedules, selfies or group pictures, and links to upcoming content showcasing a more relatable image. Companies use successful marketing strategies such as knowing the target audience to help regulate the time, money, and energy put into marketing efforts and account for the growth of both fans and artists (Stec, 2013). "In an attempt to make themselves appear as dreamy and accessible as possible, they use social media as a vehicle to drive engagement and increase fan loyalty. People expect 24/7 access and social media makes it easy to monitor comments, questions, and concerns in a timely manner" (Stec, 2013). Online presence strengthens the loyalty of their fans, and by engaging with fans on platforms they use regularly for updates, they remain in the public eye (Sturge, 2022).

One explanation for the formation of these relationships is the parasocial compensation hypothesis, which predicates "parasocial relationships (PSRs) with media personae can not only extend viewers' perceived social circles but also serve as functional alternatives to social relationships" (Bond, 2022). The person the connection has been formed with will never be mean, unkind, or reject the other party due to not knowing them in real life, which can help with feelings of disconnect or loneliness in populations at an increased risk. As with everything, the beneficial features also have a downside. "A distortion takes place with those we admire at a distance: These objects are much, much farther away than they appear. We don't know the whole person, just a slice of them blown all out of proportion" (Boyce, 2022, para. 5).

Chronic Illnesses and Social Vulnerability

The technological age that the human race has created also means the continuous evolution of medical advances and a long lifespan for individuals with chronic conditions and disabilities due to medicine and science that was not previously available. Chronic conditions are defined as anything lasting longer than 6 months and often requiring extended periods of care and supervision, affecting physical, cognitive, social, and emotional aspects of development that can also have repercussions for those around them. According to the Centers for Disease Control and Prevention, in America, 6 out of 10 adults have a chronic illness and 4 out of 10 have two or more (Watson, 2022). Out of 74.3 million children and adolescents in the United States, 10–20 million have some form of a chronic illness or disability, with numbers continuing to steadily rise. They are the leading cause of death and further disability, along with being responsible for the nation's $4.1 trillion annual healthcare cost (CDC, 2022).

Chronic illnesses are generally characterized by at least three important features: they last for an extended duration, they do not resolve on their own without intervention, and they are very rarely cured completely (Compas et al., 2012). Along with these illnesses and diseases, "psychological and behavioral disturbances in children suffering from a severe and debilitating medical condition are common and compound the distress and impairment they are enduring," with anxiety, depression, and delirium being the most prominent (Nibras et al., 2022, p. 11). Chronic illnesses during childhood and adolescence can result in a lifetime of chronic stress, and visible signs or treatment marks can cause alienation from peers, resulting in lower levels of emotional well-being due to this alienation (Yeo & Sawyer, 2005). Frustration with the constant care needed for their conditions, several stressors leading to mental health disorders, and social isolation are also seen in chronically ill children (Yeo & Sawyer, 2005).

Chronically ill children also face a greater vulnerability to psychosocial problems in childhood and adolescence (Secinti et al., 2017). By facing significant challenges due to their conditions, they may experience disruptions to their psychological well-being, and psychological problems in childhood are known to be precursors of poor mental health in adulthood. Research has previously suggested that as children with chronic conditions age, their psychosocial problems will either decrease or persist and become more severe (Secinti et al., 2017). Overall, individuals with a history of childhood chronic physical illnesses are more likely to have depression and anxiety but not post-traumatic stress disorder (PTSD) or unspecified emotional problems (Secinti et al., 2017). The psychological distress of having an illness and going through treatment, such as feeling like one has lost control of their body and maladaptive illness cognitions, may contribute to the development of these emotional problems and possibly put these individuals at a higher risk of developing parasocial relationships.

Vulnerabilities in Chronically Ill Individuals and Parasocial Relationships

As already established, chronically ill individuals are more vulnerable to emotional and social challenges when compared to "healthy" peers. One of the challenges that may surface from this absence of social stimulation is a lack of emotional vulnerability (Brown, 2010). Emotional vulnerability is defined as the willingness and ability to address and articulate emotions. To develop emotional vulnerability, one must acknowledge their emotions and deal with them in a healthy, productive manner. While painful emotional experiences will take place across the lifespan, through socialization and habit, a tendency to suppress and hide uncomfortable emotions develops. Avoiding and denying the existence of painful emotions, such as shame, frustration, anxiety, hurt, and grief can create a strain on mental well-being creating uncertainty (Brown, 2012).

By acknowledging and sharing the emotions experienced, emotional and mental well-being can be significantly improved. A problem arises when individuals feel they cannot share their experiences with anyone, either due to self-isolation or barriers to establishing close relationships with others. This lack of relationships creates fewer opportunities to build empathy, improve self-awareness, lower anxiety around unpleasant emotions, and strengthen trust within a relationship (Masterclass, 2022).

When individuals engage in parasocial relationships, they can talk about their experiences with their idols (for better or for worse). Despite being completely one-sided, they have formed a bond and feel understood in a way that is nonexistent in their real life. Due to the lack of reciprocation, they will not be rejected, and this could help ease anxiety surrounding talking about their emotions. As a result of this engagement in a parasocial context, individuals may become more anxious regarding real-life confrontations and unpleasant experiences. There is a reliance on the relationship to function as a friend or community would, but a one-way connection cannot provide what the individuals are looking for resulting in a disconnect between relational expectations.

Social isolation, considered a reduced social network and lack of social contact, can increase feelings of loneliness and leave individuals more susceptible to vulnerabilities not experienced by those who are not lonely (Yanguas et al., 2018). These vulnerabilities range from health issues to being victims of crime, abuse, or exploitation due to the lack of support from those around them. This vulnerability is also closely linked to the concept of scarcity relating to sustainability, development, social exclusion, poverty, and the lack of social support resources (Yanguas et al., 2018). Additionally, social vulnerability is closely tied to physical frailty and mortality as "one's health and development is marked by involvement in community social activities, the ability to take care of oneself, the level of control over circumstances in one's life, and the context to which relationships with those around us take place" (Yanguas et al., 2018, p. 303).

Social isolation resulting from constant symptom management can leave individuals exposed to a variety of complications, such as the development and worsening of health issues, and lead to social vulnerabilities. In a study investigating the relationship between social vulnerability and chronic health conditions, an increased level of social vulnerability was associated with an increased number of chronic health conditions (Nguyen et al., 2019). To assess social vulnerability, Andrew et al. (2008) used an index focused on communication with the wider community, living situation, social support and engagement, socially oriented daily activities, leisure activities, and socioeconomic status. The study focused on individuals with multimorbidity (three or more chronic conditions) and had 19 categories of self-reported conditions including metabolic/hormone disorders, gastrointestinal problems, cancer of any type, musculoskeletal conditions, and cardiovascular disease. Among these, obesity, depression/anxiety, and cardiovascular disease were independently associated with the most social vulnerability among patients (Nguyen et al., 2019).

Loneliness

The need to feel connected to others has been demonstrated across the lifespan, but sometimes there can be a disconnect, resulting in loneliness (Qualter et al., 2015). Loneliness can be defined as the "perception of being alone or isolated and feeling disconnected from others" (Tiwari, 2013). It has been associated with objective social isolation (lack of contact/interaction with others), depression, introversion, or poor social skills. There also exists research suggesting that loneliness is a unique condition in which an individual perceives themself to be socially isolated, even when surrounded by others. In industrialized countries, 1 in 12 people are severely affected and this number continues to increase, resulting in an individual being irritable, depressed, and self-centered (Cacioppo & Cacioppo, 2018). Loneliness is further associated with a 26% increase in the risk of premature death (Cacioppo & Cacioppo, 2018). It is often stigmatized, trivialized, or ignored, but a rapidly growing number of people are facing loneliness. With an increased likelihood of premature death and deleterious effects discovered in human and animal models: loneliness is an emerging public health problem (Cacioppo & Cacioppo, 2018). Further, human and animal studies indicate that the effects of loneliness are not attributable to a certain trait of individuals who are lonely but are due to the effects of loneliness on ordinary people.

Differences in the source of loneliness exist depending on the age of the individual and these differences are associated with changes in belonging needs. The first source of loneliness is peer friendship. While friendship quantity may be more important for predicting loneliness in young children, it shifts to friendship quality during late childhood and adolescence. This is due to children moving away from friends formed from proximity and more toward friendships characterized by validation, understanding, self-discourse, and empathy (Qualter et al., 2015). The second source of loneliness is the peer group; as children age, they become increasingly aware and concerned with being accepted by a peer group and peer rejection can lead to loneliness. At this age, the absence of friendship, low friendship quality, peer rejection, and victimization are all predictors of loneliness in adolescence (Qualter et al., 2015). In late adolescence, focus on social status decreases but the need for an intimate connection remains, making romantic relationships the third source of loneliness. When changes in the social environment are accompanied by major physical and psychological developmental shifts, the highest loneliness prevalence has been found. The percentage of people that feel lonely "sometimes" and "often" peek at two specific times: adolescence and old age. During adolescence, individuals experience puberty and face challenges surrounding social identity, and increased frailty and decreased mobility paired with the loss of loved ones during old age create more chances to feel lonely (Qualter et al., 2015).

Interdependence

Loneliness and social isolation have a strong influence on an individual's physical and mental health. Social isolation is commonly associated with depression as low mood, fatigue, and loss of interest and motivation make it difficult to maintain social connections, resulting in individuals feeling lonely. As previously mentioned, loneliness also serves as a predictor of depression, and both loneliness and depression are linked to chronic illnesses such as diabetes and cardiovascular disease (Theeke et al., 2018). Some degree of loneliness in our production-based, individualistic society is normal; it can also be traumatic due to significant social stigma, inactivity, and substance use, all of which can make preexisting health conditions worse. Long-standing illnesses and disabilities can also increase feelings of loneliness and have negative effects on one's health, including the worsening or development of physical and mental conditions (Mushtaq et al., 2014).

It is suggested that chronically ill young adults face more barriers to establishing and maintaining satisfactory peer relationships throughout adolescence and into adult life. Factors include the burden of symptoms and treatment, the time needed to attend hospital appointments, and fear of rejection from peers due to their illness (McGlone & Long, 2020). With all of these factors playing off of one another, there is no surprise that many individuals may gravitate toward parasocial relationships in the place of real-life connections. Research has shown there exist meaningful associations between PSRs and loneliness in the context of specific populations (Woznicki et al., 2021).

In a study investigating whether or not chronically ill and disabled young adults aged 16–24 are at an increased risk of loneliness compared to "healthy" peers, results showed a significant correlation between the two (McGlone & Long, 2020). Predominant theories for this association focus on periods of absence from school due to ill health, physical impairment, and reduced ability to partake in opportunities to socialize with peers. When separating the age brackets, younger participants (16–21 years of age) were lonelier than older participants (22–24 years of age), highlighting that transition periods commonly encountered, such as graduating and leaving high school, starting work, and furthering education as more vulnerable periods for loneliness especially when paired with a chronic illness (McGlone & Long, 2020).

Loneliness and parasocial relationships have been studied with mixed results. Significant positive associations were found when looking at specific dimensions of loneliness [such as emotional (family, romantic), social, chronic, situational, and transient loneliness] or sampling socially vulnerable populations (such as LGBTQ+ adolescents). With these mixed results but associations found with specific dimensions of loneliness and socially vulnerable populations, the "parasocial compensation hypothesis may predict the value of PSRs in times of crisis," with chronic illness, constant symptom management, and feeling isolated from others possibly being considered as such (Bond, 2022).

The highest prevalence of loneliness can be found when changes in the social environment are accompanied by major physical and psychological developmental shifts. It has also been found that loneliness peaks during adolescence, regardless of whether the individual has a chronic condition. This period also comes with its share of transitional periods that can create challenges for some individuals; graduating high school or college, moving out, entering the workforce, and navigating romantic relationships. These milestones can also create disruption or distress for some as their conditions may be keeping them from reaching them. On top of puberty and challenges surrounding emerging social identity, constant symptom management can cause adolescents and emerging adults to feel severely isolated from others. These barriers could manifest in decreased emotional vulnerability as they have no one to share their experiences with.

Future Research and Implications

Like all technology, social media is a neutral interface that relies on an individual's behavior: it can be used for healthy and unhealthy purposes. Though inherently neutral, it has proved helpful for chronically ill individuals when accessible to them and can be used to their advantage (Patel et al., 2015). The Internet allows these individuals to find others with similar struggles and create a community that provides support, disease management tips, and a safe place where they do not feel alienated. Though most of the research currently available focuses on individuals with cancer, obesity, and depression, it is suggested that "targeting specific social media technologies to specific diseases may be most valuable to improve clinical care" (Patel et al., 2015). Facebook, X (previously known as Twitter), and online forum sites were at the center of these studies as some of the bigger platforms out there were nonexistent at the time. With this in mind, future research needs to be done on the usefulness of applications such as Instagram, TikTok, Tumblr, Reddit, and YouTube for chronically ill individuals and whether they have a positive, neutral, or harmful effect.

During adolescence and emerging adulthood, social media can start to feel like an obligation and create negative behaviors. Individuals may find themselves feeling envious and distressed because they are not meeting the same milestones as their "healthy" peers. This could further lead to unhealthy comparisons revolving around body image, achievements, and relationships, all of which may advance distress. With a parasocial relationship, individuals are investing time, money, and emotions into someone they do not know to help with feelings of loneliness. The difference between being a fan and having a parasocial relationship is constant association and a meaningful bond, and being aware of this distinction could be helpful even working with this population. These relationships start healthy but can quickly develop into an intense attachment built on emotional dependence and act as a form of escapism. Instead of being used for enjoyment, more time is spent keeping up with content, no matter the personal expense. Currently, there are no scales or questionnaires to evaluate the intensity and effects of parasocial relationships. To accurately measure these relationships, future research should be done to create an instrument that can be used in a clinical setting.

As mentioned previously, blogs and forums can be utilized as a way to develop meaningful social connections away from parasocial relationships. Online environments are usually sought out to find others who are experiencing the same events or transitions, such as disease/illness-specific support groups. Behind the usernames and profile pictures are real people going through the same challenges but unlike a parasocial relationship, communication and emotional connection are reciprocated. Individuals may also find it easier to be vulnerable on social media with online friends than in real life. In an online space, there exists a greater sense of anonymity and less concern about what the other person thinks of the individual (Degges-White, 2020). It is very unlikely they will ever meet face-to-face, so there is less fear surrounding shame and retroactive embarrassment about what was shared. These confessions or secrets are limited to a confined space and shared with others they do not have to engage with ever again if desired.

For adolescents and emerging adults, open communication surrounding social media and parasocial relationships may be the best approach. While some individuals will shy away from talking about it, others may appreciate the opportunity to talk about things and people that are of interest to them. The important areas to cover for this population are how the content makes them feel, whether it is for enjoyment or escapism, and what to look out for in terms of the negative effects of social media. By opening this channel of communication, they can be aware of what they are consuming and elect to find other media when needed.

Conclusion

Due to the current digital age, information is more accessible than ever, and for many, parasocial relationships are practically unavoidable. These relationships can be perfectly healthy and function as an extension of the individual's social circle, but they can also cause real emotional turmoil despite being completely one-sided. While simply an extension of ordinary social cognition, or the result of loneliness and disconnection, the true nature of these relationships and their effect remains largely speculated. With loneliness on its way to becoming a public health crisis and millions of Americans living with chronic illnesses, research must explore using the technology at one's disposal to establish connections that decrease vulnerabilities.

References

Andrew, M. K., Mitnitski, A. B., & Rockwood, K. (2008). Social vulnerability, frailty and mortality in elderly people. *PLoS One, 3*(5). https://doi.org/10.1371/journal.pone.0002232

Bond, B. J. (2022). Parasocial relationships as functional social alternatives during pandemic-induced social distancing. *Psychology of Popular Media, 11*(3), 250–257. https://doi.org/10.1037/ppm0000364

Boyce, B. (2022). The truth about parasocial relationships. *Mindful*. https://www.mindful.org/the-truth-about-parasocial-relationships

Brown, B. (2010, June). The power of vulnerability [Video]. *TED Conferences*. https://www.ted.com/talks/brene_brown_the_power_of_vulnerability

Brown, B. (2012, March). Listening to shame [Video]. *TED Conferences*. https://www.ted.com/talks/brene_brown_listening_to_shame

Cacioppo, J. T., & Cacioppo, S. (2018). The growing problem of loneliness. Lancet (London, England), 391(10119), 426. https://doi.org/10.1016/S0140-6736(18)30142-9

Chronic diseases in America | CDC. (2022, November 8). https://www.cdc.gov/chronicdisease/resources/infographic/chronic-diseases.htm

Compas, B. E., Jaser, S. S., Dunn, M. J., & Rodriguez, E. M. (2012). Coping with chronic illnesses and childhood and adolescence. *Annual Review of Clinical Psychology, 8*(455), 455–480. https://doi.org/10.1146/annurev-clinpsy-032511-143108

Degges-White, S. (2020, May 29). Do online friendships differ from face-to-face friendships? *Psychology Today*. https://www.psychologytoday.com/us/blog/lifetime-connections/202005/do-online-friendships-differ-face-face-friendships

Espinal, V. (2021, February 21). Parasocial relationships in k-pop: Emotional support capitalism. *EnVi Media*. https://www.envimedia.co/parasocial-relationships-k-pop/

fontainexpert. (2022). *Tumblr*. https://www.tumblr.com/fontainexpert/695661364105101316/hi-this-is-a-text-for-my-delulu-fans-but

Giles, D. C., & Maltby, J. (2006). Praying at the altar of the stars. *The Psychologist, 19*(2). https://www.bps.org.uk/psychologist/praying-altar-stars

Hoffner, C. A., & Bond, B. J. (2022). Parasocial relationships, social media, & well-being. *Current Opinion in Psychology, 45*. https://doi.org/10.1016/j.copsyc.2022.101306

Horton, D., & Wohl, R. R. (1956). Mass communication and para-social interaction. *Psychiatry, 19*(3). https://doi.org/10.1080/00332747.1956.11023049

Kim, J., & Song, H. (2016). Celebrity's self-disclosure on Twitter and parasocial relationships: A mediating role of social presence. *Computers in Human Behavior, 62*, 570–577. https://doi.org/10.1016/j.chb.2016.03.083

Masterclass. (2022). Emotional vulnerability: How vulnerability helps relationships. *Masterclass Articles*. https://www.masterclass.com/articles/emotional-vulnerability

McGlone, M., & Long, E. (2020). Are young adults with long-standing illness or disability at increased risk of loneliness? Evidence from the UK longitudinal household study. *Journal of Public Health Research, 9*(4), 544–549. https://doi.org/10.4081/jphr.2020.1861

Murray, W. (2022a) New thriveworks research shows abundance of parasocial relationships in us. *ThriveWorks*. https://thriveworks.com/blog/new-thriveworks-research-shows-abundance-of-parasocial-relationships-in-the-us/

Murray, W. (2022b) Parasocial relationships: The good, the bad, and the boy bands. *ThriveWorks*. https://thriveworks.com/blog/parasocial-relationships-boy-bands/

Mushtaq, R., Shoib, S., Shah, T., & Mushtaq, S. (2014). Relationship between loneliness, psychiatric disorders and physical health ? A review on the psychological aspects of loneliness. *Journal of Clinical and Diagnostic Research: JCDR, 8*(9), WE01–WWE4. https://doi.org/10.7860/JCDR/2014/10077.4828

Nguyen, T. N., Ngangue, P., Bouhali, T., Ryan, B. L., Stewart, M., & Fortin, M. (2019). Social vulnerability in patients with multimorbidity: A cross-sectional analysis. *International Journal of Environmental Research and Public Health, 16*(7). https://doi.org/10.3390/ijerph16071244

Nibras, S., Kentor, R., Masood, Y., Price, K., Schneider, N. M., Tenenbaum, R. B., & Calarge, C. (2022). Psychological and psychiatric comorbidities in youth with serious physical illness. *Children, 9*(7), 1051–1065. https://doi.org/10.3390/children9071051

Patel, R., Chang, T., Greysen, S. R., & Chopra, V. (2015). Social media use in chronic disease: A systematic review and novel taxonomy. *The American Journal of Medicine, 128*(12), 1335–1350. https://doi.org/10.1016/j.amjmed.2015.06.015

Qualter, P., Vanhalst, J., Harris, R., Van Roekel, E., Lodder, G., Bangee, M., Maes, M., & Verhagen, M. (2015). Loneliness across the lifespan. *Perspectives on Psychological Science, 10*(2), 250–264. https://doi.org/10.1177/1745691615568999

Secinti, E., Thompson, E. J., Richards, M., & Gaysina, D. (2017). Research review: Childhood chronic physical illness and adult emotional health - a systematic review and meta-analysis. *Journal of Child Psychology and Psychiatry, 58*(7), 753–769. https://doi.org/10.1111/jcpp.12727

Stec, C. (2013). What boy bands can teach your business about effective marketing practices. *IMPACTPlus*. https://www.impactplus.com/blog/what-boy-bands-can-teach-your-business-about-effective-marketing-practices

Sugue, M. (2022). 10 things marketers can learn from k-pop marketing strategies. *Spiralytics*. https://www.spiralytics.com/blog/learn-from-k-pop-marketing-strategies/

Theeke, L., Carpenter, R. D., Mallow, J., & Theeke, E. (2018). Gender differences in loneliness, anger, depression, self-management ability and biomarkers of chronic illness in chronically ill mid-life adults in Appalachia. *Applied Nursing Research, 45*(2019), 55–62. https://doi.org/10.1016/j.apnr.2018.12.001

Tiwari, S. C. (2013). Loneliness: A disease?. *Indian journal of psychiatry, 55*(4), 320–322. https://doi.org/10.4103/0019-5545.120536

Watson, K. B. (2022). Chronic conditions among adults aged 18—34 years—United States, 2019. *MMWR. Morbidity and Mortality Weekly Report, 71*. https://doi.org/10.15585/mmwr.mm7130a3

Woznicki, N., Arriaga, A. S., Caporale-Berkowitz, N. A., & Parent, M. C. (2021). Parasocial relationships and depression among LGBQ emerging adults living with their parents during Covid-19: The potential for online support. *Psychology of Sexual Orientation and Gender Diversity, 8*(2), 228–237. https://doi.org/10.1037/sgd0000458

Yanguas, J., Pinazo-Henandis, S., & Tarazona-Santabalbina, F. J. (2018). The complexity of loneliness. *Acta Bio Medica, 89*(2), 302–314. https://doi.org/10.23750/abm.v89i2.7404

Yeo, M., & Sawyer, S. (2005). Abc of adolescence: Chronic illness and disability. *BMJ: British Medical Journal, 330*(7493), 721–723. https://www.jstor.org/stable/25459266

Part II
Psychological Vulnerability

Psychosocial Predictors of Suicide Risk in Medical Students

Alejandro Daniel Domínguez-González and Susana Castaños-Cervantes

Introduction

Suicide is a major public health problem that has a significant economic, social, and psychological impact on a global scale. Worldwide, one person dies every 40 s from suicide (World Health Organization [WHO], 2019). It is also the leading cause of death among young people aged 15–29 years old, after road injury (WHO, 2018). The age-adjusted suicide rate increased from 10.4/100,000 to 14.2/100,000 between 2000 and 2018, representing a steady increase of 36.7% (Curtin et al., 2016; Xu et al., 2020). This trend may be even more serious as the 40.7% increase in the rate of unintentional deaths from 2000 to 2017 is mostly attributed to unspecified falls (with an increase of 86.5%) and unintentional poisonings (with an increase of 98.5%), both of which may include misclassified suicide cases (Mann et al., 2021). In Mexico, each 90 min a person commits suicide. Moreover, the suicidal rate has doubled in 25 years, and it is the second cause of death among teenagers ages 15–19 years old, and the fifth for those between 10 and 14 years old (Instituto Nacional de Estadística y Geografía [INEGI], 2018). Recently, the American Psychological Association has indicated that suicide prevention should be a public health priority. Suicidal ideation appears as a key variable in suicide prevention.

Suicide is defined as death caused by self-directed injurious behavior with the intent to die because of such behavior. Suicide attempt is a nonfatal self-directed, potentially injurious action with intent to die as a consequence of those actions, and

A. D. Domínguez-González (✉)
Faculty of Medicine, La Salle University, Mexico City, Mexico
e-mail: alejandro.dominguez@lasalle.mx

S. Castaños-Cervantes
Escuela de Psicología, Facultad de Ciencias de la Salud, Universidad Panamericana, Ciudad de México, Mexico
e-mail: scastanos@up.edu.mx

S. Castaños-Cervantes et al. (eds.), *Working with Vulnerable Populations*,
https://doi.org/10.1007/978-3-031-67710-6_7

suicide ideation refers to thinking about, considering, or planning suicide (National Institute of Mental Health [NIMH], 2019a). Some of the main risk factors for suicide are depression, anxiety, other mental disorders, and substance abuse disorder (NIMH, 2019b).

Notes on the History of Suicide

The word suicide is a Latinism, which comes from the Latin expressions "sui" (oneself) and "caedere" (to kill) (suicide | Search Online Etymology Dictionary, n.d.). Apparently, it was the physician and philosopher Sir Thomas Browne who used this term for the first time in his work *Religio Medici* in 1642, distinguishing between the act of killing another person and the "homicide of oneself."

It is an intricate challenge to pinpoint the origins of the first act of suicide or to unravel the myriad causes that may have led to such profound decisions. Professor Yuval Noah Harari (Harari, 2014) postulates that the human cognitive revolution dawned approximately 70,000 years before Christ, marking a pivotal moment in intellectual and linguistic advancement. This transformative period facilitated abstract thinking and the capacity to plan for the future, thereby introducing the ability to envision various destinies, including the choice to persist in life or to exercise one's free will in ending it.

Throughout the annals of history, an array of factors emerges, potentially steering individuals toward the contemplation of suicide. This spectrum encompasses using suicide as an escape from the dehumanizing clutches of brutal slavery as a conscious resolution to confront the agony of pain and suffering induced by injury or chronic illness, as seen in ritual suicides by samurai seeking to purify their honor after military defeat in ancient Greece. Suicide has also been embraced as a sacrificial act for a cause, exemplified by kamikazes and suicide bombers, as well as an avenue chosen to alleviate unrelenting anguish. Notably, mental health professionals frequently grapple with severe emotional distress, the most prevalent precursor to suicide, diligently striving to provide intervention and treatment (Khan & Fuad, 2020). In exploring the multifaceted tapestry of human experience, the complexities surrounding suicide unfold, echoing the profound impact of historical, cultural, and psychological influences on this intricate facet of existence.

The first written text referring to suicide can be found in an Egyptian document currently in the Berlin Museum, dating from the time of the ancient Middle Kingdom of Egypt (1991–1786 BC). In 1896, Professor Adolf Erman translated this papyrus, which he called "The Dispute with His Soul of One Who Is Tired of Life," considered the first suicide note. It is a set of four poems that can be considered the writings of a severely psychotically depressed man with feelings of persecution and self-depreciation, who undoubtedly also shows strong suicidal tendencies (Thomas, 1980).

The concept and representation of suicide has changed throughout history, revealing itself to be a malleable social construct, susceptible to social influences and, above all, to the cultural characteristics of each era.

In the context of ancient Greco-Roman culture, perspectives on suicide manifested themselves in complex and nuanced ways. Within mythology, stories were woven that explored the emotions thought to trigger suicidal behavior, such as despair, guilt, shame, and madness itself. Notable examples include the suicides of Jocasta, Aegeus, and Ajax. However, it was the transcendental act of Socrates in 399 BC that left an indelible mark in the history of the philosophy of voluntary death. Likewise, the case of Seneca the Younger, tutor of the Roman Emperor Nero, who was forced to take his own life after being accused of conspiring against Nero, adds significant chapters to this narrative.

On the other hand, in ancient times suicide was also considered a crime against the state, punishable by law, since it deprived the polis (the community) of one of its members and his contribution to collective progress. It was also considered by a significant portion of Greek society to be an impious act against the gods. This approach reflected a deep appreciation of life as an integral part of the social and spiritual structure, emphasizing the perspective that the individual was not the exclusive owner of his existence, but rather an essential component of the community and its relationship to the divine.

The Middle Ages marked a radical shift in the perception of suicide, heavily influenced by prevailing religious doctrines. The Christian view of suicide was that it was a mortal sin with consequences beyond life on earth. Those who took their own lives were often excluded from funeral rituals and faced the confiscation of their possessions.

In medieval Europe, suicide was shrouded in a veil of moral condemnation, considered a mortal sin. Augustine of Hippo (354–430), a prominent figure in medieval Catholic thought, emerges as the foremost exponent on the subject of suicide. Drawing inspiration from Scripture, Augustine argues that he finds no authorization for the act of taking one's own life, even as a means of escaping pain or suffering. The author adheres to the divine commandment "Thou shalt not kill" and concludes that this principle applies directly to suicide. He conceptualizes it as a form of homicide and asserts that there is no true freedom of choice in one's life and death since these aspects belong to the domain of the divine will (San Agustín, 2014).

In the Renaissance, humanist philosophers courageously challenged the entrenched theological positions surrounding suicide. In this scene of intellectual inquiry, Michel de Montaigne (1533–1592) stands as a trailblazer by proclaiming that the moral evaluation of suicide cannot be derived from divine dictates but must emanate from the realm of personal choice. Over the course of the eighteenth century, there was a gradual achievement of the secularization and definitive decriminalization of suicide, although it persisted associated with mental illness and various states of "madness."

With the arrival of the nineteenth century and the advent of romanticism, suicide undergoes a transformation in its connotation. Psychological motivations take precedence over ethical considerations, elevating emotions and regarding suicide as the ultimate act of freedom or an expression of desperate states.

By the late nineteenth century, the French sociologist Emile Durkheim made a monumental contribution to the study of suicide in his work *Suicide* (published in the year 1897). Durkheim posits that suicides are inherently individual phenomena linked to social causes, arguing that spikes in suicide rates reveal the lack of norms and the weakness of existing ones (Durkheim, 1982).

Death by Suicide Among Physicians and Medical Students

The life of physicians often involves facing situations of illness and the risk of death, as well as making difficult personal decisions in the fulfillment of their professional responsibilities. Although there is a widespread perception that the medical community is somewhat protected against the risk of death by suicide due to their knowledge, access to healthcare, conflict resolution skills, and appreciation of self-preservation, data shows that, despite extensive training and awareness in this field, suicides among physicians have been on the rise (Bhatia et al., 2023).

It might be assumed that physicians have some degree of protection against death by suicide, given their knowledge, access to healthcare, conflict resolution skills, favorable socioeconomic status, and commitment to self-preservation, among other factors. However, despite extensive academic and professional training and awareness within the medical community, the ratio of suicide among physicians compared to the general population has been documented to be 1.41 for men and 2.27 for women (Duarte et al., 2020). In addition, the overall suicide mortality rate was approximately the same for male and female physicians (Lindeman et al., 1996), unlike the general population in America, where 79% of suicides occur among men, a trend that defies statistical patterns (ONU, 2023).

Another distinctive feature regarding suicide among physicians was uncovered in a 10-year prospective study. The findings revealed that the average age of suicide among physicians was 44 years, with a range spanning from 30 to 65 years. This discovery contrasts with the general population, where the age most commonly associated with suicide falls between 25 and 34 years (Freire et al., 2020).

In the transition from adolescence to adulthood, the university population is vulnerable to developing emotional disorders. Among them, medical students are the ones who present higher levels of anxiety, depression, and suicidal ideation (Domínguez- González, 2023).

A meta-analysis study of suicidal ideation prevalence in medical students extracted from 24 cross-sectional studies (n = 21 002) from 15 countries shows that the overall pooled crude prevalence of suicidal ideation was 11.1% (2043/21 002 individuals; 95% CI, 9.0% to 13.7%, I2 = 95.8%), prevalence estimates ranged across assessment modalities from 7.4% to 24.2% (Rotenstein et al., 2016).

A cross-sectional and longitudinal cohort study (Dyrbye et al., 2008) shows that 11.2% (CI, 9.9% to 12.6%) reported suicidal ideation within the past year. In a sensitivity analysis that assumed all nonresponders did not have suicidal ideation, the prevalence of suicidal ideation in the past 12 months would be 5.8%. A meta-analysis conducted by Puthran et al. (2016) also shows that the mean frequency of suicide ideation was 5.8%.

In medical students, the prevalence of suicidal ideation ranges from 1.8% to 53.6% (Coentre & Góis, 2018). However, medical student rates are infrequently reported in the research literature, and data collection techniques are inconsistent (Blacker et al., 2019). As such, gaps exist in knowledge of medical student's suicide rates, risk factors, and targets for intervention. Nonetheless, there still are no current statistics about the number of physicians that die from suicide (Nájar, 2010).

Some of the most frequent factors associated with suicidal ideation that increase the risk of suicide in medical students are depression (Gishen, 2019; Zeng et al., 2018), anxiety (Yang, 2014), substance use and abuse and poor mental health (Barrimi et al., 2019), and a previous diagnosis of a psychiatric disorder. Amongst psychoactive substance use, alcohol use is a potential risk factor predisposing to suicidal ideation (Carrasco et al., 2019).

A cross-sectional analytical study conducted by Akram et al. (2018) on Pakistani medical students shows that self-distraction, active coping, use of emotional support, use of instrumental support, positive reframing, planning, humor, acceptance, and religion were negative predictors of suicidal ideation, whereas denial, substance use, venting, and self-blame were positive predictors of suicidal ideation.

Furthermore, current research has shown that the use of maladaptive coping strategies (e.g., rumination, venting, avoidance, behavioral disengagement, suppressive, and reactive) (Ong & Thompson, 2019) and dysfunctional emotion regulation skills (e.g., denial, avoidance, suppression, and rumination) are linked to increasing risk of suicide (Hatkevich et al., 2019).

A systematic overview of risk factors for suicidal ideation (SI) and suicide attempt (SA) among medical students by Seo shows poor mental health outcomes including depression (OR 6.87; 95% CI [4.80–9.82] for SI; OR 9.34 [4.18–20.90] for SA), burnout (OR 6.29 [2.05–19.30] for SI), comorbid mental illness (OR 5.08 [2.81–9.18] for SI), and stress (OR 3.72 [1.39–9.94] for SI) presented the strongest risk for SI and SA among medical students (Seo et al., 2021).

A study that we conducted among students of the Mexican Faculty of Medicine reveals a noteworthy direct impact of anxiety and emotional dysregulation on depression. Furthermore, amidst the COVID-19 pandemic, a longitudinal study aimed to assess the prevalence of emotional disorders during lockdown. The findings indicated a substantial rise in the prevalence of depression from 19.84% to 40.08% between April and December 2020. Remarkably, the suicide ideation rate remained relatively stable, hovering around 18% during this period (Domínguez-González et al., 2022).

In Mexico, the academic and clinical hospital shifts that medical intern undergo can extend up to 36 uninterrupted hours, considering the night shifts that occur every three or four days. Extended hospital shifts, especially those exceeding 36 h, can have various consequences. Constant exposure to prolonged workdays may contribute to the development of physical health problems, such as sleep disorders, metabolic disturbances, and cardiovascular issues. Emotionally, these extended shifts generate high levels of stress and anxiety, leading to the loss of empathy and emotional exhaustion. These factors impact interpersonal relationships, both professionally and personally.

On the other hand, fatigue and exhaustion can affect concentration and decision-making in the diagnosis and treatment of patients, increasing the likelihood of medical errors. This phenomenon has serious implications for patient safety and underscores the importance of addressing working conditions to ensure the health and well-being of healthcare professionals and those they serve.

To develop and refine interventions to prevent youth suicide, knowledge is needed about specific processes that reduce risk at a population level. Concerning medical students, the extent to which gender differences in suicide risk factors remains unclear.

Moreover, previous research on Latin American medical students and suicide risk has focused on suicide attempt as a risk factor for major depressive disorder (Romo et al., 2019), suicide stigma (Rivera et al., 2018), psychopathology screening (Galván et al., 2017), suicide risk, anxiety and depression (Jiménez et al., 2015), psychiatric symptoms (Heinze et al., 2008), and prevalence of suicide ideation (Alexandrino et al., 2009) and suicide rates (Meleiro, 1998; Millan et al., 1990). Therefore, in order to add to the body of growing literature on suicide risk in medical students, particularly in the context of Latin American cities, we sought to examine some psychosocial factors in shaping suicide risk and plausible pathways that may explain its effects based on the Interpersonal Theory of Suicide (Van Orden et al., 2010). Consequently, relationships between suicide risk, depression, anxiety, coping skills, alcohol problems, and emotional dysregulation were assessed. As such, the path model tested was based on the following hypothesized model (Fig. 1).

Understanding these psychosocial factors in Mexican medical students is imperative to invest effectively and efficiently in the promotion of their well-being, thus contributing to preventing school dropout, strengthening their capabilities, promoting their adequate performance, and improving their quality of life and career success.

Regarding rates of the psychosocial factors explored, Mexican medical students exhibit a lower degree of alcohol use, suicide risk, anxiety, and depression, which is consistent with previous research that indicated that first-year medical students presented lower levels of depression, anxiety, and burnout (Goel et al., 2016), with prevalence rates of 9.09% or less (Reddy et al., 2015). Medical students in the latter years tend to exhibit higher scores in suicide risk, depression, anxiety, and stress.

This may be attributed to greater fear of not attaining their goal of being a doctor or may be due to excessive load of both paraclinical and clinical subjects compared to first years (Shawaz et al., 2015).

In a Mexican study carried out with medical students (Palma et al., 2018), it was found that less than 3.2% of the participants presented mild depression and less than 16% anxiety. In fact, Jiménez et al. (2015) found that at the beginning of the academic year, a group of Mexican medical students reported low depressive symptoms (3.7%), low anxiety symptoms (3.8%), and low degree of suicide risk (1.9%).

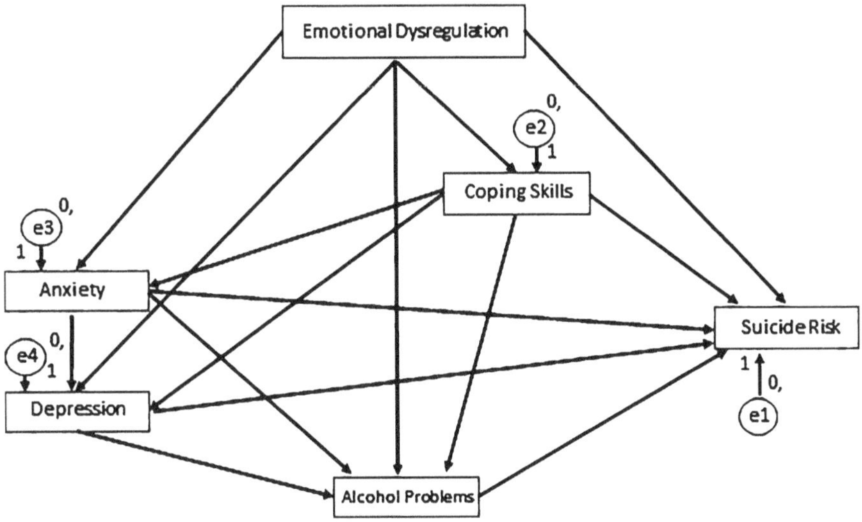

Fig. 1 Hypothesized version of the path model analysis of suicide risk in a group of Mexican medical students with anxiety, depression, alcohol problems, emotional dysregulation, and coping skills as psychosocial correlates. (Source: Authors' elaboration)

Besides, there seem to be no gender differences regarding coping strategies in Mexican medical students, thus being congruent with prior studies (Sepúlveda et al., 2012). Lastly, rates of alcohol use are low also coinciding with previous research (Puig et al., 2011).

Concerning our path model tested, outcomes revealed that emotional dysregulation and depression were significant direct predictors of suicide risk, while anxiety had an indirect effect on suicide risk with depression as the mediating variable (Fig. 2).

According to the Interpersonal Theory of Suicide (Van Orden et al., 2010), intrapersonal factors as would be the emotional states of a person may be relevant for causing suicidal ideation. Likewise, impulsivity and a mental state of agitation play an important role in suicidal attempt. Previous research has demonstrated the effect of lack of self-control, outburst of emotions, and mental instability in suicide ideation. Therefore, suicide risk is usually predicted by emotion regulation and depression (Gómez et al., 2018). Furthermore, in a Latin American sample, suicidal ideation was predicted by depressive symptoms (Pinzón-Amado et al., 2013).

Although anxiety has been related to suicidal thinking in medical students (Rosiek et al., 2016), the fact that anxiety does not seem to directly predict suicide risk in Mexican medical students may be explained because anxiety sensitivity is more associated with suicide risk than anxiety by itself (Stanley et al., 2018). In addition, anxiety usually precedes the onset of depression (Moriarity et al., 2018), as it can substantially increase stress and interfere with daily functioning, thus leading to depression (Kendall, 2012).

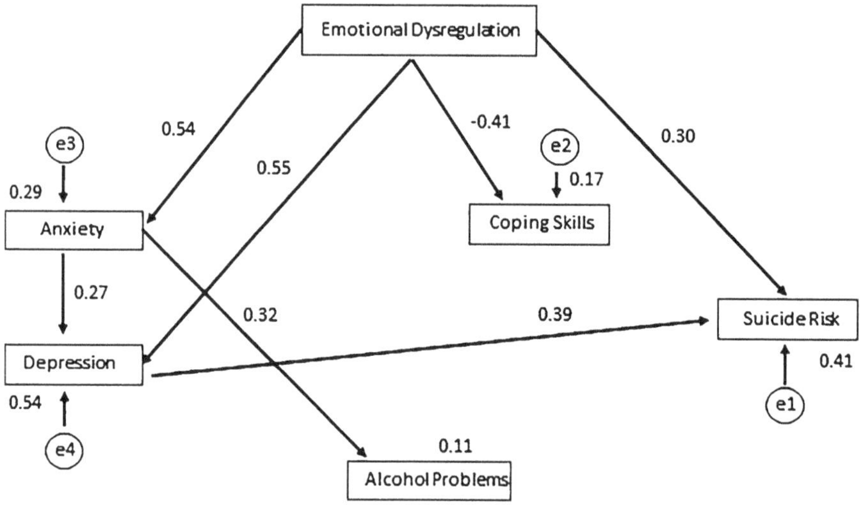

Fig. 2 Final version of the path model analysis of suicide risk in a group of medical students. Standardized regression weights are shown. $p < 0.01$. (Source: Authors' elaboration)

Moreover, coping skills seem to be a less relevant protective factor against suicide risk since they were not a significant predictor.

Finally, it is necessary to be more thorough while examining the effects of emotional dysregulation on suicide risk, because additional information can be provided such as which emotion regulation strategies are associated with suicide risk. These data can be useful when identifying risk and protective factors of suicide risk, particularly in Mexican medical students, and while designing efficient and sustainable intervention programs aimed at targeting such emotion regulation strategies. Consequently, we discovered that the emotional dysregulations strategies of denial and suppression positively and negatively predict suicide risk, respectively. However, in Mexican male students the only strategy linked to suicide risk was denial, while in females both emotional dysregulation strategies of denial and suppression.

Suicidal behavior has been associated with maladaptive strategies for emotion regulation (Harris et al., 2018). An Argentinian study found that negative cognitive emotion regulation strategies predict suicidal thoughts (Flores et al., 2019). As such, prior studies have also found that denial predicts suicidal ideation (Akram et al., 2018; Rajappa et al., 2012).

The fact that denial seems to be the only emotional dysregulation strategy that positively predicts suicide risk in Mexican male medical students may be because men are working to alter their own experience of negative emotions and events resulting from stressful sources in a way in which their manliness is not compromised or threatened, hence avoiding social disapproval and fitting social expectations. Ideals of masculinity often discourage males from awareness and expression of psychic pain and admission of weaknesses and vulnerabilities. The masking of emotional distress or problems may be a face-saving strategy for many men who are less skilled at emotional expression and bound by expectations that men must be strong and invincible (Falicov, 2003).

Contrastingly, in Mexican medical female students, suppression is also a significant negative predictor of suicide risk. Women have a higher mean suppression score compared to males (Vasudeva & Singh, 2017). From a cultural point of view, in collective cultures and male-oriented societies such as Mexican culture, women are oriented toward placing the needs of others ahead of themselves, in a manner that results in a "silencing of the self" (Jack, 1991). Consequently, women sacrifice to adapt to cultural specifications for their behavior while simultaneously interpreting their inferior positions as due to internal shortcomings (Stoppard, 2000). As such, females may feel coerced to suppress themselves unconsciously. Thus, psychological and moral pressures, severe discipline, threats, punishment, and limitations and constraints cause children to become submissive, lacking the courage to express themselves.

Our path model of suicide risk helps develop effective and sustainable interventions addressing specific psychosocial risk and protective factors in Mexican medical students and pave the way for future research involving the promotion of their mental well-being. Particularly, intervention programs should target emotion regulation and depression, focusing too, on emotion regulation strategies. In Mexican medical male students, interventions must include techniques to address the emotional dysregulation strategy of denial, while in females they should also incorporate the emotional dysregulation strategy of suppression.

Therapeutic interventions such as cognitive-behavioral therapy (CBT) have been shown to be effective in reducing the risk of suicidal behavior. In adults and adolescents with depression, as well as in adults with borderline personality disorder, this therapy has demonstrated significant benefits in reducing the risk associated with suicidal behavior and has successfully halved the recurrence rate in patients who have recently attempted suicide and sought emergency services (Brown et al., 2005).

The use of CBT with individuals at risk for suicide focuses on empowering them to use more effective coping strategies, such as cognitive restructuring, especially in situations of stress and triggers that may lead to suicidal behavior. CBT can have a positive impact by improving negative problem orientation and emotional regulation (Slee, et al., 2008b), reducing impulsivity in problem-solving (Ghahramanlou-Holloway et al., 2012), and decreasing suicidal ideation (Slee, et al., 2008a).

In the field of pharmacological therapeutic interventions, ketamine has been shown to reduce suicidal ideation within a few hours. This rapid and robust reduction in suicidal ideation can have a significant impact on patient safety. However, the impact of this reduction on suicidal behavior is still unknown, making it a priority for suicide prevention research. The combination of medication and individual psychotherapy does not provide any discernible advantage (Mann et al., 2021).

The transition to adulthood involves significant social challenges that can lead to interpersonal conflicts, breakups, and family problems. In addition, this period has the highest incidence of issues related to identity or sexual orientation.

According to a Canadian study, the prevalence of suicidality (suicidal ideation, suicide plans, and suicide attempts) was higher in sexual minority populations than in the heterosexual population, particularly in the bisexual population, regardless of gender or age.

Prior to the pandemic, the prevalence of recent suicidal ideation was 14.0% in the bisexual population, 5.2% in the gay/lesbian population, and 2.4% in the heterosexual population. The rates of lifetime suicide attempts were 16.6%, 8.6%, and 2.8%, respectively. More than 40% of the sexual minority population aged 15–44 had experienced suicidal ideation at some point in their lives. In addition, 64.3% and 36.5% of the gender minority population had suicidal ideation and attempted suicide at some point in their lives. These populations had a lower prevalence of protective factors related to social support and access to healthcare (Liu et al., 2023).

On the other hand, numerous medical students exhibit perfectionistic personality traits, which, combined with intense academic competition and fear of failure, drive them to strive tirelessly to excel, significantly sacrificing sleep hours. This physical exhaustion, coupled with a lack of social interaction and recreational time, has a significant impact on mental health, thus contributing to the emergence of anxiety and depression within the student community.

The hospital environment also exerts significant pressure. The strenuous workload during extended academic and work periods, the high number of patients, and deficiencies in infrastructure and security within medical facilities generate stress and exhaustion among the assigned staff, as well as among clinical cycle students (Athié Gutiérrez et al., 2016; Martinez-Fierro et al., 2022). Exposure to the hospital hierarchy often involves facing workplace and sexual harassment. A study that explored the perception of sexual harassment among female medical and nursing students revealed a high prevalence of verbal harassment by health personnel (assigned staff, residents, and other medical professionals), leading these students to feel threatened, humiliated, or embarrassed (De Sio et al., 2020; Waryam Singh Malhi et al., 2021).

Despite their knowledge of mental health, both physicians and medical students face mental health stigma. Perceptions of weakness or fear of professional repercussions can lead some physicians to avoid seeking help when they need it. In many cases, physicians choose to self-medicate with prescription drugs, alcohol, and a variety of other substances (Ventriglio et al., 2020).

The issue of suicide risk among medical students is a complex one with multiple biological, psychosocial, cultural, and societal causes.

Numerous neurochemical alterations amenable to pharmacological treatment have been shown to be effective in reducing suicide risk. In addition, psychosocial determinants can be addressed through therapies and workshops designed to cultivate emotional coping skills that protect and support students in managing their emotions in stressful situations. Mindfulness workshops and other wellness activities also play an important role in emotional health.

It is critical to address the stigma associated with mental health within the medical community. Mental health awareness campaigns, supported by institutional policies that promote leisure and self-care, can create an environment conducive to open dialogue.

The overall well-being of healthcare workers also requires attention, including appropriate nutritional standards and guidance from culinary experts on hospital food offerings to ensure the presentation of healthy and tasty meals that promote a balanced diet. There is also a need to develop artificial intelligence-based applications to streamline administrative tasks for physicians, one of the most time-consuming activities in hospitals that is often delegated to medical trainees.

An integrated approach that includes these and other initiatives can go a long way toward improving the quality of life and well-being of healthcare professionals.

References

Akram, B., Ahmad, M., & Akram, A. (2018). Coping mechanisms as predictors of suicidal ideation among the medical students of Pakistan. *Journal of the Pakistan Medical Association, 68*(11), 1608–1612.

Alexandrino, C., Pereira, M., Bustamante, C., Ferraz, A., Baldassin, S., De Andrade, A., & Alves, T. (2009). Suicidal ideation among students enrolled in healthcare training programs: A cross-sectional study. *Revista Brasileira de Psiquiatria, 31*(4), 338–344.

Athié Gutiérrez, C., Cardiel Marmolejo, L., Camacho Aguilera, J., & Avellaneda, M. (2016). Burnout en médicos internos de pregrado del Hospital General de México Dr. Eduardo Liceaga. *Investigación en Educación Médica, 5*(18), 102–107.

Barrimi, M., Maazouzi, M., Malakt, S., Lazaar, S., & Khaoulani, H. (2019). Suicidal thoughts and suicide attempts among medical students in Morocco: Results of a multicenter study. *Annales Medico-Psychologiques, 178*, 481–486. https://doi.org/10.1016/J.AMP.2018.11.012

Bhatia, G., Sharma, P., Pal, A., & Parmar, A. (2023). The silent epidemic: Death by suicide among physicians. *Asia-Pacific Psychiatry, 15*(1), e12522. https://doi.org/10.1111/appy.12522

Blacker, C., Lewis, C., Swintak, C., Bostwick, J., & Rackley, S. (2019). Medical student suicide rates: A systematic review of the historical and international literature. *Academic Medicine, 94*(2), 274–280. https://doi.org/10.1097/ACM.0000000000002430

Brown, G. K., Ten Have, T., Henriques, G. R., Xie, S. X., Hollander, J. E., & Beck, A. T. (2005). Cognitive therapy for the prevention of suicide attempts: A randomized controlled trial. *JAMA, 294*(5), 563–570. https://doi.org/10.1001/jama.294.5.563

Carrasco, C., Álvarez, D., Vilchez, J., Lizana, M., Durand, P., Rengifo, J., Rebatta, A., Cubas, W., Arroyo, H., & Toro, C. (2019). Alcohol consumption and suicide risk in medical internship: A Peruvian multicentric study. *Drug and Alcohol Review, 38*(2), 201–208.

Coentre, R., & Góis, C. (2018). Suicidal ideation in medical students: Recent insights. *Advances in Medical Education and Practice, 9*, 873–880. https://doi.org/10.2147/AMEP.S162626

Curtin, S. C., Warner, M., & Hedegaard, H. (2016). Increase in suicide in the United States, 1999-2014. *NCHS Data Brief, 241*, 1–8.

de Freire, F. O., Marcon, S. R., Espinosa, M. M., Santos, H. G. B. D., Kogien, M., de Lima, N. V. P., & Faria, J. S. (2020). Factors associated with suicide risk among nurses and physicians: A cross-section study. *Revista Brasileira de Enfermagem, 73*(Suppl 1), e20200352. https://doi.org/10.1590/0034-7167-2020-0352

De Sio, S., Cedrone, F., Buomprisco, G., Perri, R., Nieto, H. A., Mucci, N., & Greco, E. (2020). Bullying at work and work-related stress in healthcare workers: A cross sectional study. *Annali di Igiene: Medicina Preventiva e di Comunita, 32*(2), 109–116. https://doi.org/10.7416/ai.2020.2335

Domínguez-González, A. D. (2023). *Suicidal ideation, socioemotional disorders and coping strategies in medical students*. IntechOpen. https://doi.org/10.5772/intechopen.1002612

Domínguez-González, A. D., Guzmán-Valdivia, G., Ángeles-Téllez, F. S., Manjarrez- Ángeles, M. A., & Secín-Diep, R. (2022). Depression and suicidal ideation in Mexican medical students during COVID-19 outbreak. A longitudinal study. *Heliyon, 8*(2), e08851. https://doi.org/10.1016/j.heliyon.2022.e08851

Duarte, D., El-Hagrassy, M. M., Couto, T. C. E., Gurgel, W., Fregni, F., & Correa, H. (2020). Male and female physician suicidality: A systematic review and meta-analysis. *JAMA Psychiatry, 77*(6), 587–597. https://doi.org/10.1001/jamapsychiatry.2020.0011

Durkheim, E. (1982). *El Suicidio (First ediction).* Ediciones Akal. (Published in 1897).

Dyrbye, L. N., Thomas, M. R., Massie, F. S., Power, D. V., Eacker, A., Harper, W., Durning, S., Moutier, C., Szydlo, D. W., Novotny, P. J., Sloan, J. A., & Shanafelt, T. D. (2008). Burnout and suicidal ideation among U.S. medical students. *Annals of Internal Medicine, 149*(5), 334–341. https://doi.org/10.7326/0003-4819-149-5-200809020-00008

Falicov, C. (2003). Culture, society and gender in depression. *Journal of Family Therapy, 25*, 371–387. https://doi.org/10.1111/1467-6427.00256

Flores, P., García, Z., Moretti, L., & Medrano, L. (2019). Towards an explanatory model of suicidal ideation: The effects of cognitive emotional regulation strategies, sffectivity and hopelessness. *The Spanish Journal of Psychology, 22*(4), E43.

Galván, J., Jiménez, M., Hernández, J., & Arellano, J. (2017). Psychopathology screening in medical school students. *Gaceta Medica de Mexico, 153*(1), 75–87.

Ghahramanlou-Holloway, M., Bhar, S. S., Brown, G. K., Olsen, C., & Beck, A. T. (2012). Changes in problem-solving appraisal after cognitive therapy for the prevention of suicide. *Psychological Medicine, 42*(6), 1185–1193. https://doi.org/10.1017/S0033291711002169

Gishen, F. (2019). Suicide among medical students. *BMJ (Clinical Research Ed.), 366*, l5465. https://doi.org/10.1136/bmj.l5465

Goel, A., Akarte, S., Agrawal, S., & Yadav, V. (2016). Longitudinal assessment of depression, stress, and burnout in medical students. *Journal of Neurosciences in Rural Practice, 7*, 493–498. https://doi.org/10.4103/0976-3147.188625

Gómez, M., Limonero, J., Toro, J., Montes, J., & Tomás, J. (2018). Relationship between emotional intelligence and negative affect on suicide risk in young university students. *Ansiedad y Estrés, 24*(1), 18–23.

Harari, Y. (2014). *Sapiens: A brief history of humankind.* Random House.

Harris, L., Chelminski, I., Dalrymple, K., Morgan, T., & Zimmerman, M. (2018). Suicide attempts and emotion regulation in psychiatric outpatients. *Journal of Affective Disorders, 232*, 300–304.

Hatkevich, C., Penner, F., & Sharp, C. (2019). Difficulties in emotion regulation and suicide ideation and attempt in adolescent inpatients. *Psychiatry Research, 271*, 230–238.

Heinze, G., Vargas, B., & Cortés, J. (2008). Psychiatric symptoms and characteristics of personality in two opposing groups of the UNAM Faculty of Medicine. *Salud Mental, 31*(5), 343–350.

Instituto Nacional de Estadística y Geografía. (2018). *Estadísticas a propósito del día mundial para la prevención del suicidio (datos nacionales) [World day suicide prevention 2018 statistics (national data)].* Retrieved from: https://www.inegi.org.mx/contenidos/saladeprensa/aproposito/2018/suicidios2018_Nal.pdf

Jack, D. C. (1991). *Silencing the self: Women and depression.* Harvard University Press.

Jiménez, J., Arenas, J., & Angeles, U. (2015). Depression, anxiety and suicide risk symptoms among medical residents over an academic year. *Revista Médica del Instituto Mexicano del Seguro Social, 53*(1), 20–28.

Kendall, P. (2012). *Child and adolescent therapy. Cognitive-behavioral procedures.* The Guildford Press.

Khan, F., & Fuad, M. (2020). *Suicide: A biography.* https://www.psychiatrictimes.com/. https://www.psychiatrictimes.com/view/suicide-a-biography

Lindeman, S., Laara, E., Hakko, H., & Lonnqvist, J. (1996). A systematic review on gender-specific suicide mortality in medical doctors. *The British Journal of Psychiatry: the Journal of Mental Science, 168*(3), 274–279. https://doi.org/10.1192/bjp.168.3.274

Liu, L., Batomen, B., Pollock, N. J., Contreras, G., Jackson, B., Pan, S., & Thompson, W. (2023). Suicidality and protective factors among sexual and gender minority youth and adults in

Canada: A cross-sectional, population-based study. *BMC Public Health, 23*(1), 1469. https://doi.org/10.1186/s12889-023-16285-4

Mann, J. J., Michel, C. A., & Auerbach, R. P. (2021). Improving suicide prevention through evidence-based strategies: A systematic review. *The American Journal of Psychiatry, 178*(7), 611–624. https://doi.org/10.1176/appi.ajp.2020.20060864

Martinez-Fierro, M. L., Ramirez-Madrigal, M. A., Covarrubias-Carrillo, R. M., Avila- Carrasco, L., Flores-Morales, V., Meza-Zavala, O. G., de León-Sigg, M., Vázquez- Reyes, S., Mauricio-González, A., Velasco-Elizondo, P., & Garza-Veloz, I. (2022). Security and violence perception of medical interns during social service practice in Mexico. *International Journal of Environmental Research and Public Health, 19*(1). https://doi.org/10.3390/ijerph19010318

Meleiro, A. (1998). Suicide among physicians and medical students. *Revista da Associação Médica Brasileira, 44*(2), 135–140.

Millan, L., Rossi, E., & De Marco, O. (1990). Suicide among medical students. *Revista do Hospital das Clínicas, 45*(3), 145–149.

Moriarity, D., McArthur, B., Ellman, L., Coe, C., Abramson, L., & Alloy, L. (2018). Immunocognitive model of depression secondary to anxiety in adolescents. *Journal of Youth and Adolescence, 47*(12), 2625–2636. https://doi.org/10.1007/s10964-018-0905-7

Nájar, A. (2010). *Preocupa a México suicidio de médicos [Suicides in physicians worry Mexico].* Retrieved from: https://www.bbc.com/mundo/cultura_sociedad/2010/03/100318_0325_suicidio_me dicos_mexico_mz

National Institute of Mental Health. (2019a). *Suicide.* Retrieved from: https://www.nimh.nih.gov/health/statistics/suicide.shtml

National Institute of Mental Health. (2019b). *Suicide prevention.* Retrieved from: https://www.nimh.nih.gov/health/topics/suicide-prevention/index.shtml

Ong, E., & Thompson, C. (2019). The importance of coping and emotion regulation in the occurrence of suicidal behavior. *Psychological Reports, 122*(4), 1192–1210.

ONU. (2023, febrero 23). *El suicidio aumenta en América mientras disminuye en el resto del mundo.* https://news.un.org/es/story/2023/02/1518852

Palma, F., Ricaño, K., Palma, J., Martínez, M., Puig, A., & Puig-Lagunes, A. (2018). Síntomas depresivos y rendimiento académico en estudiantes de medicina. *CIMEL, 23*(2). https://doi.org/10.23961/cimel.v23i2.1053

Pinzón-Amado, A., Guerrero, S., Moreno, K., Landínez, C., & Pinzón, J. (2013). Suicide ideation among medical students: Prevalence and associated factors. *Revista Colombiana de Psiquiatria, 43*(1), 47–55.

Puig, A., Cortaza, L., & Pillon, S. (2011). Alcohol use among Mexican medical students. *Revista Latino-Americana de Enfermagem, 19*(SPEC. ISSUE), 714–721.

Puthran, R., Zhang, M. W. B., Tam, W. W., & Ho, R. C. (2016). Prevalence of depression amongst medical students: A meta-analysis. *Medical Education, 50*(4), 456–468. https://doi.org/10.1111/medu.12962

Rajappa, K., Gallagher, M., & Miranda, R. (2012). Emotion dysregulation and vulnerability to suicidal ideation and attempts. *Cognitive Therapy and Research, 36*(6), 833–839.

Reddy, E., Raju Srijampana, V., Rajana, B., & Muddana, S. (2015). Perceived stress and prevalence of depression among first-year medical students. *Journal of NTR University of Health Sciences, 4*, 209–213. https://doi.org/10.4103/2277-8632.171689

Rivera, E., Rosario, E., Carminelli, P., & Tollinchi, N. (2018). Suicide stigma among medical students in Puerto Rico. *International Journal of Environmental Research and Public Health, 15*(7), 1366.

Romo, N., Bobadilla, R., Tafoya, S., Guízar, D., Gutiérrez, J., Carriedo, P., & Heinze, G. (2019). Major depressive disorder in Mexican medical students and associated factors: A focus on current and past abuse experiences. *Journal of Affective Disorders, 245*(15), 834–840.

Rosiek, A., Rosiek-Kryszewska, A., Leksowski, L., & Leksowski, K. (2016). Chronic stress and suicidal thinking among medical students. *International Journal of Environmental Research and Public Health, 13*(2).

Rotenstein, L. S., Ramos, M. A., Torre, M., Segal, J. B., Peluso, M. J., Guille, C., Sen, S., & Mata, D. A. (2016). Prevalence of depression, depressive symptoms, and suicidal ideation among medical students: A systematic review and meta-analysis. *JAMA, 316*(21), 2214–2236. https://doi.org/10.1001/jama.2016.17324

San Agustín. (2014). *La ciudad de Dios*. Porrúa.

Seo, C., Di Carlo, C., Dong, S. X., Fournier, K., & Haykal, K.-A. (2021). Risk factors for suicidal ideation and suicide attempt among medical students: A meta-analysis. *PLoS One, 16*(12), e0261785. https://doi.org/10.1371/journal.pone.0261785

Sepúlveda, A., Romero, A., & Jaramillo, L. (2012). Coping strategies and their relation with depression and anxiety in pediatric residents in a third level pediatric hospital. *Boletín Médico del Hospital Infantil de México, 69*(5), 347–354.

Shawaz, I., Sandhya, G., & Venkatarao, E. (2015). Stress, anxiety & depression among medical undergraduate students & their socio-demographic correlates. *The Indian Journal of Medical Research, 141*, 354–357.

Slee, N., Garnefski, N., van der Leeden, R., Arensman, E., & Spinhoven, P. (2008a). Cognitive-behavioural intervention for self-harm: Randomised controlled trial. *The British Journal of Psychiatry: the Journal of Mental Science, 192*(3), 202–211. https://doi.org/10.1192/bjp.bp.107.037564

Slee, N., Spinhoven, P., Garnefski, N., & Arensman, E. (2008b). Emotion regulation as mediator of treatment outcome in therapy for deliberate self-harm. *Clinical Psychology & Psychotherapy, 15*(4), 205–216. https://doi.org/10.1002/cpp.577

Stanley, I., Boffa, J., Rogers, M., Hom, M., Albanese, B., Chu, C., Capron, D., Schmidt, N., & Joiner, T. (2018). Anxiety sensitivity and suicidal ideation/suicide risk: A meta- analysis. *Journal of Consulting and Clinical Psychology, 86*(11), 946–960.

Stoppard, J. (2000). *Understanding depression: Femininist social constructionist approaches*. Routledge.

Suicide | Search Online Etymology Dictionary. (s. f.). (n.d.). Online Etymology Dictionary. Recuperado 11 de diciembre de 2023, de https://www.etymonline.com/search?q=suicide

Thomas, C. (1980). First suicide note? *British Medical Journal, 280*(6214), 284–285.

Van Orden, K., Witte, T., Cukrowicz, K., Braithwaite, S., Selby, E., & Joiner, T. (2010). The interpersonal theory of suicide. *Psychological Review, 117*(2), 575–600. https://doi.org/10.1037/a0018697

Vasudeva, N., & Singh, H. (2017). A study of emotional regulation process among patients with current suicide attempt. *Minerva Psichiatrica, 58*(3), 113–117.

Ventriglio, A., Watson, C., & Bhugra, D. (2020). Suicide among doctors: A narrative review. *Indian Journal of Psychiatry, 62*(2), 114–120. https://doi.org/10.4103/psychiatry.IndianJPsychiatry_767_19

Waryam Singh Malhi, F. S. A., Sugathan, S., Binti Azhar, N. A. S., Binti Wan Roslan, W. I. N., Abu Bakar, H. A. B., & Binti Zolkaine, S. M. (2021). Self-perception of sexual harassment: A comparison between female medical and nursing students during clinical practice. *Education for Health (Abingdon, England), 34*(2), 55–63. https://doi.org/10.4103/1357-6283.332958

World Health Organization. (2018). *Global health estimates 2016: Deaths by cause, age, sex, by country and by region, 2000–2016*. World Health Organization.

World Health Organization. (2019). *Suicide: One person dies every 40 seconds*. Retrieved from: https://www.who.int/news-room/detail/09-09-2019-suicide-one-person-dies-every-40-seconds

Xu, J., Murphy, S. L., Kockanek, K. D., & Arias, E. (2020). Mortality in the United States, 2018. *NCHS Data Brief, 355*, 1–8.

Yang, L. (2014). Risk and risk factors of suicide attempt after first onset of suicide ideation: Findings from medical students in grades 1 and 2. *Journal of Hygiene Research, 43*(1), 47–53.

Zeng, B., Zhao, J., Zou, L., Yang, X., Zhang, X., Wang, W., Zhao, J., & Chen, J. (2018). Depressive symptoms, post-traumatic stress symptoms and suicide risk among graduate students: The mediating influence of emotional regulatory self-efficacy. *Psychiatry Research, 264*, 224–230.

Art Therapy: Focus to Decrease Vulnerability Condition and Increase Sense of Community

Angélica Ojeda García and Gabriela A. González Ruíz

Definition and Scope of the Concept of Vulnerability

"Vulnerability" is a concept that contains a remarkable complexity. There are at least two types of human vulnerabilities: anthropological vulnerability, understood as a condition of fragility unique and intrinsic to the human being, by its biological and psychic being; and sociopolitical vulnerability, which derives from cultural belonging either to a group, by gender, locality, or socioeconomic condition and culture (Delor & Hubert, 2000).

The polysemia of this term refers to a common denominator: the harm. Not for nothing, the origin of the term "vulnerability" is, in Latin, "vulnus," meaning wound, blow, pang, and misfortune, or affliction. Similarly, the semantic field is "vulneratio," wound or injury, and the verb "vulnero," hurt or harm. However, the damage can also be psychic or emotional, in which case it opens the way to suffering. And there is also moral damage, which is caused by a situation of evil, injustice, contempt, or any other form of harm that will affect identity as a group. Thus, the analysis of the conditions of victims of natural disasters, situations of marginality and crime, racial or gender discrimination, social exclusion, mental health problems, among others, leads to the claim that there are spaces that induce you to a condition of vulnerability (Delor & Hubert, 2000). This exposes people to greater risks and situations of lack of power or control, the impossibility of changing their circumstances, and therefore, to unprotection (Ricoeur, 2008).

A. O. García (✉)
Universidad Iberoamericana, Ciudad de México, Mexico
e-mail: angelica.ojeda@ibero.mx

G. A. González Ruíz
Universidad Iberoamericana, Puebla, Mexico
e-mail: gabriela.gonzalez.ruiz@iberopuebla.mx

S. Castaños-Cervantes et al. (eds.), *Working with Vulnerable Populations*,
https://doi.org/10.1007/978-3-031-67710-6_8

For Chambers (1983), vulnerability has two dimensions: exposure to constant contingencies/stressors and the difficulty of dealing with them. Vulnerability is a term that refers to a three-coordinate point of confluence: "exposure," or risk of being exposed to crisis situations; "capacity," or risk of not having the necessary resources to deal with such situations; and "potentiality," or risk of serious consequences as a result of crises, which leads to a condition of helplessness on the part of the person and lack of resources to contain the risks that live. In other words, the condition of vulnerability emphasizes the relational, the contextual, and the processual and invites to act to decrease or minimize the conditions favorable to damage; therefore, this constitutes the environment for vulnerability (Nussbaum, 2002). Among which stands out, certainty in the face of challenges, as it is the factor that allows for the structuring of social support networks and the integration of those who form them into society.

The family plays an important role in anyone's subjective life and well-being. This is the axis of organization and confluence of various social processes. Rodrigo et al. (2008) defined families in psychosocial vulnerability as those in which those responsible for the care and education of the child, due to personal and relational circumstances, as well as adverse influences of their environment, neglect their parental functions or make improper use of them, committing to the development of the child, but without achieving the gravity that justifies a measure of protection, in which case it is considered the separation of the child from his family. So social welfare is part of the interrelationship of people, situations, and circumstances of vulnerability, which will depend on the adaptation and psychological well-being of its members within and outside this system. However, everything that happens in it—good and bad, positive or negative—can be translated to the community, as it is seen as an extension of feeling and family experiences and, vice versa, the family reflects what is appreciated in the context of the community where it is inserted (Vargas et al., 2017). Meza (2009) emphasizes precisely that a community grows and consolidates its collective identity from a sharing of the interrelationship between its members and their shared stories.

Then, studying the communities and their interactions in vulnerable conditions, this implicates understanding their social communication, that is, observing their level of proximity between people and the meaning they attribute to their messages (Yanes, 2007). Simon et al. (2016) see the community as a human conglomerate that goes beyond a geographical location, where its common history, interesting spiritual and physical reality, customs, habits, norms, symbols, and shared codes are what generate that sense of belonging. According to this definition, the sense of community (a) has an important core around social interaction between the members of a collective and is complemented by (b) the perception of territorial roots and (c) a general feeling of mutuality and interdependence (Malchioni, 2014). It is also a subjective experience that has an inverse relationship with the sense of privacy (Gómez & Hombrados, 1992).

Yanes (2007) refers to the sense of community being built on what he calls the visual narrative of meaning. This is a methodology that applies in group experiences, where stories shared through art have transformed the process of formation and shaping of the self (identity). Every individual builds his self from the access and mastery skills of the symbolic resources to which he has access according to his economic and cultural context; however, it takes on a personal and subjective meaning if in the light of the reference group this thinking and feeling are shared. For this author, group social processes convey the meaning of everything is best captured in essence through art-making, where it forms a visual support that shows the group's identity and culture, especially if it was done through collaborative participatory means. Hence, it is called communities of meaningful production, interpretation, and reresigning of daily life. They are groups that start with very different ideas but that in the confrontation of the symbolic and significant produces emotion and incites collective action in order to organize ideas and respond to the need in common (Cueto et al., 2016; Gomez & Hombrados, 1992). It is to reflect critically on the living conditions themselves and seeking a sense of reality through the birth of dreams, recognition of fears, ways to bring it down, and the resurgence of hope. So, the sense of community is a co-construction of meanings of things and reflects the daily lifestyle, where group work culminates in

- Go back to a narrative of "me" in front of the other "social world."
- The past of a "world of objects" to own "subjective world" experience.
- Reflects quality in their family and neighborhood interpersonal relationships, based on describing social support, solidarity, mutual exchange, mutual help, and concern for others since their introspection.

Doing an analysis process of the concept, Jariego (2004) and Cueto et al. (2016) refer to the psychological sense of community as a subjective experience of belonging, that is, it is the feeling or perception of being part of a network of mutually supportive relationships of trust. It is done from a personal assessment to perceive a similarity with others in recognition, willingness of interdependence, and commitment to the group to allow yourself to feel part of a broader, stable, and reliable structure. For the above, identifying and/or fostering a sense of community is of great value as it integrates not only the group in general but the individual with their community. So, this is a feeling created by the others and shared with those who make up the group in question. Already McMillan and Chavis (1986) defined it as "a feeling that members have of belonging, that members are important to others and to the group, and a shared faith that *the needs of members will be met through a commitment to be together*" (p. 9). According to these authors, there are four elements that must be present to talk about a sense of community:

- Membership refers to a feeling that you have invested part of yourself in the community by providing an emotional security experience, personal investment in the community, and identification with group members.
- Influence refers to the power that members wield over the group and vice versa. Individuals with a stronger sense of community are the most active in the dynamics of the group and become a reference for the rest of the participants.
- The development and satisfaction of needs are important to consider the exchange of resources that exist in the group to meet the needs of the members, linked to the values and cohesion of the group.

- A shared emotional connection and the link of prolonged positive contact and participating in common experiences and stories.

Empower the community in personal resources with impact on improvements for the group as a unit (Fernández et al. 2020). It is therefore also of paramount importance to seek, facilitate, or promote citizen-social participation. Ramos-Vidal and Maya-Jariego (2014) explain that citizen participation is an effective mechanism for strengthening social cohesion and keeping community members together. It is a process in which community members get involved in decision-making, trying to improve their lives by engaging in community organizations. Participation is a process that involves a transformative action, especially when art is included, which has the characteristic of being able to generate a thought from emotion (Carnacea, 2012).

Jariego (2004) and Cueto et al. (2016) refer to community empowerment as a collective process that develops "from the bottom up" as it is common for it to originate in the base groups in the community. In the study presented here, this point will be addressed from the social role of mothers, of the participants, since this is a motivating, fighting, and constancy role to achieve certain goals in what Mexican culture can be defined as the object of study. However, according to this author, the empowerment varies depending on the context (it is influenced by history, experiences, and cultural diversity). In this sense, it takes a positive approach, and focuses on adaptation, and health, not disease. On the other hand, it replaces the role of the professional and expert with the population with that of facilitator and confers an active role on the participants of the community.

In the literature, you can find some work with group and art therapy that seeks to potentialize the collective. Miret and Jove's research (2011) carried out an innovative project with art therapy in an educational community at the primary level to implement during student school hours. Participants were chosen through third parties and not by personal addition as teachers were asked to supplement questionnaires (SDQs) on students'strengths and weaknesses. The project aimed to monitor the presence, participation, and progress of those students with some emotional affection to direct them toward a quality education. The group gave multiple meanings to the art of the participants; hence, the art therapy project was named for all, that is, they sought common needs and concerns, by age group, school year, and gave it a shared meaning. This is very similar to what is raised in this study. Catalan (2015) agrees with this and advocates that collective (group) practice is a methodology that potentials through sharing among its members individual experiences toward collective experiences and these can be the engines of many benefits for the social progress of their community.

On their part, Ojeda and Serrano (2008) conducted a study with Cadiz women who were discriminated against and faced violence by their family environment, providing them with a space for emotional expression, where they could disassemble and rebuild a whole series of emotional defensive structures that transcend their low self-esteem and loss of identity to enable them with changes and pathways to personal growth. According to art therapy, it has enormous potential as an engine and vehicle so that through symbolic and meaningful dialogue it places them and integrates them into a situation of life less loaded with traumatic and more positive meanings. By confronting themselves and their circumstances through art, you can take them to a second level; this is in relation to their personal situations and experiences. Thus, when such experiences are understood and assimilated by the group, there is a work of observation, listening, analysis, and commitment, where demands, haste, or the search for clarifying answers flow and stand out through the pictorial forms, images, words, strokes, and movements. These are aspects that, when identified, reinforced their individual identity.

The means of reaching the potentializing side of a community is to generate a reflection of a personal or group character to generate a sense of belonging. Previous studies refer that shared stories and participation among the members of the group are the means to enhance them individually toward generating others, such as family resilience (Miret & Jove, 2011; Ojeda & Serrano, 2008; Yanes, 2007).

According to Martínez and Lopez (2005), art therapy is a discipline that works therapeutically using artistic means, images, the creative process, and thoughtful dialogue to promote change. The art generated from collective groups manages to combat social fragmentation and highlights social–community participation. Its purpose is not to achieve a beautiful result but to mobilize and achieve a transformation around a concern and problem, which, in general, is the result of a communality in sharing meanings, so empathize, solidarity, and act as a way to participate with the group turn out to be the generating agent of a sense of community (Carnacea, 2012). In every group, a space must be created in which not only its members can express their own emotions, but also identify with each other and learn from the experiences of others by identification (Ojeda & Serrano, 2008). They add how it is that through shared symbolization and the process of identification by reciprocity that occurs among the members of a group it is that art as an intermediary is the one that functions as the agent of change.

In this sense, the objective of this study was to empower the group of women to build common goals and from their mother's or wife's role in their family and women's role, through re-meaning the practice of living and feeling in community, of creating in them an attitude, seeing possibilities, taking an interest in others, helping each other, and supporting and facilitating the growth of the group. In addition, as a result, a sense of belonging, collective identification, and a bond created through shared experiences and stories is expected to be achieved.

Method

Participants

According to Freyermuth (2004, p. 617), women are a fundamental factor both in the individual, family, and social aspects in terms of well-being of a society, and it was decided to work with a group of 10 women, all mothers and residents of an area classified as extreme poverty (according to the parameters of CONEVAL) known as "Barranca El Cilantro" in Santa Fe and with high rates of danger (Ms. Carmen, leader, gives the community) and vulnerability. Women in this community were characterized as being between 24 and 35 years of age with one or five children between "newborns" and 13 years of age. All women were dedicated only to the home, to raising children, and meet all the domestic needs of hygiene, food, and education. Women's attendance ranged from 15 to 10 women over 20 sessions covering the two pre-work phases reported here.

Design

Using techniques taken from art therapy, a workshop of 15 sessions was designed with this group of mothers from the community referred to above, so that within the context of the working group they would find a point of support that would allow them to reflect and make changes in their life situation.

Instrument

The construction method proposed by Dr. Landgarten (1981), consisting of five stages or phases described below, was used for data collection.

Phase 1: Initial Evaluation

This phase includes the diagnostic process not in terms of looking for some pathology, but exploring and familiarizing yourself with the group of participants in question. It uses some art production technique, where the generated art is any second product that allows the participant to express some individual or group need.

Phase 2: Policy Planning Through Dialogue

This is a phase in which dialogue between the process facilitator and the participants is promoted in order to understand in his words his feeling, perception, and context of life, and, on the other hand, establish a "metaphorical" conversation that can be resumed for art directives in subsequent sessions. A metaphor is any word that condenses certain content in terms of emotions or sensations and makes sense of the whole group. At the same time, recognize among the content of the dialogue the messages both expressed and not expressed since the interpretation made by each participant (or author of his art) from his context. This stage is commonly referred to as "sharing," and each participant is invited to express their feeling and perception.

Phase 3: Metaphor Management

The metaphor will become the strategic means of provoking integration and identification among participants; at the same time, confrontation will establish the guidelines of the path toward possible change in a nondirect way. Distinguishing the right metaphor for each case depends on the active listening of the narrative of the case, as well as the understanding of the content of the art given by its author.

Phase 4: Establish Work Goals for or Without Therapeutic Purposes

Having identified the needs or concerns of the participants, the subsequent "directives" for intervention through art may be inferred. The policy is the goal you are looking for; it is created based on the need to be resolved. That is, understanding the group context generates the first policy, which in this case was to explore its role as a mother in the participants. From the results of this first exploration, the second directive was drawn out; in this case, it was to strengthen those resources that can facilitate the process of resolution and family integration. From the results of this phase, you get the third directive, which was essentially what can change from her role as a mom and that this serves the means to offer other moms in the community. In this sense, art therapy is built as it is applied, not planned. Once the work goals have been identified, they direct the actions of the participants toward possibilities of action and/or support links as a valuable strategy to make the change. Based on the data being collected, the process sequence is constructed.

Phase 5: Close

At this stage, the facilitator should be attentive to integrating the reflections, dialogues, and arts generated by the participants, so that they lead each participant to realize, discover from what resources a new attitude can be adopted (especially of flexibility, openness, and change), and put into practice by trial and error until it generates a new dynamic in daily life.

Materials to Develop Art Directives

Corrugated strip paper, liquid glue, scissors, clippings of various images from magazines, colored paper, stamen, colored downs, glitter, foot cleaner, fabric patch, fabric padding, medium-sized unicell spheres, colored clay, cold silicone, colored fabrics, colored slats, wire, corrugated paper, colorful Chinese paper, and wooden sticks.

Procedure

The sessions were characterized by regular development, expressing at the beginning of the session their mood during the week as well as who have discovered themselves in the family dynamics, expressing and sharing their feeling. From this same exchange, the directive is built to work, emerging questions, doubts, concerns, and topics that give direction to the work of art therapy through the different materials that are presented. The facilitators manage to frame the directives according to the methodology set out at this stage to achieve the intended objectives. Women have freedom of choice of materials and expression of their thinking and feeling, deciding to make collage, painting, drawings, among others. It is a moment of encounter with themselves where they contact their needs, thoughts, and emotions managing to capture their "being" and "being" initiating an internal dialogue of recognition and expression. At the end of this task, they manage to share their art result among all women. As Garcia (2006) points out, it is a time for individuals to connect with their work, recognise the challenges, and listen to feedback from peers and the art therapist, who offer unique perspectives. This study's findings, analysed and integrated using Yanes's (2007) visual narrative of meaning technique, underscore the valuable role of the art therapist in the process.

Results

The results are presented by phase, according to the methodology of construction and data collection.

Phase 1 This first stage was taken as a diagnosis and evaluation stage, the data generated from a previous work phase by means of the technique of analyzing a line of life generated by participants, based on three questions: Who taught you to be a mom? What do you want to change to improve your role as a mom? In response to the first question, they expressed repetitive patterns that reflect how motherhood is built.

- "They learn" to be moms in practice, taking care of brothers, nephews, and cousins because there was no one else. Later because they get pregnant (they don't decide to get pregnant) in adolescence. They fail to complete life cycles in childhood/adolescent/adulthood stages.
- They fall in love, without thinking about the consequences of exercising unprotected sexuality and let themselves be carried away in the name of love for the promises and illusions they build like any young man beside their loved one, that is,
- Idealization of romantic and couple love conditioned by the media. This could also denote some infantilization of the relationship.

In response to the second question, they expressed repetitive patterns in ways that reflect how motherhood is exercised:

- Female conceptions: Women are the ones who manage the economy of the home, provide their resources of food, order, and cleanliness such as parenting.
- Domestic violence: Most coincide with previous family stories of domestic violence from a paternal partner, such as mother to daughter. This denotes structural problems of violence related to issues of poverty, gender beliefs, lack of opportunities, etc.
- The sense of being a mother, where the narrative of the attendees was loaded with a different emotion at the time of sharing their work, being expressed between laughter and jokes the frustration and exhaustion that comes with being a mom. The endless form of household chores that no one appreciates being necessary routine work, wearers, and little considered important to the family such as cleaning the house, having food prepared, and achieving order and neatness in their home.
- Construction of a healthy parenting style. Women synthesized boundaries, authority, love (heart), and feelings of anger and frustration at home obligations, which are the obstacles that prevent them from being "better moms with children here and now." Women agreed to cite the need to return to the essential values of the family, to assess the dynamics of the family through what is needed more than is needed, than is right without the democratic. It is important to consider these meaningful and positive learnings to get them up and running with your children, evaluating that they may not have been learned in the best way in their nuclear family, and that they now have the possibility to experience and teach them in their own style and, yes to teach them! not to avoid them, not to override them because of the personal experience that entails, but to put them on an immediate plan of action because they are the ones who teach by example, those who model these values and attitudes from their role as a mother. They concluded that educating through values is transmitting to the family a healthy coexistence, always being aware of why they are doing it.

The answer to the third question expressed fears, but at the same time some possibilities for action and change from this role of mom:

- As the workshop progressed, they became aware of themselves, their possibilities, and action skills; they decided to do so to facilitate improvements in their person or family (see Fig. 1).
- It was noted that women struggled in their family situation and sometimes expressed frustration at their marital situation, their occupation in the house, and their poor relationship with their children (see Fig. 2).

Phase 2 To plan the directives, the technique of group art therapy of "identification of actions by participants" was used. The facilitator had questioned each of the attendees in the exhibition of his art, pointing out the symbolism with which he had been elaborated. It was here that women were questioned in a group way ... "They have all shared their difficulty in setting boundaries or being authority with their

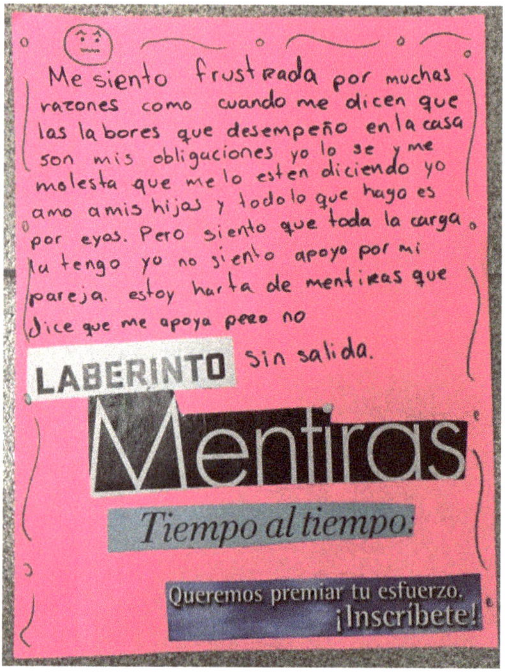

Fig. 1 Letter written by a participant that reflects how frustrated she is to not enjoy her role as a mother and must practice every day

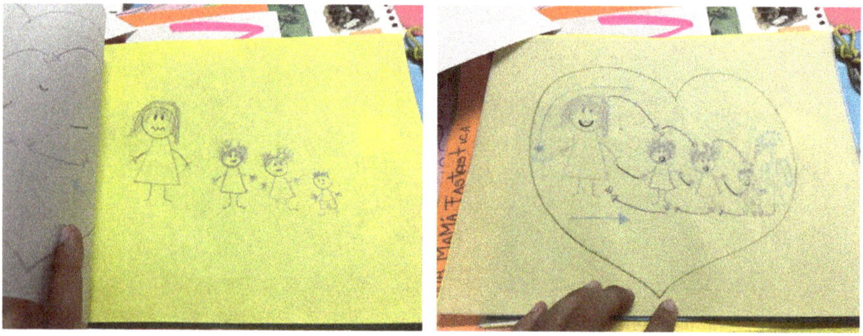

Fig. 2 Art in 2D and modified by another participant by means of the technique of appreciation and advice by means of adding Albanian paper, in which case it sends the message that there is a lack of love among the drawn members

children, as well as detracting from their husbands' authority before their children, by *disagreeing with the way they rebuke them, how could they change it?"* They were asked to select a single color and draw a problem that in the immediate past would have happened with their children, something that would give them sadness, anger, fear, and frustration. They were asked to try to make it as clear as possible using symbols, not words. At the end of the drawing, the drawings would be rotated with the other participants and each, using Albanian paper, would finish the drawing

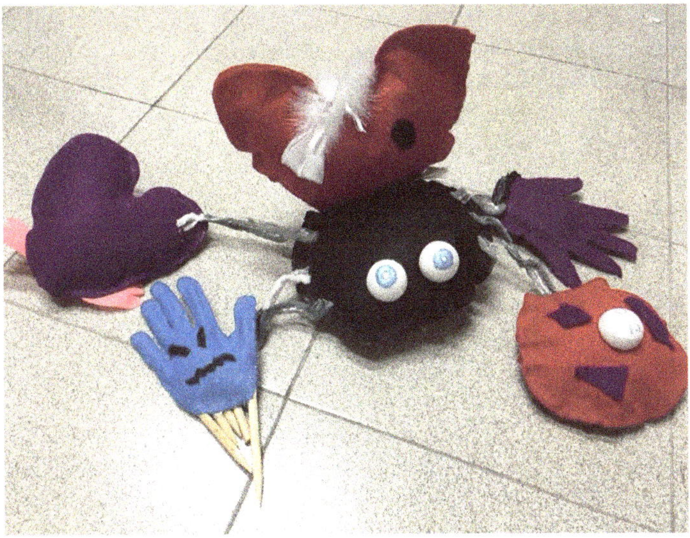

Fig. 3 3D art created by all participants, where each figure represents a particular fear and all decided to join in the fear that seemed to them in common: the spider, which represents the black, the dark, fear of change

by adding or contributing how they would improve that expressed conflict. From the analysis of the proposals made by the rest of the group, each participant shared how he now saw.

Phase 3 This phase took a little longer, working with metaphors. They began by raising awareness, asked them to think of an uncomfortable situation they have experienced and how they felt about not acting the way they would have wanted, to identify where in their body they feel that emotion. Subsequently, with the material provided, they were asked to represent that part of the body that contained such emotions; thus, they were taught that it was a metaphor and how it synthesizes many times what is thought, what is felt, and gives the possibilities of action (see Fig. 3).

The results showed that each participant generated a symbol of their greatest concern and need to change, which condensed a cluster of feelings and emotions. So, we find that

Participant 1 [P1]: "... draw a heart that represents my partner, I don't want him to be so strong with his words, it's angry I'd like to change it that his words are sweeter towards me... towards my son, I want him to understand that there is no need to be so hard ..."

Participant 2 [P2]: "I'd like to have more hands to do more things ... in addition to feeding them, helping them with schoolwork ... I would like to be able to carry out activities such as living with my children, playing with them ... because they reproach me."

Participant 3 [P3]: "It is a hand mine I made an evil face since I cannot protect myself from my angry reactions either. I recognize that I can become more aggressive, I have to contain myself for it when I explode I overflow, the sticks that I put inside my hand represent that hardness, anger not controlled in me ... something that can frustrate me a lot ... I take an attitude of intolerance and it makes me very bad."
Participant 4 [P4]: "I made a spider that represents the awkward situations at home, since I am very afraid and being a mother is a challenge and I am afraid to face some situations, I am going through a very complicated stage that is already diminishing my health, the spider represents things that I have handled in a certain way like having a couple that are sometimes violent , uncompromising, part of my faults, things that one is dragging and in times of crisis comes out for me that spider lost my temper."
Participant 6 [P6]: "I didn't represent anything from me, but I identify with both hands and heart, hands, the effort you make for the family, the spider problems."
Participant 7 [P7]: "It is a purple heart, because it is color that identifies me and is angel-shaped, for it represents the weak one I am to set limits when it comes to my children. if they put a face on me or beg me so much, I agree easily."

By sharing them, the group made associations of what the art-work symbolized:

- A spider that symbolized the fears of not being able to see in children all the efforts of wanting to be a good mom, or of not even having any evidence of it.
- Various gesticulated hearts/hands that represented the hard feeling of the mother by setting limits or, on the contrary, the softness with which children are treated with an excess of permissiveness. So, the whole group of women joined their arts with that of the spider as a central symbol in which rotates all the family dynamics and of course their role as a mother.
- Art work allowed them to recognize themselves as moms who feel similar things and need to do, create, build, and implement what has worked with each other as tools of action or thought to deal with and generate changes in their family dynamics. One of the most important elements by which a sense of community was achieved in the women's group was the fact that they had in common the experience of motherhood.

Phase 4 As this phase is the sequence and result of the three, they were asked to exemplify what they had made conscious and that they wanted to change to improve their role as mothers because they were in a learning process for it. The goal was that what they described should be taken as homework to be implemented at home with their family. The results showed that while the diversity of goals that a mother has in mind for the family to form and function, this time her collages were more structured and integrated, that is, she was not represented as a woman with her different roles or roles that play within the family, but in her different family facets integrating aspect of personal care, family coexistence, and improvements for the family in general.

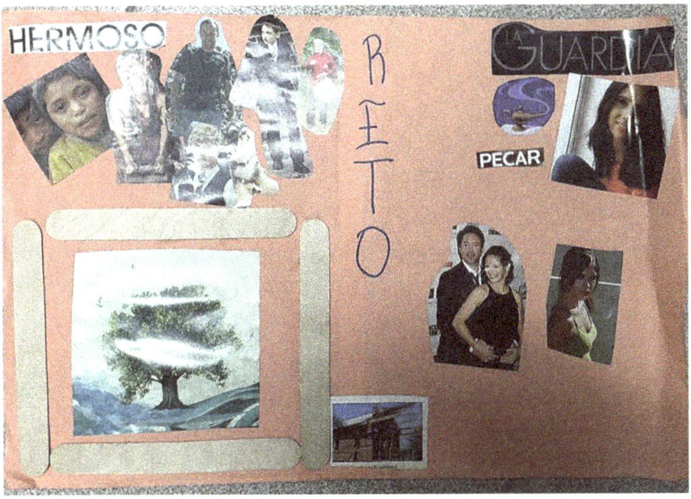

Fig. 4 Collage generated by a participant but representing the post-reflection work on fears and looking for how to diminish them through defining a challenge to follow and fear of overcoming

The results helped redirect sequential acts to generate changes at home from her role as a mom. To close this last part of the lifeline, all participants identified and expressed their sense of being mothers now, recognizing the gains of having left their homes and sharing their own experiences with other women, managing to stand in solidarity with each other, and providing and facilitating strategies to solve those difficulties of their lives. All the women assistants agreed that "the mother they can be" is already present and is in self-description through their companions who observe, reflect, accompany, and contribute to their own, achieving communion in the group of women where they mirror each other in that it involves being a mom here and now (see Fig. 4).

Phase 5 The women expressed the changes they made from attending the group and creating bonds with their peers, sharing the concern of other mothers in the community, who had approached the group's protagonists, to find out what they had learned and how they had achieved it. The group of women commented on the importance of this "discovery of themselves among themselves" and how relevant it would be to make an impact on other breasts. The women's trust was realized, in making different proposals to invite and benefit more mothers. The sense of community was made present.

Later—as a group—they decided to invite and attract women who may be living in the same situation: "*Women realized* that *by inviting other women it was a strategy to be more aware of themselves and children. Recognizing the importance of looking at themselves and making it easier for other women is to generate greater value with themselves by learning to value themselves, recognizing the strength to continue, just as effective as giving themselves things that make them feel.*"

Women were participatory and receptive to the proposal, having doubts about what and how to do so. So, the facilitator emphasized *"you can organize to find and create a symbolism that identifies you with other mothers and can convey to you how you have discovered and achieved certain changes with the family. And in this way invite them to participate and integrate into the work that is done in the workshop through art therapy."* They were provided with various materials where they had to create their art as a group:

Q5: "You have to make a doll that represents women, us as breasts, like when I made the doll that represented me myself with my hair standing."
Q3: "You have to start by drawing the head of what the doll would be like."
Q1: "I make the doll blouse they're building."

Sense of Community

As noted in theory, part of the sense of community is to have a sense of belonging, collective identification, and a bond created through shared experiences and stories. One of the most important elements by which a sense of community was achieved in the mothers' group was the fact that they had a common experience, motherhood. Each of the participants individually and assuming the appropriation of their experience shared their experiences as a mother, coinciding and resembling experiences, indicating the lack of expert and prior to learning in their maternal role, generating a feeling of identification in the account of each of the protagonists, and a feeling of solidarity and cohesion in the group.

It is important to mention that in the group of mothers a union and solidarity were achieved between them, a link through which they have been able to share difficult experiences that each lived on their side and catalyze them in a positive way and together (see Table 1).

Discussion

Giving a sense of community to women through art is when a profound process of reflection and inner dialogue begins in which art therapy has enormous potential as an engine and vehicle for a symbolic and meaningful work that places them face to face with themselves, with their experiences, and emotions (Casasola & Sánchez-Guzmán, 2011; Ojeda & Serrano, 2008).

These women forged strong bonds with each other for the benefit of the entire community. They now intend to become wellness promoters within the Coriander Barranca. Through art, experiences arise in common, achieving identification with the experience or perception of the other members of the group. It was facilitated to have an environment of safety and emotional containment, having established

Table 1 Verbalization of the sense of belonging following the parameters in which the visual narrative of meaning is given

P1	P2	P3	P4	P5
"... now I'm not lonely, I'm part of a group ... feeling accompanied has changed the way I see things..."	"... I have absorbed so much of all. I feel very sensitive."	"... I get to know my companions and I know what each one expresses ... what I can learn from each other."	"... Today I realized that if you can... thanks to the group I have been able to see the problems differently."	"I don't miss the workshop no matter what, I've learned so much. I was lonely and I saw my dead and problems, now I don't know how but I see them differently."
P6	**P7**	**P8**	**P9**	**P10**
"For me it is a challenge, I have learned from all and above all from me, I have tested myself."	"Now I am no longer such a heavy hand, I have learned from A and from you. it's important to let them learn and not give so much importance to an idea of mine."	"Thanks to what I have learned from all of them I am putting on the challenge of letting my children get dirty, because I have learned that coexistence would help me put limits with them and with me."	"It saddens me that many moms pretext the work of the house and I have really learned that if you organize you can, I have learned a lot."	"I leave everything, this day we eat anything but with the workshop I have been able to reflect on how to do to be a better mom."

Source: Authors' elaboration

meeting times once a week during an hour and a half of work, which created a link between the members. It was found as the group of mothers built a union and solidarity between them, a bond, through which they have been able to share difficult experiences that each person lived and catalyzed them in a positive way together.

Participating mothers expressed their motivation and compensation only for attending, knowing, sharing, and building a group of women who collaborate with a common purpose: self-knowing, being better "mothers," and achieving a group with whom to share. Women, having space, time, and organization within reach to attend the sessions on average, managed to generate a network of support among themselves, noting how they sought and expressed their interest in the absentee companions to the sessions, being aware of each other with themselves.

Groups generate a space to link to others, and this generates growth. It is thanks to this space that the beneficiary can clarify his identity by revealing himself (Casasola, 2011; Linesch, 1988; Marchioni, 2014; Yanes, 2007). When a group, within a community, achieves stability, it begins a healing process among its members, that is, because the sense of community increases strength and effectiveness by causing each member to commit to the other members of the group. They explain that art is an activity that allows a social sense of belonging through group participation by allowing people to communicate and work on their identity (Thomas et al., 2011).

References

Carnacea, M. (2012). Arte para la transformación social: desde y hacia la comunidad. *I Congreso Internacional de Intervención Psicosocial, Arte Social y Arteterapia. Community Psychology, 14*, 6–23.

Casasola, R. G. & Sánchez-Guzmán, E. S. (2011). Arteterapia y subjetividad femenina: construyendo uncollage. Arteterapia. *Papeles de arteterapia y educación artística para la inclusión social, 6*, 87–103. https://doi.org/10.5209/rev_ARTE.2011.v6.37086

Catalán Villalobos, Y. (2015). Creación de experiencias colectivas a través del arte (Doctoral dissertation, Universitat Politècnica de València). https://riunet.upv.es/bitstream/handle/10251/58704/CATALÁN%20-%20CREACIÓN%20DE%20EXPERIENCIAS%20COLECTIVAS%20A%20TRAVÉS%20DEL%20ARTE.pdf?sequence=3

Chambers, D. W. (1983). Stereotypic images of the scientist: The draw-a-scientist test. *Science education, 67*(2), 255–265. https://www.researchgate.net/profile/David-Chambers-11/publication/229689208_Stereotypic_images_of_the_scientist_The_Draw-A-Scientist_Test_Science_Education_672_255-265/links/5c64c0d445851582c3e6e67f/Stereotypic-images-of-thescientist-The-Draw-A-Scientist-Test-Science-Education-672-255-265.pdf?_sg%5B0%5D=started_experiment_milestone&origin=journalDetail

Consejo Nacional de Evaluación de la Política de Desarrollo Social (CONEVAL). https://www.coneval.gob.mx/Medicion/MP/Paginas/Lineas-de-bienestar-y-canasta-basica.aspx

Cueto, R. M., Espinosa, A., Guillén, H., & Seminario, M. (2016). Sentido de Comunidad Como Fuente de Bienestar en Poblaciones Socialmente Vulnerables de Lima. *Perú Psykhe, 25*(1), 1–18. https://doi.org/10.7764/psykhe.25.1.814

Delor, F., & Hubert, M. (2000). Revisiting the concept of 'vulnerability'. *Social science & medicine, 50*(11), 1557–1570. https://doi.org/10.1016/s0277-9536(99)00465-7

Fernández, A. G., Waldmüller, J., & Vega, C. (2020). Comunidad, vulnerabilidad y reproducción en condiciones de desastre. Abordajes desde América Latina y el Caribe Presentación del dossier. *ÍCONOS Revista de Ciencias Sociales, 66*(XXIV), 7–29. https://doi.org/10.17141/iconos.66.2020.4156

Freyermuth Enciso, G., & Fernández Guerrero, M. (2004). El material etnográfico como instrumento de factores de riesgo y la generación de propuestas en relación con el problema de la muerte materna. *AGATHOS: Atención Sociosanitaria y Bienestar, 3*, 34–51.

Freyermuth, G. (2004). Maternidad Peligrosa. Evaluación de la atención Institucional a la urgencia Obstétrica en Los Altos de Chiapas. SEDESO-INDESOL; ForoNacional de Mujeres yPolíticas de Población; CIESAS.

García, R. (2006). Sistemas complejos: conceptos, métodos y fundamentación epistemológica de la investigación interdisciplinaria. Gedisa. https://secat.unicen.edu.ar/wpcontent/uploads/2020/03/GARCIA-Sistemas-complejos1.pdf

Gómez, L. & Hombrados, M. (1992). Sentido de comunidad y privacidad. *Revista de Psicología Social, 7*(2), 213–226. https://d1wqtxts1xzle7.cloudfront.net/90667099/Dialnet-SentidoDeComunidadYPrivacidad-111772-libre.pdf?1662349312=&response-contentdisposition=inline%3B+filename3DSentido_de_comunidad_y_privacidad.pdf&Expires=1724529619&Signature=XkcSIeNyTQfqX~dCkg00dG9TfOmJAI482ZAsIfs~8wYqprHkEGuC1HJjiMjGr78Ja2GW~9fl6nBK1n~6KPCUdg42CdHff-BZd8DrScYcSmJ7tcGUz12BmwJzm8eSHSL8I46mJbxVBOTkRQZyNvkpbUzMOfjjNCcg-GZcT1~4TxKaE7-2vla683yjtXrepswT9KLWE-NRfUqsiZ7fJsQ~QD9jFocHhhmywqmyqh3upz7Ct8nfp2s8RXNFG-Rj7AYim7GjchgvBQ6DmcfiYr5~yibkHabZv7yC5Q__&Key-Pair-Id=APKAJLOHF5GGSLRBV4Z

Jariego, M. (2004). Sentido de comunidad y potenciación comunitaria. *Apuntes de Psicología, 22*(2), 187–211.

Landgarten, S. (1981). Skilled medical director can turn conflict into collaboration. *The Hospital Medical Staff, 10*(5), 2–9.

Linesch, D. (1988). *Adolescent art therapy*. Brunner/Mazek.

Marchioni, M. (2014). De las comunidades y de lo comunitario. *Revista Espacios Transnacionales* [En línea], 3, Julio-Diciembre. https://dialnet.unirioja.es/servlet/articulo?codigo=5419932

Martínez, N., & López, M. (2005). Arteterapia, Principios y ámbitos de aplicación: El Arte como Terapia en España.

McMillan, B., & Chavis, D. M. (1986). Sense of community: A definition and theory. *Journal of Community Psychology, 14*, 6–23. https://scirp.org/reference/referencespapers.aspx?referenceid=1494195

Meza, G. (2009). *Comunidad y Sentido de Comunidad: La intervención del Programa Puente en seis familias en situación de extrema pobreza en la comuna de La Florida*. Universidad de Chile. Escuela de Psicología.

Miret Latas, M. À., & Jové Monclús, G. (2011). Arteterapia para todos: La clave está en la diferencia. https://repositori.udl.cat/server/api/core/bitstreams/87c4fa9d-1c4d-4bc5-a6e6-a79620f68616/content

Nussbaum, M. (2002). *Las mujeres y el desarrollo humano*. Herder.

Ojeda, M., & Serrano, A. (2008). Mujer y Arteterapia, una visión sobre la violencia de género. *Papeles de arteterapia y educación artística para la inclusión social, 3*, 157–164.

Ramos-Vidal, I., & Maya-Jariego, I. (2014). Sentido de comunidad, empoderamiento psicológico y participación ciudadana en trabajadores de organizaciones culturales. *Psychosocial Intervention, 23*(3), 169–176.

Ricoeur, P. (2008). *Autonomy and vulnerability. Just 2. Studies, readings and exercises of applied ethics*. Trotta.

Rodrigo, M. J., Maiquez, M. L., Martín, J. C., & Byrne, S. (2008). Preservación familiar: Un enfoque positivo para la intervención con familias. In *Family preservation: A positive approach to intervention with families*. Pirámide.

Simón, C., Giné, C., & Echeita, G. (2016). Escuela, Familia y Comunidad: Construyendo Alianzas para Promover la Inclusión. *Revista Latinoamericana de Educación Inclusiva, 10*(1), 25–42. https://doi.org/10.17141/iconos.66.2020.4156

Thomas, Y., Gray, M., McGuiny, S., & Ebringer, S. (2011). Homeless adults engagement in art: First steps towards identity, recovery and social inclusion. *Australian Occupational Therapy Journal, 58*(6), 429–436. https://pubmed.ncbi.nlm.nih.gov/22111645/

Vargas Rubilar, J., Lemos, V., & Richaud, M. C. (2017). Parental strengthening program in social vulnerability contexts: A proposal from the interdisciplinary school area. *Inter-American Center for Psychological Research and Related Sciences, 34*(1), 157–172. https://www.redalyc.org/pdf/180/18052925010.pdf

Yanes Córdoba, V. (2007). La narrativa visual como metodología del sentido: Articulación metodológica e implicaciones terapéutico-educativas. *Papeles de Arteterapia y educación artística para la inclusión social, 2*, 233–246. https://revistas.ucm.es/index.php/ARTE/article/view/ARTE0707110233A

A Literature Review on Autism Spectrum Disorders Treatment

Niceta W. Ireri

Autism Spectrum Disorder (ASD) Characteristics and Diagnosis According to DSM-5

In previous editions of the Diagnostic and Statistical Manual of Mental Disorders (DSM), autism disorder was classified as one of the pervasive developmental disorders (including Rett's disorder, autism disorder, Asperger's disorder, pervasive developmental disorder—not otherwise specified [PDD-NOS], and childhood disintegrative disorder). These disorders are typically diagnosed in childhood or adolescence. However, in the fifth edition of DSM (DSM-5), autism spectrum disorder (ASD) was reclassified under the neurodevelopmental disorder category, completely separate from the pervasive developmental disorder classification (American Psychiatric Association, 2013). Diagnostic and statistical manual of mental disorders (5th ed.), (APA, 2013).

The DSM-5 conceptualizes ASD as dimensional rather than categorical, encompassing previous diagnoses like Asperger's disorder, autistic disorder, and PDD-NOS.

ASD is now characterized by two main symptom clusters instead of the previously described triad of social interaction, communication, and restricted, repetitive patterns of behavior, interests, and activities. Diagnosis in the DSM-5 requires impairments in two domains: social communication and interaction, and restricted, repetitive patterns of behavior, interests, or activities.

Under category A, deficits in social communication and social interaction are delineated by three diagnostic criteria. Individuals must exhibit all three criteria, either currently or historically, for an ASD diagnosis. These criteria include: (1) deficits in social-emotional reciprocity, (2) deficits in nonverbal communicative

N. W. Ireri (✉)
Africa International University, Nairobi, Kenya
e-mail: niceta.ireri@aiu.ac.ke

S. Castaños-Cervantes et al. (eds.), *Working with Vulnerable Populations*,
https://doi.org/10.1007/978-3-031-67710-6_9

behavior, and (3) deficits in developing, maintaining, and understanding relationships. The DSM-5 provides illustrative examples for each criterion, such as abnormal social approach and difficulty in engaging in back-and-forth conversations (A1).

Category B addresses restricted, repetitive patterns of behavior, interests, or activities, specifying four criteria. To be diagnosed with ASD, individuals need to meet at least two of these criteria, either currently or historically. These criteria include: (1) stereotyped movements, use of objects, or speech; (2) insistence on sameness, inflexible adherence to routines, or ritualized patterns of verbal or nonverbal behavior; (3) restricted interests that are unusually intense or focused; and (4) hyper- or hypo-reactivity to sensory input or unusual interest in sensory aspects of the environment.

The DSM-5 provides illustrative examples for each criterion, such as B1, which includes behaviors like lining up toys, flipping objects, and echolalia. Additionally, three overarching diagnostic criteria are outlined. Criterion C specifies that symptoms must appear early in development, though impairments may only become evident later in life when demands increase. Criterion D requires symptoms to cause significant impairment in functioning. Criterion E states that deficits should not be better explained by intellectual disability or global developmental delay, despite the potential co-occurrence of intellectual disability and ASD.

According to DSM-5 guidelines, individuals previously diagnosed with autistic disorder, PDD-NOS, or Asperger's disorder should now receive an ASD diagnosis. This diagnosis includes two sets of specifiers: severity specifiers indicating the level of support needed for each symptom domain—rated independently as Level 1 (needing support), Level 2 (needing substantial support), or Level 3 (needing very substantial support).

Severity levels can change throughout a person's lifetime, and while DSM-5 defines three severity levels, the accompanying text acknowledges that symptoms may occasionally fall below Level 1, indicating minimal need for support. The second set of specifiers requires clinicians to note whether ASD is present with or without additional intellectual or language impairments, in conjunction with any known medical, genetic, or environmental factors, and if catatonia is also present.

Lastly, it's important to note that the DSM-5 includes the diagnosis of social (pragmatic) communication disorder. This condition is classified under communication disorders rather than neurodevelopmental disorders and serves as a potential alternative diagnosis for individuals with impairments in social communication but without symptoms of restricted, repetitive behaviors either currently or historically. However, it's worth noting that research on the diagnostic validity of social communication disorder is inconclusive (Ozonoff, 2012; Skuse, 2012), and further studies are needed in this area.

The Severity of Symptoms in Children with Autism

Evidence suggests that no biological markers reliably identify autism in specific patients (Arky, 2016; Ecker et al., 2010; Posey et al., 2008). This is because ASD is a neurological condition, and no blood or tissue samples have ever confirmed its presence in affected individuals (Arky, 2016). Instead, ASD is diagnosed through a series of assessments that include parental reports, medical histories, psychological evaluations, and speech and language assessments. These evaluations are conducted by qualified professionals trained in ASD diagnosis.

Children with ASD struggle to form and maintain healthy social relationships (Bellin, 2006; Reaven, 2009; White et al., 2013). Research indicates that these children lack the skills necessary to interact effectively with typically developing peers due to neurological impairments that affect their sensory processing, thereby impacting their social participation (Herbert, 2005; Shriber, 2010). Further studies confirm that in autism, different parts of the brain appear to function uniquely (Just et al., 2004), leading to challenges in information processing.

The DSM-5 (APA, 2013) outlines social difficulties experienced by individuals with ASD, including deficits in social-emotional reciprocity such as difficulty in engaging in typical back-and-forth conversations, reduced sharing of interests or emotions, and challenges initiating or responding to social interactions. There are also deficits in communicative gestures, such as limited eye contact, difficulties integrating verbal and nonverbal communication, and a lack of gestures and expressions. Additionally, there are struggles in developing, maintaining, and understanding relationships, which manifest in difficulties regulating behavior across different social settings, challenges in imaginative play and forming friendships, and a lack of interest in peers. Anxiety symptoms and social challenges are linked to episodes of depression and can significantly impact social relationships and academic performance in children with ASD.

Treatment of ASD

There is no cure for ASD, but there are interventions designed to manage symptoms and help individuals with ASD lead fulfilling lives (Huerta et al., 2012). Early interventions are particularly encouraged to assist individuals in acquiring skills, communicating effectively, managing household tasks, and achieving success in school (White et al., 2013). Various approaches have been developed to support individuals with ASD, discussed below.

Cognitive-Behavioral Approaches

Cognitive-behavioral approaches, also known as comprehensive psychosocial interventions, are the most widely used nonmedical treatments for ASD. Specific techniques include applied behavior analysis (ABA) and Treatment and Education of Autistic and Related Communication-Handicapped Children (TEACCH). Other approaches that involve family or community participation in the treatment of children with ASD include cognitive-behavioral therapy (CBT), Denver Health Sciences, the DIR/Floortime method, the LEAP program, and the Miller method. Initiating these interventions early in life, once the diagnosis is confirmed, is recommended to have a positive impact on children with ASD.

Cognitive-Behavioral Therapy (CBT)

CBT was initially developed as a nonpharmacological treatment for mood and anxiety disorders in children and adolescents with ASD. This method includes emotional training and cognitive restructuring. Emotional training aims to help individuals with ASD understand that emotions vary in intensity, individual capability, and expression (Kalyva, 2011).

Among behavioral modification treatments, CBT has shown considerable success. CBT utilizes graded exposure to gradually confront anxiety-inducing situations, teaches relaxation techniques, and employs cognitive restructuring to identify and modify irrational thought patterns through modeling appropriate thinking. CBT operates on the premise that restructuring maladaptive thinking, such as amplifying negatives or overgeneralizing, can lead to changes in maladaptive behavior. However, using traditional CBT with children with ASD may present challenges related to their cognitive and communication skills.

In their study, Lickel et al. (2012) evaluated cognitive abilities in children with ASD compared to typically developing children. The research confirmed that children with ASD generally possess the cognitive abilities necessary for CBT. They can differentiate between thoughts, feelings, and behaviors and can work toward modifying their thoughts. Their primary challenge lies in identifying emotions. However, modified CBT approaches tailored for children with ASD emphasize repetitive practice, involve parents, utilize visual aids, and focus on concreteness (Reaven, 2009; Wood et al., 2009a, b). For instance, instead of verbally rating their anxiety levels on a scale, a child with ASD might point to a visual thermometer indicating their anxiety level in a specific situation. Alternatively, focusing on the individual's strengths and preferences helps maintain engagement and motivation.

CBT has been effective in alleviating anxiety symptoms in empirical research (Moree & Davis, 2010; Reaven, 2009). Studies indicate that individuals with higher cognitive functioning in ASD may experience more pronounced anxiety symptoms (Lemmon, 2013). Further analysis by Mazurek and Kanne (2010) suggests that individuals with ASD are more prone to anxiety disorders compared to those without intellectual disabilities. As individuals with ASD become more aware of themselves and their environment, anxiety levels may increase (White et al., 2009).

In Africa, there is limited documentation on anxiety in young people, especially among those with ASD. However, anxiety is generally recognized as a significant motivator in human behavior and a normal response to both threatening and non-threatening situations in the environment (Ndetei et al., 2011).

The impact of anxiety extends beyond the child with ASD to affect parents and teachers, a common occurrence in households (Gona, 2016). Teachers who lack the skills to manage these children may refer them elsewhere, not necessarily for assistance but to avoid responsibility for poor academic performance, as noted in preliminary surveys by researchers. Withdrawing these children from social interactions or confining them at home does not alleviate their anxiety (Riccio, 2011). Furthermore, parents often sacrifice their livelihoods to care for these children, which in the Kenyan context can exacerbate ASD symptoms and lead to the development of anxiety.

In cognitive restructuring, children with ASD are guided to correct their distorted self-perceptions and taught appropriate ways to handle social interactions, which are often sources of stress for them. Managing anxiety through classic relaxation techniques involves identifying social situations that provoke anxiety and providing necessary support with the child's involvement (Kalyva, 2011).

CBT combines effective psychological and behavioral techniques to help individuals with ASD reduce their anxiety, manage emotions like anger, and overcome self-injurious behaviors (Sze & Wood, 2007; White et al., 2009; Wood et al., 2009a, b). Studies have shown that CBT can decrease anxiety levels and improve social behaviors such as sharing and participating in group activities (Reaven, 2009; Wood et al., 2009a, b).

Applied Behavior Analysis (ABA)

ABA has been the most widely used method for over 40 years in treating children with ASD, demonstrating significant success (Foxx, 2008). This approach focuses on replacing undesirable behaviors with more desirable ones by understanding the function of behavior. There is ample research supporting the efficacy of ABA for individuals with ASD (Foxx, 2008), and the technique has evolved over time.

Treatment and Education of Autistic and Related Communication-Handicapped Children (TEACCH)

TEACCH, similar to ABA but with some distinct differences, emphasizes structured educational settings for children with ASD. It integrates diagnostic assessment, management, professional training, and daily living skills in a systematic approach designed to create a predictable environment that fosters independence and security (Kalyva, 2011). Longitudinal studies have shown improvements in areas such as daily living skills and relationships among children with autism when TEACCH is combined with other programs like ABA and CBT.

Developmental, Individual Difference, Relationship-Based (DIR)/Floortime Method

The DIR/Floortime method emphasizes the importance of normalizing interactions and communication timeframes for children with ASD to reduce self-stimulation behaviors. It focuses on nurturing meaningful interactions based on the child's emotions and interests, facilitating the acquisition of skills in gestures, persistence, language, and play (Kalyva, 2011).

Learning Experiences: An Alternative Program for Preschoolers and Parents (LEAP)

LEAP involves children with ASD and their families in an integrated preschool setting and behavior modification training for parents. It aims to develop fundamental skills globally, including personalized educational plans, behavior management, social skills, and smooth transitions between educational levels. While research on LEAP's effectiveness is limited, its inclusive approach involving parents and educators underscores its potential impact, though comparative studies with other treatments are lacking.

Miller Method

The Miller method targets individuals with ASD struggling with sensory integration, social relationships, and communication in educational or clinical settings. It emphasizes direct interaction with people and objects to facilitate learning.

These approaches represent a range of strategies aimed at supporting individuals with ASD, tailored to address their specific needs and challenges. There are other techniques of ASD intervention that are notably different in that they lean heavily and exclusively on the improvement of social and communication skills (e.g., "social stories" and "circle of friends" or the "friendship club").

Multimodal Anxiety and Social Skills Intervention (MASSI)

MASSI is grounded in the principles of behavioral, cognitive, and learning psychology (Dobson & Dobson, 2009). Central to cognitive-behavioral therapy (CBT) is the idea that thoughts influence emotions and behavior. By restructuring maladaptive thoughts, emotional distress can be reduced and social skills improved (Beck, 1972; Ireri et al., 2019; White et al., 2010). The implementation of MASSI techniques is rooted in CBT principles, particularly operant conditioning (Skinner, 1953).

Operant conditioning principles advocate for using positive reinforcements, such as praise, and negative reinforcements to modify behavior based on consequences (Rao et al., 2008). For instance, praising a child serves as a positive reinforcement to increase the likelihood of the desired behavior recurring, while negative consequences like being ignored or mocked can decrease the chances of undesirable behaviors. MASSI incorporates response cost methods to reduce problematic behaviors and foster skill acquisition (Lopata et al., 2008; White et al., 2013).

Social learning theory helps integrate cognitive and behavioral elements in MASSI. This theory suggests that learning occurs through modeling and observing others' behaviors, consequences, and outcomes. Motivation and self-efficacy are critical components that mediate cognition, including goal-setting, evaluating activities, and self-monitoring (Bandura, 1973). Thus, MASSI incorporates social skills training, which involves collaborative efforts in cognitive, behavioral, and learning domains to enhance individuals' understanding of complex situations (cognitive) and expand their repertoire of responses (social learning) to various circumstances.

While these intervention strategies are effective in addressing specific aspects of ASD, they do not comprehensively manage all symptoms (White et al., 2009). Therefore, there is a recognized need to complement these approaches with more integrative treatment strategies, as noted by White et al. (2013). In response, MASSI was developed as a nonmedical, physiotherapy-based approach to managing and caring for adolescents primarily diagnosed with ASD (White et al., 2013). This structured cognitive-behavioral intervention targets anxiety symptoms and social skills deficits among adolescents with ASD.

Research evaluating nonmedical, psychosocial treatments for anxiety in youth with ASD remains limited (Scarpa & Reyes, 2011). Children with ASD could benefit significantly from social and behavioral interventions similar to those observed in regular classroom settings (Riccio, 2011), which encompass programs targeting anxiety behaviors and involving parents and teachers.

In conclusion, an effective intervention strategy should comprehensively address anxiety and social deficits in school children, involving collaboration among parents, teachers, and the children themselves. Addressing issues like delayed diagnosis and inadequate treatment is crucial in mitigating the impact of anxiety in children with ASD (Stichter et al., 2007).

References

American Psychiatric Association. (2013). *Diagnostic and statistical manual of mental disorders* (5th ed.). Author.

Arky, B. (2016). *Autism and medication: Why are so many kids on the spectrum taking it? And is it being misused?* Retrieved from http://childmind.org/article/autism-and-medication

Bandura, A. (1973). *Aggression: A social learning analysis*. Englewood Cliffs, Prentice Hall.

Beck, A. T. (1972). *Depression: Causes and treatment*. University of Pennsylvania Press.

Bellini, S. (2006). The development of social anxiety in adolescents with autism spectrum disorders. *Focus on Autism and Other Developmental Disabilities, 21*, 138–145.

Dobson, D., & Dobson, K. S. (2009). *Evidenced-based practice of cognitive behavioural therapy*. Guildford Press.

Ecker, C., Marquand, A., Mourão-Miranda, J., Johnston, P., Daly, E. M., Brammer, M. J., & Murphy, D. G. (2010). Describing the brain in autism in five dimensions: Magnetic resonance imaging. Assisted diagnosis of autism spectrum disorder using a multiparameter classification approach. *Journal of Neuroscience, 30*, 10612–10623.

Foxx, R. M. (2008). Applied behaviour analysis treatment of autism: The state of the art. *Child and Adolescent Psychiatric Clinics of North America, 17*(4), 821–834.

Gona, J. K. (2016). *Autism and other neurodevelopmental disabilities on the Kenyan coast: Challenges, perceived causes and rehabilitation options*. Springer.

Herbert, M. R. (2005). Large brains in autism: The challenge of pervasive abnormality. *The Neuroscientist, 11*(5), 417–440.

Huerta, M., Bishop, S. L., Duncan, A., Hus, V., & Lord, C. (2012). Application of DSM-5 criteria for autism spectrum disorder to three samples of children with DSM-IV diagnoses of pervasive developmental disorders. *American Journal of Psychiatry, 169*(10), 1056–1064.

Ireri, W. I., White, S., & Mbwayo, A. (2019). Treating anxiety and social deficits in children with autism spectrum disorder in two schools in Nairobi, Kenya. *Journal of Autism and Developmental Disorders, 49*, 3309–3315. https://doi.org/10.1007/s10803-019-04045-6

Just, M. A., Cherkassky, V. L., Keller, T. A., & Minshew, N. J. (2004). Cortical activation and synchronization during sentence comprehension in high-functioning autism. Evidence of underconnectivity. *Brain, 127*(8), 1811–1821.

Kalyva, E. (2011). *Cognitive-behavioural approaches in autism: Educational and therapeutic approaches*. SAGE Publications Ltd.

Lemmon, K. (2013). Alleviating anxiety in children and adolescents with autism spectrum disorders: Exploring the effectiveness of cognitive-behaviour therapy. *New Zealand Journal of Teachers' Work, 10*(1), 67–86.

Lickel, A., Maclean, W. E., Jr., Blakeley-Smith, A., & Hepburn, S. (2012). Assessment of the prerequisite skills for cognitive behavioural therapy in children with and without autism spectrum disorders. *Journal of Autism and Developmental Disorders, 42*(6), 992–1000.

Lopata, C., Thomeer, M. L., Volker, M. A., Nida, R. E., & Lee, G. K. (2008). Effectiveness of a manualized summer social treatment program for high functioning children with autism spectrum disorders. *Journal of Autism and Developmental Disorders, 38*, 890–904.

Mazurek, M. O., & Kanne, S. (2010). Friendship and internalizing symptoms among children and adolescents with ASD. *Journal of Autism and Related Disorders, 40*, 1512–1520.

Moree, B. N., & Davis, T. E. (2010). Cognitive-behavioural therapy for anxiety in children diagnosed with autism spectrum disorders: Modification trends. *Research in Autism Spectrum Disorders, 4*, 346–354.

Ndetei, D. M., Khasakhala, L. I., Mbwayo, A. W., & Mutiso, V. (2011). Epidemiological patterns of anxiety disorders in Kenya. *Anxiety and Related Disorders, 5*, 254–258.

Ozonoff, S. (2012). Editorial perspective: Autism spectrum disorders in DSM-5: An historical perspective and the need for change. *Journal of Child Psychology and Psychiatry, 53*, 1092–1094.

Posey, D. J., Stigler, K. A., Erickson, C. A., & McDougle, C. J. (2008). Antipsychotics in the treatment of autism. *Journal of Clinical Investigation, 118*, 6–14.

Rao, P., Beidel, D., & Murray, M. (2008). Social skills interventions for children with asperger's syndrome or high-functioning autism: A review and recommendations. *Journal of Autism and Developmental Disorders, 38*, 353–361.

Reaven, J. A. (2009). Children with high-functioning autism spectrum disorders and co-occurring anxiety symptoms: Implications for assessment and treatment. *Journal for Specialists in Pediatric Nursing, 14*, 192–199.

Riccio, A. (2011). *Autism in Kenya: A social, educational and political perspective*. Independent study project (ISP) collection paper no. 1203.

Scarpar, A., & Reyes, N. M. (2011). Improving emotion regulation with CBT in young children with high functioning autism SD: A pilot study. *Behavioural and Cognitive Psychotherapy, 39*, 495–500.

Shriber, L. (2010). Autism: A neurological and sensory-based perspective. *International Encyclopedia of Rehabilitation, 6*(3), 211–218.

Skinner, B. F. (1953). *Science and human behaviour*. Macmillan.

Skuse, D. H. (2012). DSM-5's conceptualization of autistic disorders. *Journal of the American Academy of Child and Adolescent Psychiatry, 51*, 344–346.

Stichter, J., Randolph, J., Gage, N., & Schmidt, C. (2007). A review of recommended social competency programs for students with autism spectrum disorders. *Exceptionality, 15*(4), 219–232.

Sze, K. M., & Wood, J. J. (2007). Cognitive behavioural treatment of comorbid anxiety disorders and social difficulties in children with high-functioning autism: A case report. *Journal of Contemporary Psychotherapy, 37*, 133–143.

White, S. W., Oswald, D., Ollendick, T., & Scahill, L. (2009). Anxiety in children and adolescents with autism spectrum disorders. *Clinical Psychology Review, 29*(3), 216–229.

White, S. W., Albano, A., Johnson, C., Kasari, C., Ollendick, T., & Klin, A. (2010). Development of a cognitive-behavioural intervention program to treat anxiety and social deficits in teens with high-functioning autism. *Clinical Child and Family Psychology Review, 13*, 77–90.

White, S. W., Ollendick, T., Albano, A. M., Oswald, D., Johnson, C. R., & Southam-Gerow, M. A. (2013). Randomized controlled trial: Multimodal anxiety and social skill intervention for adolescents with autism spectrum disorder. *Journal of Autism and Developmental Disorders, 43*, 382–394.

Wood, J. J., Drahota, A., Sze, K., Har, K., Chiu, A., & Langer, D. A. (2009a). Cognitive behavioural therapy for anxiety in children with autism spectrum disorders: A randomized, controlled trial. *Journal of Child Psychology and Psychiatry, 50*, 224–234.

Wood, J. J., Drahota, A., Sze, K., Van Dyke, M., Decker, K., & Fujii, C. (2009b). Effects of cognitive behavioural therapy on parent-reported autism symptoms in school-age children with high-functioning autism. *Journal of Autism and Developmental Disorders, 39*, 1608–1612.

Multicultural Therapy with Vulnerable Populations: A Narrative Case Study

Nicole M. Vélez Agosto and María C. Almario-Zgheib

Introduction

The World Health Organization (2010) considers people with severe mental illness (SMI) as a vulnerable group due to noted risks for human rights abuses and the lack of opportunities to experience agency and participate in important social and economic activities. Women with mental illness experience significant rates of physical and sexual victimization and are rarely protected by systems that afford them a sense of safety (Goodman et al., 2001). Having a sense of safety is a basic cornerstone of psychological functioning and a threshold beneath which real human functioning is not possible (WHO, 2010; Nussbaum, 2000; Worell & Remer, 2003). Research suggests a bidirectional relationship exists between mental health symptoms and victimization (Maniglio, 2009). SMI places individuals at risk for victimization, and victimization leads to increased symptoms and impairment. In comparison to the general population, individuals with both SMI and trauma exposure are likely to present a complex clinical picture and prolonged course of illness that requires specialized treatment (Grubaugh et al., 2011).

SMI intersects with other aspects of social stratification, such as race, ethnicity, gender, class, or sexual orientation, which compounds the stigma of living with a mental illness (Jackson-Best & Edwards, 2018). SMI diagnoses include schizophrenia spectrum disorders or mood disorders coupled with severe and persistent social and occupational impairments (Grubaugh et al., 2011). What furthers the

N. M. Vélez Agosto (✉)
University of Texas Rio Grande Valley, Edinburg, TX, USA
e-mail: nicole.velezagosto@utrgv.edu

M. C. Almario-Zgheib
Counseling Psychology Program, Department of Educational, School, & Counseling Psychology, College of Education, University of Kentucky, Lexington, KY, USA
e-mail: maria.almario@gmail.com

S. Castaños-Cervantes et al. (eds.), *Working with Vulnerable Populations*,
https://doi.org/10.1007/978-3-031-67710-6_10

vulnerability is the need for assistance with daily living increasing the risk for frequent institutionalization to manage primary symptoms and prevent relapse and/or hospitalization (Grubaugh et al., 2011). Consequences of vulnerability for people with SMI are both the experience of trauma itself and the subsequent development of PTSD. Considering intersectionality in people with SMI, women are more vulnerable to experiencing development of PTSD and complex PTSD due to the impact of sexism and the significant rate of sexual abuse and violence that impacts this population (Latalova, et al., 2014). They also constitute a significant proportion of the population served in community mental health centers (National Alliance of Mental Illness, 2019) and are in increasing need of culturally competent treatments.

Vulnerability Theories and Conceptualizations

The Latin root of the word vulnerability is *wound*. Underlying this concept is the idea of enhanced risk or the probability that an individual will become sick in a period of time (Aday, 1994). Public health discourse defines a vulnerable subject as determined by the assets, capacities, or resilience gained through a complex set of interactions with societal institutions (Rich, 2018). The line between public and private institutions, as well as the autonomy of individuals, is blurred when people are considered vulnerable (Rich, 2018). "People are heavily intertwined and dependent upon institutions, and it is through these institutions that people gain autonomy" (Rich, 2018, p. 15).

There are different conceptualizations about vulnerable people. In general, they are conceived as people at risk of abuse because of their condition of social, economic, cultural, or psychological disadvantage. Factors related to the emergence of vulnerability are developmental problems, personal disabilities, disadvantaged social statuses, poor interpersonal networks, degraded social environments, and a complex interaction between these factors (Mechanic & Tanner, 2007). Vulnerability is experienced as social exclusion (Vázquez et al., 2016) leading to increased susceptibility to harm (Mechanic & Tanner, 2007) due to the interaction between the amount of resources available to marginalized people and the life challenges they face.

Mechanic & Tanner (2007) identified two dimensions of vulnerability. Vulnerability arises first from a social stress process. Social stress is the experience of challenging social circumstances potentially caused by socioeconomic deficits, social exclusion, illness, disability, and increase of traumatic events, such as physical and sexual violence. This foundational social stress is mediated by coping, or how people respond to the hardships within a social context. Coping is enhanced by quality and quantity of social support and the individual's sense of control and mastery over difficult situations. Therefore, vulnerability is a dynamic concept, with both risk and strengths involved in navigating of a wider cultural context of privilege and oppression.

Gender and Vulnerability

As the World Health Organization (2019) states: "gender determines the differential power and control men and women have over the socioeconomic determinants of their mental health and lives, their social position, status and treatment in society and their susceptibility and exposure to specific mental health risks" (p. 2). Therefore, women with SMI encounter gender disparities in mental health; in their outcomes, in treatment experiences, and in barriers to care (Mizock & Brubaker, 2019; Borba et al., 2012; Mowbray et al., 1992; Cogan, 1998). Women with SMI are significantly more likely to experience sexual violence than men (Grubaugh et al., 2011) in both childhood and adulthood. Exposure to trauma, in particular to gender-based violence, including intimate partner violence, rape, sexual assault, and stalking, may contribute to women developing severe mental disorders, having greater and more severe comorbidity and general disability, and significantly lower quality of life (Nguyen et al., 2017).

Women diagnosed with a serious mental illness have been stigmatized as poor parents regardless of their circumstances and the characteristics of the individual mother (Cogan, 1998). For instance, in spite of growing evidence that abusers often use custody battles to retain control over their former partners and that domestic violence dynamics often involve the systematic use of terror and enforced dependency, women are often penalized by having their children removed, even when engaged in a process of domestic violence emancipation (Fauci & Goodman, 2019). The experience of having a child removed would be overwhelming for almost anyone. However, gender disparities place women at increased risk for emotional distress. Therefore, gender plays a significant additional role in adding a vulnerability layer to an already vulnerable population.

Community Mental Health and Vulnerable Women

Vulnerable populations lack adequate access to mental health services in the United States (Saxena et al., 2007). Stigma about mental disorders constrains the use of available resources, which further reduces access for vulnerable people (Saxena et al., 2007). Although community mental health centers provide services to those with government assistance and public health insurance, quality of services may be compromised by institutional barriers and systematic oppression, exacerbated by stigma, prejudice, and discrimination (Mechanic & Tanner, 2007). Federal and state governments are more likely to provide assistance to those who are not perceived as responsible for their vulnerability, such as children, the blind, Veterans with disabilities, and the elderly (Mechanic & Tanner, 2007). When people are seen as responsible for their life circumstances, such as substance use disorders, single mothers, or ex-offenders (formerly incarcerated), they tend to experience less compassion and more stigma. Also, the fragmentation and selective focus of many of these NGO agencies addressing the needs of vulnerable populations inevitably result in vulnerable individuals and communities "falling through the cracks" (Mechanic & Tanner, 2007) and multiplying the burden for vulnerable women.

There is a tendency for mental health providers and researchers to treat people with SMI as genderless despite their different mental health experiences, life trajectories, and needs (Mowbray et al., 1992; Toth et al., 2013). A gender-blind paradigm overlooks important experiences that are central to women's lives and psychological well-being (Cogan, 1998). Many providers appear to lack training in working with women with SMI and are unaware of the life experiences shared by this group (Mizock & Brubaker, 2019). Moreover, the existent treatment literature indicates that women with SMI experience sexism and gender bias from their mental health providers (Borba et al., 2012; Mizock & Brubaker, 2019). Although there are ample critiques of the supposed psychopathologic vulnerability of women (Roselló-Peñazola & Cabruja-Ubach, 2019), emotional reactions continue to be pathologized (Mizock & Brubaker, 2019). For instance, research on gender bias in personality disorders suggests that practitioners tend to overly diagnose women with histrionic personality disorder, even while histrionic features such as seductiveness and excessive need for approval are behaviors that are often reinforced for women in some cultural environments (Samuel & Widiger, 2009). Women that are socioeconomically disadvantaged suffer more depression than the rest of the population. Therefore, disparities in healthcare can even result in worse outcomes (Toth et al., 2013).

Common Therapeutic Approaches

Cognitive-behavioral therapy (CBT) is the most common approach in community mental health centers and has shown effective results in controlled studies. Exposure therapy (ET) has also been found to be effective in the treatment of PTSD in community mental health centers (Grubaugh et al., 2011). Despite the effectiveness of therapy, philosophical assumptions that underline these theories have been questioned by critical psychology theorists and other scholars (Leder, 2017; Pilgrim, 2011). CBT suggests that the individual is responsible for their distorted thoughts, emotions, and behaviors. This can lead to downplay the role of context and culture, and the lived experiences of the person whose environments have been profoundly invalidating. Common factors such as the reparative influence of the therapeutic alliance are rarely accounted for in the effectiveness of treatment in vulnerable women (Scheyett & McCarthy, 2006). Women tend to value a sense of caring, empathy, and mutuality in their providers (Scheyett & McCarthy, 2006) and often develop strong alliances with their providers, which can enhance their satisfaction with care (Mizock & Brubaker, 2019). Therefore, there is a need for culturally competent approaches that capitalized on these observed strengths of vulnerable women in therapy.

Alternative Therapeutic Approaches

Vulnerable women in community mental health centers present a challenge for providers. Many present with complex trauma, including the aftermath of sexual abuse and domestic violence, among other traumatic events. When working with this population, there is a need for contextualized treatment that capitalizes on vulnerable women's strengths. We argue that narrative therapy with the inclusion of a critical multicultural analysis is such an approach.

Narrative therapy assumes that people organize their experience of events in temporal sequences to obtain a coherent account of themselves and the world around them. The person selects what is included in their narrative. This selection is defined as the dominant narrative. Dominant narratives limit the person and their possibilities; therefore, the person comes to therapy when they feel confined within them. Dominant narratives are informed not only by the experience of the person but from a wider cultural context. Thus, narrative therapy brings the world of the client into the session by integrating context and using techniques to elucidate meanings through language and construct alternative stories. Narrative therapy is about allowing clients to experience the therapist's respect. Experiencing respect is a relational aspect; a shared experience; and thus, it is a fundamental part of the therapeutic relationship. Empathy is interwoven in the theoretical and technical aspects of narrative orientations (White & Epston, 1990; White, 2007).

Narrative therapy has numerous approaches and critiques within the practice, but its core elements are shared: therapy is a power relationship, language is the medium for therapeutic work, and the subjectivity of both therapist and client is multicultural and part of a wider context. Narrative practitioners insert themselves into the participant's world, using their language, and participating in their assumptions. However, the relationship created with the participant is not devoid of power. As therapists are always placed in the position of the expert, they also bring dominant narratives about what is psychopathology and mental health with a scientific-technical vocabulary that can be alienating to participants.

Integrating context in psychotherapy is one of the purposes of a multicultural practice. Multiculturalism is an emergent trend in psychotherapy that focuses on how social identity locations, such as race, ethnicity, language, sexual orientation, gender, age, disability, class status, education, religious/spiritual orientation, and other cultural dimensions intersect in mental health. Multicultural psychotherapy pays attention to how notions of identity are integrated into clients' narratives, learns and engages with clients about their cultural context and beliefs, encourages therapists' self-assessments of privilege and oppression, and aims for social justice (Goodman & Gorski, 2014). This study explores the benefits of adopting critical multiculturalism as a framework and explores how integrating narrative perspectives benefits the treatment of a vulnerable cisgender Puerto Rican woman served in a community mental health center.

Methods

Design

The study used a narrative case study design to explore themes in the client's psychotherapy experience and acknowledges researcher reflexivity. Reflexivity is part of qualitative research designs and refers to making visible the researcher's subjectivity (Parker, 1999). Qualitative inquiry is an interpretative endeavor (Parker, 1999) and, thus, relies on the co-construction of narratives between the researcher and the participant. Narrative or descriptive case studies seek to tell the story of what happened in therapy, from the point of view of the client or the therapist or both McLeod (2010). The primary goal of this form of case study is to extend and widen our understanding of therapy by providing memorable accounts that transcend current professional categories (McLeod, 2010).

Recruitment of Participant

Purposive sampling was used to recruit the participant because the case itself is of primary interest in the exploration (Grandy, 2009). The participant was recruited by the principal investigator from a mental health community center. A written informed consent form was signed by the participant prior to the interview. The researcher participated as participant observer (Kawulich, 2005) because of her role as the therapist.

Materials

The material for this case study was a triangulation of two data sources. The first one, a narrative interview with the participant about her story and what has worked for her in therapy. Narrative interviews are unstructured and less restrictive approaches to gathering data. Informants are encouraged to tell their stories and then questions are phased after the story to clarify or extend themes expressed by the informant (Bauer, 1996; DiCicco-Bloom & Crabtree, 2006). The other source was the therapist's case formulation derived from psychotherapy notes and impressions of therapy, such as dimensions of transference and counter-transference and themes observed in the first 16 sessions. None of the material identifies the client and a fictional name is used to protect her confidentiality. The interview transcript was translated from Spanish to English by the principal investigator and then revised for content by the second investigator.

Analysis

Although there is no single way of analyzing a narrative interview (Clandinin & Huber, 2010), they required a process of co-creation and meaning-making of a story between the researcher and participant. The principal investigator read the transcript two times to get an overall theme in her story. A summary of Rosa's story integrating some verbatim quotes was conducted. Afterward, themes related to transference and countertransference, as well as multicultural themes embedded in her narrative, were highlighted. Then, a summary of her perspective was drafted regarding what has worked with her in therapy, providing verbatim quotes of her responses. A review of literature was done after her story was portrayed to contrast themes that emerged in her narrative with those in scientific literature. Clinical supervision was obtained throughout the process.

Findings

The main findings will be divided into sections, and since the therapist assumed the researcher role, sections were written with an active voice (first person).

Rosa's Story

Rosa[1] is a 62-year-old woman and mother of eight adults between the ages of 30 and 40. She has a partner who resides with his mother and during the day visits Rosa at her house. Rosa has never worked outside her home and helps out her daughters and sons as the caregiver of her 27 grandchildren. Rosa describes her childhood in Puerto Rico as "difficult" and "traumatic." She reported that she was raised by her paternal grandmother and an uncle. "I saw my father every Mother's Day for a few hours and never had a relationship with him beyond that." She also stated that she met her mother and another sibling when she was an adult but did not maintain contact after that. Her mother went to live in New York when she was a child and took her sister with her.

Rosa indicated that she was verbally and physically abused by her grandmother and uncle. She also reported that her uncle sexually molested her every day and sometimes ran her off with a *machete* (large knife with a broad blade). As a result of this, when she was a child, she would often hide inside a kitchen cabinet whenever she came home from school, so he couldn't find her. She also didn't finish elementary school. She was put to work daily, beginning at 4:00 a.m. she had to pick up water from the river to bring home. She carried it in her head for a long distance.

[1] Name was changed to maintain confidentiality.

Rosa was 16 or 17 when a young man was attracted to her and her grandmother decided that she should live with her father if she was going to be courted by this young man. While living with her father, the young man visited, but Rosa told her father she didn't like him. When Rosa was 17 her father arranged for her to marry this person who she identifies today as her ex-husband. "For sixteen days I didn't want to be intimate with him and he respected that, but returned me to my father. I told him no, I wanted to stay, anything but going back, so I let him have sex with me, it was rape." She described her relationship as "abusive" and reported that he was physically abusive, an alcoholic, and raped her for every pregnancy she had. When her daughters were old, she divorced him because he threatened her life with a gun. First, she moved to New York and lived with his aunt, but he came for her a month later. She tried things again, until finally, after the gun incident she went to a shelter and asked for help.

Rosa raised her children on her own and "like a hen with her chickens" they followed her everywhere. She moved to another state in her thirties and later met her current partner. She has been 27 years in this relationship, which she describes as a "weird one." She indicated, "He seldom talks to me and he is always on the phone talking to someone else." In the last five years, they have not been intimate because "I found out he tells everything to his mother, including our sex life." She said that her partner is "good" with her daughters and sons, but that she doesn't feel like he is in a relationship with her.

Rosa shares a home with one of her daughters and grandchildren. She also helps raise a one-year-old grandchild from her daughter who is diagnosed with schizophrenia. She describes her son and daughters as being good workers and living close by, although she worries about a daughter's abusive relationship. During the holidays, all her family gets together and helps out to make a dinner.

Rosa sought out therapy when she was 28 following a suicidal attempt. She reported that she was in a car with her partner and they had a discussion, and she thought "I rather not live" and jumped out of the car. She began therapy and was diagnosed with depression and schizophrenia in her late twenties. She indicated that because she "sometimes sees things moving in her house and hears spirits" the doctors thought she was presenting with hallucinations and deliriums. She indicated also that has had these experiences since she was a child and that her grandmother was in "Santeria." She indicated feeling as though she also has the "gift" of being able to hear spirit voices. Rosa reported that she sometimes has premonitions in her dreams and if she tells them "they often come true," so she prays for protection. She tried psychiatric medication but said she didn't like who she was with medications and stopped them. Rosa had been attending therapy for 22 years.

Treatment Summary/Transference and Countertransference (Themes and Patterns)

At the beginning of therapy, Rosa was willing to share her story and answer all my questions. I was very curious and felt saddened by all the suffering she recounted in her childhood. My chest tightened remembering what happened in our sessions and I started feeling maternal as if I could protect her.

As treatment progressed and I got to know her better, I began feeling excited to see her and she confided she expressed also feeling this way. She stated that she could talk to me about things that she couldn't talk about before, including to other therapists. As sessions progressed, I sensed a comfort in our interactions, like people who have known and appreciated each other for a long time.

I still felt deep sadness sometimes after our interactions. I noticed when she talked about her past with a detached tone of voice but gave away a lot of details in her memories. She smiled often when remembering and making comments, sometimes attributing responsibility to herself, such as "I was ignorant" or "I was young." Such comments prompted me to intervene and remind her that it wasn't her fault. But often I stayed quiet just listening. I wondered, how did she survive such cruelty and was able to lift a whole family, like a matriarch or how does she continue to care for others.

DSM-5 Diagnosis

I gave Rosa the diagnosis of Persistent Depressive Disorder (PDD) from the *Diagnostic and Statistical Manual of Mental Disorders, Fifth Edition* (DSM-5) (American Psychiatric Association, 2013). She met the criteria because of her prolonged sadness of more than two years, her negative conceptions about herself, her hopelessness, and her interpersonal conflicts. PDD is not necessarily considered an SMI, despite the condition leading to significant impairment in mood and daily functioning lasting for years and often associated with great suffering. This is only one of the many limitations associated with diagnostic criteria when attempting to capture the complex picture of the mental health struggles of marginalized women, their traumas, and their lack of social support. Rosa, more accurately, could be diagnosed with complex PTSD, which is not recognized in the DSM-5-TR as an official disorder but is defined by symptom clusters mainly resembling an enhanced PTSD, with symptoms such as shame, feeling permanently damaged and ineffective, feelings of threat, social withdrawal, despair, hostility, somatization, and diversity from the previous personality (Giourou et al., 2018). Her prior history of being diagnosed with schizophrenia was not included in my conceptualization as her presentation of experiencing what others deemed hallucinations was rooted in a cultural and religious practice shared by same-cultured peers. Following DSM-5-TR diagnostic criteria, if the experiences would be considered normative by same-cultured peers, a diagnosis of psychosis is contraindicated. Rosa did not describe any psychotic experiences that were not culture-bound, so a diagnosis of schizophrenia is not clinically accurate. However, her complex trauma was compounded by the stigma associated with her being diagnosed with SMI and the generalized marginalization of women who share similar social identities.

Intervention

Narrative tools were useful with Rosa because of her comfortableness with the use of metaphors and her willingness to share a detailed experience in her narratives. I employed two of the common tools in narrative therapy, externalizing conversations and re-authoring practices. Externalizing the problem or externalizing conversations are questions and interpretations that help the clients see the problem as outside of them by naming them and personifying them externalizing conversations can lead to further exploration of the problem and looking for exceptions. Re-authoring practices involve searching for exceptions within a dominant narrative and constructing alternative stories from them (White, 2007).

Rosa described a lot of incidents she named "supernatural." She described using prayers to ward off the impact of these incidents. I lead our conversations exploring ways in which she challenges the supernatural and manages to continue with her daily commitments. Instead of challenging her beliefs, I looked for exceptions to her powerlessness under them.

Multicultural Themes: Identities and Social Locations

Multicultural therapy is a framework that helps the therapist locate our clients in a cultural context (Goodman & Gorski, 2014). It is assumed that our clients are a multiplicity of identities integrated and developed in a particular social context. This theory explores the impact of two crucial concepts on a given individual's development of identity (i.e., social location and social identity). Social locations are the identity categories that are constructed and recognized by a given culture and that place individuals into discrete social groups. In other words, how a given society views and treats an individual. Social identities are individuals' acknowledged and unacknowledged identifications with their personally important social locations in a given culture and/or situation. This is how individuals perceive their social locations (Worell & Remer, 2003). Social identity and social location are two dialectic concepts that shape how a person experiences their mental health. In our social arrangement, identities are located as gender, race, sexual orientation, disability, socioeconomic status (SES), migration, among others.

Assuming a critical multicultural framework means helping clients situate their stories in larger cultural narratives to question dominant perspectives that locate the problems in the individual and affect how their narrative is told. This is particularly crucial in Rosa's treatment in which she forms a perspective of self as a Puerto Rican woman living in rural Puerto Rico and then had to navigate her social location as a Puerto Rican woman living in the United States.

Rosa's socioeconomic status (SES) was described as low. She only finished elementary school. She benefited from governmental assistance because of her income. Her trauma and mental health issues further violated her ability to have her basic physical and psychological integrity. In addition, Rosa grew up practicing Santeria, which is a spiritual practice misunderstood and often demonized in Western cultural arrangements. Therefore, her experience was perceived as pathological, which further accentuated a disjointed sense of religious affiliation characterized by imposed shame. Critical multicultural theory integrated with narrative therapy prepares the setting to enter the client's world, transcending the confinements of their cognitions and bringing culture into the sessions.

Rosa, a cisgender heterosexual woman, experienced physical and sexual abuse by her relatives and her ex-husband. From a critical multicultural perspective, all of her identities developed in the context of a traumatic and invalidating experience. The prolonged and consistent intersection of her perceived identity with the larger context has continued to reinforce a sense of defenselessness that contributes to her persistent depressive disorder. Mirroring the social feedback that she received throughout her life of what it is like to exist as a woman living in poverty, she also internalized some aspects of vulnerability, which often overwhelmed her evident resilience. It is noteworthy that even the way she experiences her family's "gift" to be in touch with the supernatural is also perceived as a "curse." At a symbolical level, the idea of existing with this "gift" is associated with danger and alienation. For many persons whose social locations are marginalized, the experience of having the gift of life is also associated with danger and alienation. In the context, of her social location, her religious experience seemed to mimic similar themes.

Rosa's gender identity, when explored in therapy, opened up her social location within the narrative of traditional womanhood in Western societies. As a cisgender woman, Rosa described herself as "defenseless" and assumed a passive role in her relationships, including her current partner. She also described her life as "a jail without walls" and her motherhood role as the only thing that she is capable of doing/being: "I am always giving my son and daughters everything, even caring for my grandchildren and great-grandchildren." Her womanhood also comes with her sexuality, where she describes herself as an attractive woman with desire: "You get old but you still want the same things, like romance." In summary, her identity as a woman was circumscribed to her passivity, motherhood role, and heterosexuality, which are dominant constructions of traditional femininity. From a symbolic perspective, her life of service, her gift, has rendered her defenseless, the curse.

Migration themes are also embedded in Rosa's story. She described her reason for leaving Puerto Rico as "to escape from my abusive husband." Therefore, her migration was motivated by trauma from a violent relationship. This has further implications as to how relocating to a majority White and English-speaking nation as a Spanish-speaking LatinX may lead to postcolonial migration distress (PCMD). M. Almario (personal communication, May 15, 2016) stated that PCMD is an emergent concept accounting for the intersecting experience of cultural gaps, socioeconomic status (SES) hardships, linguistic gaps, discrimination, and worldview shifts that often cause mental health distress in persons relocating from Puerto Rico. Rosa is a Spanish speaker, and as she stated, "because I have been caring for my children and their children, it was difficult for me to take English classes." Therefore, from a critical multicultural framework, Rosa's distress and symptoms intersect with multiple narratives in a larger context that are either enhanced or transformed by her intersecting identities and social locations.

Therapy's Effectiveness from Rosa's Perspective

What Keeps You Coming to Therapy (Appointments)?

Because I feel like "gente" (a person). I have someone to talk to … and is not about cooking or washing the dishes, I can talk to you about other things, like relief. Is like a small wound and you get cured, I feel better.

What Is the Best Thing That You Have Taken from Therapy? What Has Been the Best Lesson?

I have learned a lot, with you I have learned a lot. I used to have a bad temperament. Now I can control it more … I have learned to keep quiet when I am enraged. I used to get out of the house and go to a park to cry.

Rosa indicated that her rage was caused by the same things that happened to her now. "Is like, I finish washing the dishes and then, after a while, there are more … I barely have time for me and I feel overwhelmed." She indicated having a large family and expecting a lot from her.

Despite All Your Family Commitments, Do They Respect Your Time in Therapy?

Yes, because I am their "may" (colloquial term for mother) they don't see me as working, they just feel like I have to do this. That's what women do.

Rosa indicated that a lot of psychologists and psychiatrists don't share her beliefs in the supernatural. "Psychologists and psychiatrists think I am crazy because I see things. They (the spirits) stand behind me. Oh God, I know I can't talk about these things, because something bad happens."

Despite professionals' disbelief, Rosa stated that therapy helps, "because I let it out, I have someone to share it with." She also indicated that she liked that I gave her "opinions" because she "wants to know what is happening."

Discussion

Rosa's case is an example of the difficulties of finding appropriate treatment for vulnerable women with complex trauma. A critical multicultural approach and a narrative perspective take into consideration the different elements that constitute her meta-narrative: her conception of traditional womanhood, sexism in the form of childhood sexual, abuse, and domestic violence, and her reliance on motherhood as her sole purpose. Her childhood experience of being a child worker meets the definition of what today is referred to as human trafficking. Also, post-migration distress themes were identified, such as her linguistic gap as a Spanish speaker in an English-speaking nation. Themes that also emerged are related to mental health services such as inadequacies of capturing Rosa's rich story because of the privileging of diagnosis in the biomedical model and the silencing of spiritual matters, as well as the importance of building a therapeutic relationship with vulnerable women.

An integration of critical multicultural and narrative psychology involves a careful understanding of the time and space in which a person's life story evolved. This allows the clinician and the patient to understand how a person made decisions about the direction of their life, as well as the limitations they faced in making these decisions. It also gives a context about emotional reactions and dynamic cognitive processes that might have been valuable ways to survive in a particular context. This approach is centered on a respectful understanding of a person's story that treats them as an agent in their effort to survive and prevents them from giving up prematurely either physically or psychologically (Nussbaum, 2000).

Rosa is a 62-year-old woman who succeeded as a caretaker raising her 8 children and 27 grandchildren. She was successful to the degree that her context allowed her to be. Her childhood narrative evolved during the early sixties in an impoverished family of rural Puerto Rico. One of Rosa's complaints is that she was forced to work and prevented from attending school. Oftentimes, people experience psychological distress when their context does not afford them opportunities for the development of their inherent capabilities. Children come equipped with a desire to learn and evolve cognitively, which explains why education has become in the modern world a compulsory policy. By today's standards, Rosa would have been considered a victim of human trafficking, a modern-day slave, a person forced to live below the threshold of basic human rights and entitlements. However, chrono-systemically human trafficking laws only went into effect in the year 2000.

Addressing multicultural themes in a therapy case has been demonstrated effective and necessary. As Comas-Díaz (2017) indicated, Puerto Rican women living in the United States mainland relocate because of blatant experiences of gender and racial discrimination. Kim & Cardemil (2012) demonstrated the effectiveness of attending to social class in therapy sessions with Latina mothers of low SES. In Rosa's case, experiences of sexual abuse and the stressors associated with the motherhood role were gender-specific experiences that set the stage in which her narrative developed. Shedding a light on how multicultural contextual themes emerged in her narrative helped reduce the stigma associated with her social location, while addressing larger narratives in therapy sessions.

In addition to gender issues, Rosa's misdiagnosed SMI further distanced her from having a meaningful therapeutic interaction with prior practitioners. Such as when Rosa stated that "psychologist and psychiatrists" don't believe her supernatural concerns and think she is "crazy or schizophrenic." Women with SMI are disregarded when they express concerns about their mental health symptoms. For example, their problems are minimized or taken less seriously. This likely leads to symptom misattribution (Mizock & Brubaker, 2019). The fine line between distinguishing mental health concerns from cultural or spiritual matters is therefore obscured when a strict biomedical model is imposed on the therapeutic relationship. Also, hegemonic psychological theories conserve an ethnocentric, sexist, heteronormative character (Roselló-Peñazola & Cabruja-Ubach, 2019; Wilkinson & Kitzinger, 1993) that needs an epistemological revision through a feminist lens. By using narrative techniques, such as in the case of Rosa, her spiritual concerns could be seen as part of her "world" and, thus, served as instruments in her therapy that also help build a strong therapeutic alliance.

Conclusion

Vulnerable women with SMI are a population increasing in community mental health settings. The prevalent model for care for these women, evidenced-based practices from a biomedical model, can be limited and not take into consideration the cultural implications of their particular experiences. A critical multicultural approach and narrative therapy tools could be culturally competent models that benefit vulnerable women with SMI. Further research is needed on how to implement guidelines within this approach and examine therapeutic benefits with a large sample.

References

Aday, L. A. (1994). Health status of vulnerable populations. *Annual Review of Public Health, 15*(1), 487–509. https://doi.org/10.1146/annurev.pu.15.050194.002415

American Psychiatric Association. (2013). *Diagnostic and statistical manual of mental disorders* (5th ed.). https://doi.org/10.1176/appi.books.9780890425596

Bauer, M. (1996). The narrative interview: Comments on a technique for qualitative data collection London School of Economics and Political Science. Methodology Institute. *Papers in Social Research Methods*.

Borba, C. P., DePadilla, L., McCarty, F. A., von Esenwein, S. A., Druss, B. G., & Sterk, C. E. (2012). A qualitative study examining the perceived barriers and facilitators to medical healthcare services among women with a serious mental illness. *Women's Health Issues, 22*(2), e217–e224. https://doi.org/10.1016/j.whi.2011.10.001

Clandinin, D. J., & Huber, J. (2010). Narrative inquiry. In B. McGaw, E. Baker, & P. P. Peterson (Eds.), *International encyclopedia of education* (3rd ed., pp. 436–441). Elsevier.

Cogan, J. C. (1998). The consumer as expert: Women with serious mental illness and their relationship-based needs. *Psychiatric Rehabilitation Journal, 22*(2), 142–154. https://doi.org/10.1037/h0095253

Comas-Díaz, L. (2017). Crossing borders: Multicultural counseling with Puerto Rican migrant women. *Journal of Multicultural Counseling & Development, 45*(2), 95–110. https://doi.org/10.1002/jmcd.12067

DiCicco-Bloom, B., & Crabtree, B. F. (2006). The qualitative research interview. *Medical Education, 40*(4), 314–321. https://doi.org/10.1111/j.1365-2929.2006.02418.x

Fauci, J., & Goodman, L. (2019). "You don't need nobody else knocking you down": Survivor-mothers' experiences of surveillance in domestic violence shelters. *Journal of Family Violence, 35*(3), 241–254. https://doi.org/10.1007/s10896-019-00090-y

Giourou, E., Skokou, M., Andrew, S. P., Alexopoulou, K., Gourzis, P., & Jelastopulu, E. (2018). Complex posttraumatic stress disorder: The need to consolidate a distinct clinical syndrome or to reevaluate features of psychiatric disorders following interpersonal trauma? *World Journal of Psychiatry, 8*(1), 12–19. https://doi.org/10.5498/wjp.v8.i1.12

Goodman, R. D., & Gorski, P. C. (Eds.). (2014). *Decolonizing "multicultural" counseling through social justice*. Springer.

Goodman, L. A., Salyers, M. P., Mueser, K. T., Rosenberg, S. D., Swartz, M., Essock, S. M., Osher, F. C., Butterfield, M. I., & Swanson, J. (2001). Recent victimization in women and men with severe mental illness: Prevalence and correlates. *Journal of Traumatic Stress, 14*, 615–632. https://doi.org/10.1023/A:1013026318450

Grandy, G. (2009). Intrinsic Case. In A. J. Mills, G. Durepos, & E. Wiebe (Eds.), *Encyclopedia of case study research* (Vol. 1, pp. 499–501). Sage Publications.

Grubaugh, A. L., Zinzow, H. M., Paul, L., Egede, L. E., & Frueh, B. C. (2011). Trauma exposure and posttraumatic stress disorder in adults with severe mental illness: A critical review. *Clinical Psychology Review, 31*(6), 883–899. https://doi.org/10.1016/j.cpr.2011.04.003

Jackson-Best, F., & Edwards, N. (2018). Stigma and intersectionality: A systematic review of systematic reviews across HIV/AIDS, mental illness, and physical disability. *BMC Public Health, 18*(1), 919. https://doi.org/10.1186/s12889-018-5861-3

Kawulich, B. B. (2005). Participant observation as a data collection method. *Forum Qualitative Sozialforschung/Forum: Qualitative Social Research, 6*(2), 43. https://doi.org/10.17169/fqs-6.2.466

Kim, S., & Cardemil, E. (2012). Effective psychotherapy with low-income clients: The importance of attending to social class. *Journal of Contemporary Psychotherapy, 42*(1), 27–35. https://doi.org/10.1007/s10879-011-9194-0

Latalova, K., Kamaradova, D., & Prasko, J. (2014). Violent victimization of adult patients with severe mental illness: A systematic review. *Neuropsychiatric Disease and Treatment, 10*, 1925–1939. https://doi.org/10.2147/NDT.S68321

Leder, G. (2017). Know thyself? Questioning the theoretical foundations of cognitive behavioral therapy. *Review of Philosophy and Psychology, 8*(2), 391–410. https://doi.org/10.1007/s13164-016-0308-1

Maniglio, R. (2009). Severe mental illness and criminal victimization: A systematic review. *Acta Psychiatrica Scandinavica, 119*(3), 180–191. https://doi.org/10.1111/j.1600-0447.2008.01300.x

McLeod, J. (2010). *Case study research in counselling and psychotherapy*. Sage.

Mechanic, D., & Tanner, J. (2007). Vulnerable people, groups, and populations: Societal view. *Health Affairs, 26*(5), 1220–1230. https://doi.org/10.1377/hlthaff.26.5.1220

Mizock, L., & Brubaker, M. (2019). Treatment experiences with gender and discrimination among women with serious mental illness. *Psychological Services, 18*(1), 64–72. https://doi.org/10.1037/ser0000346

Mowbray, C. T., Herman, S. E., & Hazel, K. L. (1992). Gender and serious mental illness: A feminist perspective. *Psychology of Women Quarterly, 16*(1), 107–126. https://doi.org/10.1111/j.1471-6402.1992.tb00243.x

National Alliance of Mental Illness. (2019). *Mental health by the numbers*. National Institute of Mental Health. https://www.nami.org/Learn-More/Mental-Health-By-the-Numbers

Nguyen, T., Hauck, Y. L., Pedruzzi, R. A., Frayne, J., Rock, D., & Dragovic, M. (2017). Sexual health and sexual trauma in women with severe mental illness: An exploratory survey of Western Australian community mental health services. *Health Care for Women International, 38*(7), 705–714. https://doi.org/10.1080/07399332.2017.1313845

Nussbaum, M. C. (2000). *Women and human development: The capabilities approach* (Vol. 3). Cambridge University Press. https://doi.org/10.1017/CBO9780511841286

Parker, I. (1999). Qualitative data and the subjectivity of "objective" facts. In D. Dorling & L. Simpson (Eds.), *Statistics in society: The arithmetic of politics* (pp. 83–88). Arnold.

Pilgrim, D. (2011). The hegemony of cognitive-behaviour therapy in modern mental health care. *Health Sociology Review, 20*(2), 120–132. https://doi.org/10.5172/hesr.2011.20.2.120

Rich, P. (2018). What can we learn from vulnerability theory? *Honors Projects* 352. https://scholarworks.bgsu.edu/honorsprojects/352

Roselló-Peñazola, M., & Cabruja-Ubach, T. (2019). The feminization of psychopathology or the psychopathologization of the feminine? Discursive constructions of vulnerable bodies. *Athenea Digital, 19*(2), e2249. https://doi.org/10.5565/rev/athenea.2249

Samuel, D. B., & Widiger, T. A. (2009). Comparative gender biases in models of personality disorder. *Personality and Mental Health, 3*(1), 12–25. https://doi.org/10.1002/pmh.61

Saxena, S., Thornicroft, G., Knapp, M., & Whiteford, H. (2007). Resources for mental health: scarcity, inequity, and inefficiency. *The Lancet, 370*(9590), 878–889. https://doi.org/10.1016/S0140-6736(07)61239-2

Scheyett, A. M., & McCarthy, E. (2006). Women and men with mental illnesses: Voicing different service needs. *Affilia, 21*(4), 407–418. https://doi.org/10.1177/0886109906292114

Toth, S. L., Rogosch, F. A., Oshri, A., Gravener, J., Sturm, R., & Morgan-Lopez, A. (2013). The efficacy of Interpersonal Psychotherapy for economically disadvantaged mothers. *Development and Psychopathology, 25*(4), 1065–1078. https://doi.org/10.1017/S0954579413000370

Vázquez, M. Y. G., Sexto, C. F., Rocha, Á., & Aguilera, A. (2016). Mobile phones and psychosocial therapies with vulnerable people: A first state of the art. *Journal of Medical Systems, 40*(6), 1–12. https://doi.org/10.1007/s10916-016-0500-y

White, M. (2007). *Maps of narrative practice*. W. W. Norton & Company.

White, M., & Epston, D. (1990). *Narrative means to therapeutic ends*. W. W. Norton.

Wilkinson, S., & Kitzinger, C. (Eds.). (1993). *Heterosexuality: A feminism & psychology reader*. Sage Publications, Inc.

Worell, J., & Remer, P. (2003). *Feminist perspectives in therapy: Empowering diverse women*. Wiley.

World Health Organization. (2010). *Mental health and development: Targeting people with mental health conditions as a vulnerable group*. Mental Health and Poverty Project. https://apps.who.int/iris/bitstream/handle/10665/44257/9789241563949_eng.pdf;jsessionid=E75810355D3FF69BA0E1EE70CC482645?sequence=1

World Health Organization. (2019). *Gender disparities in mental health*. https://www.who.int/health-topics/gender#tab=tab_1

Self-Efficacy and Traumatic Events Among Palestinian Refugee Children Living in Bethlehem Refugee Camps: A Cross-Sectional Study

Ferdoos Abed Rabo Al Issa

Introduction

Forced displacement often occurs in tandem with violence, coercion, threats, intimidation, war, armed conflict, poverty, hunger, or lack of resources (Hjern et al., 1998; Basak, 2012). The resulting trauma experienced by many refugees can affect various aspects of their lives, including but not limited to family functioning, mental and physical health, behavioral well-being, and economic and social status (Hjern et al., 1998; Basak, 2012). Moreover, in places like Palestine under settler colonialism, refugee status is often prolonged, aiding in the seclusion and internal displacement of generations of Palestinians in refugee camps. The United Nations Relief and Works Agency (UNRWA) defines a Palestinian refugee as any person who resided in Palestine during the 1948 war and lost their home and means of livelihood between the period of June 1, 1946, and May 15, 1948. This definition applies to about 750,000 people. While two-thirds of these refugees fled to Jordan, Syria, and Lebanon, the rest were forced to live in refugee camps in the West Bank and Gaza. At present, there are six million registered refugees in Palestine. Approximately 190,000 of them remain in camps (UNRWA, 2019), with 39% being under 15 years of age (The Palestinian Central Bureau of Statistics, 2019).

Child refugees are particularly vulnerable to an increased prevalence of mental and psychological disorders, especially posttraumatic stress disorder (PTSD), emotional disturbances, impaired peer relationships, and behavioral issues (Bryant et al., 2018). Seventy percent of child refugees suffer from anxiety, sleep disorders, and mood disorders (Montgomery, 2011). These children frequently exhibit psychosomatic symptoms, including obsessive behaviors, concentration difficulties,

F. Abed Rabo Al Issa (✉)
Doha Institute for Graduate Studies, Doha, Qatar
e-mail: ferdoos.alissa@dohainstitute.edu.qa

S. Castaños-Cervantes et al. (eds.), *Working with Vulnerable Populations*,
https://doi.org/10.1007/978-3-031-67710-6_11

depressive symptoms, anxiety disorders, aggression, violent tendencies, paranoia, and phobias (Thabet et al., 2004, 2005, 2017). One potential means of mitigating these adverse effects is through the application of self-efficacy, as posited by Albert Bandura (1977), a psychological concept that refers to an individual's belief in their ability to successfully perform specific tasks, achieve goals, or overcome challenges in various areas of life.

This research explores Palestinian child refugee's experiences of self-efficacy in coping with the traumatic events they encounter in their daily lives. The study is grounded in data collected from 237 Palestinian children living as refugees in the Bethlehem area. The questionnaire administered to these children aimed to understand their encounters with traumatic events and their perception of their own efficacy. The findings of the study lead to several recommendations, emphasizing the need to increase efforts in seeking rights-based solutions for refugees, developing policies to protect child refugees, and establishing community-based group and individual interventions to address the unique needs of child refugees.

Literature Review

There are currently 19 refugee camps in the West Bank and Gaza (UNRWA, 2015). Among the numerous challenges faced by the residents of these camps, two of the most pressing issues are related to infrastructure and violence. In terms of infrastructure, all these camps suffer from severe overcrowding due to the typically large size of families and small houses. This overcrowding extends from households to public places, including schools and streets, making Palestinian camps some of the most densely populated areas globally (Kair et al., 2007). For instance, take Dheisheh camp, situated 4 km south of Bethlehem in the West Bank, where a staggering 15,000 people live within just 0.33 km^2, resulting in a population density of 45,454 per km^2 (UNRWA, 2015).

Following the displacement in 1947/1948, Palestinian refugees initially lived in tents, later in single-room houses for entire families, without basic amenities such as kitchens, toilets, sewage, or running water (Al-Khatib & Tabakhna, 2006). Over time, these small houses were expanded to accommodate growing families. Despite these efforts, refugee homes remain small, overcrowded, and poorly ventilated and receive minimal sunlight exposure (Al-Khatib et al., 2003).

Most of the housing units in these camps were constructed by UNRWA in 1965. Originally designed as one or two levels, these structures have now been expanded to five or six floors due to the rapid population growth (Al-Khatib & Tabakhna, 2006). In camps like Al-Am'ari in Al-Bireh, West Bank, as many as 80.9% of households mention having three or more people per room (Al-Khatib et al., 2003). In Jabaliya refugee camp, families of four or five live in houses with less than 9 m^2 of space (Badawy et al., 2013).

Overcrowding places immense strain on the already poor infrastructure, leaving residents with limited private space, particularly for women and families. The lack of recreational areas forces children to play in the streets, which can be a hazardous environment (Al-Khatib & Tabakhna, 2006). The streets in these camps are often narrow and inaccessible, with some remaining unpaved, such as in the Al-Ein refugee camp, where only the main road is paved (Al-Khatib et al., 2005). During the winter months, the unpaved streets become muddy, resulting in flooding of many homes (Badawy et al., 2013).

Access to freshwater in these camps is a persistent issue, with no regular water supply. Drinking water is stored in large containers and then manually distributed to homes, often transferred to rooftop reservoirs (Alazzeh et al., 2019). In some cases, the quality of drinking water is compromised. Tests in 2016–2017 in Aida and ‘Azza camps revealed high levels of coliforms, *Escherichia coli* (*E. coli*) bacteria, and residual chlorine (Alazzeh et al., 2019). In 2009, Dheisheh camp faced a similar problem when drinking water became contaminated with wastewater due to outdated water and waste networks (UNRWA, 2011). Water shortages in Kalandia camp have led to personal hygiene issues and increased gastrointestinal diseases (Issa et al., 2015).

Sewage management is another challenge in refugee camps. For instance, in Shu’fat camp, located in Jerusalem, the sewage system was constructed by UNRWA in the 1980s and has not been adequately maintained or renovated since then. As a result, residents have been forced to build their sewage lines, leading to issues like flooding during rainy seasons (UNRWA, 2015).

According to the Palestinian Central Bureau of Statistics (2019), a majority of refugees living in camps in the West Bank and Gaza face difficult living conditions. This includes 39% living in poverty and 23% experiencing deep poverty. In 2018, the unemployment rate for individuals aged 15 and above in these camps was as high as 40% (PCBS, 2019).

Refugee camps are also frequent sites of political violence and forced detention. Residents often face collective punishments, such as curfews and movement restrictions. For instance, during the first Intifada in 1987, the Dheisheh refugee camp was isolated by the Israelis with a fence, which was removed in 1993 by the Palestinian Authority (UNRWA, 2015). Since the second Intifada in 2000, camp residents have endured various forms of violence, including night raids, house invasions, arrests, torture, and killings by Israeli military forces. In 2002, an Israeli military invasion of Jenin camp resulted in the destruction of 400 houses, severe damage to hundreds more, and left over 2803 out of 11,213 residents homeless (UNRWA, 2015).

UNRWA reported in 2018 that Israel had continuously attacked all 19 refugee camps in 2017. These attacks resulted in the deaths of 10 individuals and injuries to 129 adults and 27 children. In 2017, the Dheisheh refugee camp alone endured 42-night raids, which resulted in 3 deaths and 55 injuries, including 13 children (UNRWA, 2018). According to PCBS (2021), approximately one million Palestinians have been arrested since 1967, though the statistics on detentions do not distinguish between refugees and non-refugees.

In Gaza, Israeli military attacks on refugee camps have exposed children to various traumatic events such as explosions and witnessing dead bodies or body parts on television. A study by Thabet et al. (2015) reported that children in Gaza experienced an average of 7 traumatic events during their early years.

The persistent stressors, including harsh living conditions and political violence, significantly impact children's mental health. While much attention is given to the negative effects of traumatic events on children, there is also a crucial need to focus on building their resilience.

Resilience of Palestinian Refugees

Resilience, as defined by the American Psychological Association (2014), refers to the "process of effectively adapting in the face of adversity, trauma, tragedy, threats, or significant sources of stress."

Over time, Palestinian refugees have developed various resilience strategies. Van Teeffelen et al. (2015), as cited in Asthana (2017), noted that the Palestinian refugees engage with media, establish local community organizations and cultural centers, and actively participate in political actions such as demonstrations. Najjar (2009) and Khoury-Machool (2007) demonstrated how Palestinian youth utilize social media, electronic resistance, and newspapers to express their identity, narratives, and social and political rights. Additionally, they employ art, wall graffiti, music, dance (like Dabke), and street theater as diverse forms of resistance against the occupation and means to enhance their resilience, often referred to as "sumud."

Education stands as another crucial tool for resilience, offering hope for a better future, a coping mechanism, and a foundation for identity formation (Alzaroo & Hunt, 2003). It serves as a vehicle for liberation and social and political transformation within society (Pherali & Turner, 2017).

Various factors influence the resilience of Palestinian refugees, including the support of family, friends, and the community, engagement in political activities, and the development of unique coping strategies. Notably, some individuals normalize traumatic events, viewing them as part of their daily lives, and carry on without allowing these events to disrupt their lives (Nguyen-Gilham et al., 2008).

Refugee Children's Mental Health

Existing literature on the psychological well-being among refugee children consistently highlights the prevalence of conditions such as PTSD, depression, and anxiety, among others. In the context of Palestine, research by Thabet & Vostanis (1999) revealed that children residing in two Gaza refugee camps, namely, Khan Younis and Jabalaya, commonly exhibit behavioral symptoms, nightmares, emotional and oppositional disorders, as well as learning disabilities. Furthermore, a cross-sectional study conducted by Thabet et al. (2001), encompassing 286 Palestinian children aged 9–18, indicated that these children had encountered an average of four traumatic events, approximately one-third (34.3%) exhibiting significant posttraumatic stress reactions. Similar findings were reported by McKell (2015) for children residing in the Baqa'a refugee camp in Jordan, where a notably high prevalence of mental health issues, including depression and anxiety, were observed. Van Teeffelen et al. (2005), as cited in Asthana, S. (2017), concluded that refugee children's lives are markedly affected by uncertainty, suffering, and pain as a result of the ongoing conflict.

Moreover, research has established a strong correlation between mental health and the challenging sociopolitical and economic circumstances prevailing in refugee camps. Basak (2012) identified that 70% of refugee children in the Dheisheh camp grapple with compromised physical and mental health due to the harsh living conditions, economic hardship, political instability, and social pressures. Vostanis (2003) similarly underscored the profound impact of socioeconomic and political factors on children's mental well-being. In the aftermath of 5 years of conflict in Gaza, a report by OCHA (2019) revealed that 14,000 Palestinians were internally displaced, with 53% of them in dire need of shelter and financial support. Additionally, 70% of Gazans who fled Gaza in 1948 are now confronted with a severe socioeconomic crisis and deep poverty, with 30% of the children experiencing poor overall well-being, including symptoms of depression.

Self-Efficacy and Traumatic Events

Self-efficacy offers a potential avenue to mitigate the adverse effects of trauma. Self-efficacy, according to Bandura (1994), is an individual's confidence, conviction, and belief in their ability to successfully influence events they encounter. Benight and Bandura (2004) argue that positive self-efficacy fosters effective adaptation and coping by instilling a sense of control over life events.

The concept of self-efficacy has evolved to encompass feelings, thoughts, and knowledge. Erel (2009) posits that self-efficacy extends to one's belief in their capacity to effect change as one develops cognitive, social, and physical skills. Gangloff and Mazilescu (2017) affirm that self-efficacy encompasses the belief in one's ability to act effectively in specific roles and contexts.

Self-efficacy exerts a profound impact on an individual's emotional state, cognition, and behavior. It can lead to feelings of security, satisfaction, strength, confidence, and the belief in one's capability to cope, adapt, perform tasks, and fulfill roles while enjoying life. It supports individuals in postponing immediate needs, enduring frustration, revising plans, and forming realistic expectations in relation to people and situations (Judge & Bono, 2001). Self-efficacy can act as a mediator facilitating recovery from childhood trauma, sexual abuse (Cieslak et al., 2008), domestic violence (Benight & Bandura, 2004), physical injuries (Flatten et al., 2008), and incidents of terrorism, such as the Oklahoma City bombing (Benight et al., 2000).

Given the inherently social nature of humans, Bandura (1999) argues that individuals not only exert personal control and representation but also engage in collective decision-making and control as part of the human agency concept (Pajares, 2002). Bandura (1999) posits that individuals and their environments interact through shared beliefs in competence, understanding, ambition, collective motivation, and collective action (Pajares, 2002). This synergy is shaped by individuals' past experiences, observations, and the behavior of others (Bandura, 1994).

Several factors influence the level of self-efficacy, including verbal persuasion, encompassing feedback, encouragement, advice, and an individual's psychological response to traumatic events (Gangloff & Mazilescu, 2017; Bandura, 1994).

Schools, as integral components of social systems, wield a significant influence over a child's capacity to develop self-efficacy. Schools contribute to cognitive and social competence, fostering the acquisition of critical thinking skills, promoting social interaction, and facilitating problem-solving, conflict resolution, and academic achievement. Through education, children gain a sense of competence, knowledge, skills, and abilities, fostering positive self-efficacy. Conversely, an unhealthy educational environment can erode self-efficacy, contributing to conditions such as depression (Bandura, 1994).

Reviewing the literature, it becomes evident that life in refugee camps presents formidable challenges. These camps are characterized by overcrowding at the household level, with public spaces, including schools and streets, suffering from poor infrastructure. Lack of private space and recreational areas forces children to engage in street play, often in hazardous conditions (Al-Khatib et al., 2003; UNRWA, 2015). Moreover, these camps serve as sites of political violence, forced detention, and collective punishments, including curfews and night raids.

Rationale for Current Study

Numerous studies have explored the psychological impact of these harsh conditions on refugee children, revealing prevalent symptoms such as PTSD, depression, and anxiety disorders (Thabet & Vostanis, 1999; Thabet et al., 2001; McKell, 2015). Remarkably, amidst these challenging circumstances, refugee children may exhibit high levels of self-efficacy. Given Bandura's (1977) theory of self-efficacy, it emerges as a potential tool to mitigate these adverse effects. Strikingly, despite the urgency of this issue, researchers in Palestinian studies have scarcely delved into this area.

Consequently, this study endeavors to explore the traumatic experiences of refugee children and their perceptions of self-efficacy. Based on the aforementioned studies, the refugee camp environment emerges as exceedingly challenging, marked by overcrowding, poor infrastructure, and political violence. Understanding the concept of self-efficacy, as posited by Bandura, holds significant potential for the

Palestinian society and mental health institutions working with refugee children to address the aftermath of trauma. This study aims to answer several key questions: Firstly, what are the most common traumatic events experienced by Palestinian refugee children in their daily lives, and how do these events relate to independent variables such as gender, age, class, school grades, and household size? Secondly, what is the level of self-efficacy among these children? Lastly, to what extent can self-efficacy mediate the impact of trauma on refugee children?

Method

Participants

Participants were recruited with the assistance of the local community activities from the three refugee camps in the Bethlehem area (Aida, Al-Aza, and Dheisheh). Two hundred and thirty-seven children participated in the study (66.2% male; 33.8% female), aged between 14 and 17 (M = 15.5 years). These children were enrolled in grades 8 through 11, with 33.3% in the 8th grade, 43.0% in the 9th grade, 15.2% in the 10th grade, and 8.0% in the 11th grade. Regarding their places of residency, 50.6% were from Dheisheh, 33.3% from Aida, and 16.0% from Al-Aza refugee camps. Family sizes varied, with 16.9% living with 3–5 family members, 66.3% residing with 6–8 family members, and 13.1% sharing a household with 9–11 family members.

Inclusion criteria included: (1) falling within the age group of 14–17 years, (2) residing in one of the three refugee camps in the Bethlehem area, and (3) possessing the ability to independently complete the questionnaires.

Ethical Considerations and Procedure

The study was granted Institutional Review Board approval by the Bethlehem University Research Council. To ensure the integrity of the data collection process, a team consisting of the researcher, two school social workers, and one sociology student was assembled. Throughout this process, the research team, who provided answers or clarifications if needed, maintained a vigilant approach to avoid leading the children toward any responses, allowing them the autonomy to discontinue questionnaire completion at any point and skip questions they were uncomfortable addressing. Completing the questionnaires took 35–40 min.

Materials

Sociodemographic questionnaire. This questionnaire was used to collect information on participants' gender, age, school grade average, number of people living in a household, and place of residence.

Life Events Checklist (LEC). The Life Events Checklist is a tool designed to measure exposure to traumatic events. It assesses participants' experiences with various traumatic incidents using a 16-item scale. Participants are asked to rate their level of exposure to each event on a 5-point nominal scale, with options ranging from 1 (experienced by me) to 5 (not applicable) (Gray et al., 2004). The scale demonstrates good internal consistency reliability, with a Cronbach's alpha of 0.85. The scale was translated and adapted for use in a prior study conducted by Alissa (2012).

Self-Efficacy Questionnaire for Children (SEQ-C). The Self-Efficacy Questionnaire is a 24-item tool designed to assess the self-efficacy beliefs or confidence levels of children in their ability to perform specific tasks or handle various situations along three different domains (academic, social, and emotional). The academic self-efficacy domain assesses children's beliefs in their ability to perform well in academic-related tasks. The social self-efficacy domain measures children's beliefs regarding social situations and interactions. The emotional self-efficacy domain assesses children's perceptions of coping with negative emotions. Participants are asked to rate their level of confidence or belief in their ability to perform activities, which often range from "not at all confident" to "very confident." A total self-efficacy score is obtained by summing all items (Muris, 2001). The scale demonstrates good internal consistency reliability, with a Cronbach's alpha of 0.82. This scale was translated into Arabic by the researcher.

Results

Traumatic Life Events

Palestinian refugee children have encountered various traumatic events. Among them, 33.0% ($n = 79$) reported experiencing physical abuse, while 30.8% ($n = 73$) found themselves in areas with armed confrontations. Conversely, the least common traumatic incidents included sexual assault, including rape, harassment, forced sex under threat, and unwanted sexual activity, which affected 9.2% ($n = 22$) of participants. Additionally, sudden deaths resulting from suicide or murder were reported by 5.1% ($n = 12$) of the children.

Traumatic Life Events and Sociodemographic Variables

Traumatic events exhibit significant correlations with gender, number of people living in a household (household size), and school grade average. Findings revealed that children experienced various forms of traumatic events, with a mean of 3.32 events (SD = 0.84). Notably, males ($M = 3.22$, SD = 1.08) reported significantly higher exposure to trauma than females ($M = 3.70$, SD = 0.87), yielding a t-value of −3.44 ($p < 0.001$). Additionally, a mean difference was observed concerning household size ($M = 2.35$, $p > 0.021$). Children residing in households with six members had a higher mean of 3.64, indicating fewer traumatic events, while those in households with 11 family members had a mean of 2.60, signifying a significant relationship between household size and traumatic events. Lastly, a statistically significant association between exposure to life events and school grade was established ($p = 0.000$). Specifically, participants in the eighth grade exhibited a higher exposure to traumatic events compared to their peers in other grades. No statistically significant relationships were observed between traumatic life events and age or place of residence.

Traumatic Life Events and Self-Efficacy

An analysis of the relationship between self-efficacy and traumatic events revealed that, among the participants directly exposed to traumatic events ($n = 8$), 2 had notably low self-efficacy, while 4 displayed very high self-efficacy. Among those who witnessed traumatic events ($n = 35$), 1 exhibited very low self-efficacy, 14 had a moderate level of self-efficacy, and 20 displayed high to very high self-efficacy. For those who heard about traumatic events ($n = 85$), 5 reported low self-efficacy, 28 had a moderate level of self-efficacy, 47 displayed a high self-efficacy, and 5 exhibited a very high level of self-efficacy. Moreover, a Chi-Square Test demonstrated a strong correlation between self-efficacy and traumatic events: as participants experienced greater direct exposure to traumatic events, their self-efficacy levels tended to increase.

Self-Efficacy

Findings indicated that 8.4% ($n = 20$) of participants exhibited a very high level of self-efficacy, 49.4% ($n = 117$) exhibited a high level of self-efficacy, 35.9% ($n = 85$) exhibited a moderate level of self-efficacy, 4.2% ($n = 10$) exhibited a low level of self-efficacy, and 2.1% ($n = 5$) exhibited a very low level of self-efficacy.

Self-Efficacy and Sociodemographic Variables

Self-efficacy exhibits significant correlations with school grade average and household size. Findings revealed that children who perceived their grades as being satisfactory ($M = 3.30$, $n = 23$) exhibited the lowest self-efficacy, while those who perceived their grades to be excellent ($M = 3.90$, $n = 61$) reflected the highest level of self-efficacy. With regard to household size, children with smaller household sizes (households with 3–4 members) exhibited the highest self-efficacy, while children with bigger household sizes exhibited the lowest self-efficacy (households with 10–11 members). No statistically significant relationships were observed between self-efficacy and the other sociodemographic variables.

Self-Efficacy Subscales

Academic Self-Efficacy. The results indicated that 59.3% of the children ($n = 140$) exhibited a high to very high level of academic self-efficacy, 28.4% ($n = 67$) displayed a moderate level, 10.2% ($n = 24$) exhibited a low level, and 2.1% ($n = 5$) reported a very low level. Scores on academic self-efficacy were significantly correlated with school grade average. For instance, the children whose grades were not bad ($M = 3.00$) portrayed the lowest academic self-efficacy, while children with good grades ($M = 3.46$), very good grades ($M = 3.60$), and excellent grades ($M = 4.18$) had higher self-efficacy. No statistically significant relationships were observed between academic self-efficacy and the other sociodemographic variables.

Social Self-Efficacy. The results indicated that 18.6% of children ($n = 44$) displayed a very high level of social self-efficacy, 39.4% ($n = 93$) exhibited a high level, 33.1% ($n = 78$) displayed a moderate level, 6.8% ($n = 16$) exhibited a low level, and 2.1% ($n = 5$) displayed a very low level. Scores on social self-efficacy were significantly correlated with grades. For instance, the children whose grades were not bad ($M = 3.17$) had lower social self-efficacy compared to children with good grades ($M = 3.60$), very good grades ($M = 3.60$), and excellent grades ($M = 3.96$). Children who perceived their academic achievement as excellent displayed the highest level of social self-efficacy. No statistically significant relationships were observed between academic self-efficacy and the other sociodemographic variables.

Emotional Self-Efficacy. The results indicated that 9.3% of children ($n = 22$) displayed a very high level of emotional self-efficacy, 26.3% (n = 62) exhibited a high level, 44.9% ($n = 106$) displayed a moderate level, 16.1% (n = 38) exhibited a low level, and 3.4% ($n = 8$) displayed a very low level. Findings showed that differences in self-efficacy in relation to gender were statistically significant. Males displayed higher levels of emotional self-efficacy than females. Moreover, scores on emotional self-efficacy were significantly correlated with household size: the smaller the household size, the lower the self-efficacy.

Discussion

Refugee children frequently encounter various traumatic events that have a profound impact on their psychological well-being. This study delved into the experiences of self-efficacy among Palestinian refugee children in light of the traumatic events they face daily. The research explored how these children perceive their own efficacy, encompassing their social, academic, and emotional self-efficacy while considering various other variables.

Traumatic Life Events

The study highlights that Palestinian refugee children are exposed to a range of traumatic events. These traumatic events encompass physical abuse, being held hostage in areas with armed confrontations, work-related accidents, sexual assault or unwanted sexual activities, and sudden deaths, including suicide or murder. These results corroborate previous research (Cieslak et al., 2008; Benight et al., 2000, 2004; Flatten et al., 2008) and emphasize the harsh and challenging environment in which these children grow up due to ongoing conflict and occupation. These children are the third generation to reside in refugee camps since the Palestinian Nakba (or Catastrophe) following the 1948 war.

Traumatic Life Events and Sociodemographic Variables

The study reveals a gender difference in exposure to traumatic events, with males reporting a higher level of exposure compared to females, consistent with the findings of Al-Sheikh & Thabet (2017). This could be attributed to various factors, such as societal roles, mobility, or activities that may expose males to more risk.

The findings also suggest a correlation between household size and traumatic events. Children in larger households tend to experience fewer traumatic events. This could be due to increased social support or protection within larger families, which might buffer the impact of traumatic events.

The study identifies a statistically significant relationship between school grade average and exposure to traumatic events. Younger children, specifically those in the eighth grade, reported higher exposure to trauma. This finding contradicts previous research (Al-Sheikh & Thabet, 2017) and may be attributed to various factors, including changes in the nature of traumatic events or differences in reporting.

Surprisingly, the study did not find significant relationships between traumatic life events and age or place of residence. This suggests that traumatic experiences are relatively consistent across age groups and locations within the refugee camps.

Traumatic Life Events and Self-Efficacy

The study examines the relationship between self-efficacy and traumatic events, revealing that children exposed to more traumatic events tend to have higher self-efficacy levels. This is an intriguing finding that suggests that, despite facing adversity, these children have developed a sense of confidence in their abilities to cope with life's challenges. This resilience is noteworthy and underscores the strength of these young individuals.

Self-Efficacy

The study's assessment of self-efficacy among Palestinian refugee children shows a range of self-efficacy levels across the sample. A substantial portion of the children exhibited high to very high self-efficacy, especially in the academic domain. This indicates that these children believe in their ability to succeed in their academic endeavors, which aligns with the idea that education can serve as a tool for personal growth and resistance against adversity.

Self-Efficacy and Sociodemographic Variables

There is a clear correlation between school grade average and self-efficacy, particularly in the academic domain. Children with better academic performance tend to exhibit higher levels of self-efficacy. This reflects the importance of academic achievement for these children and how it contributes to their confidence and belief in their abilities.

Household size appears to influence self-efficacy, with smaller households being associated with higher self-efficacy. This could be due to the availability of resources, attention, and support within smaller families.

The study identifies a gender difference in emotional self-efficacy, with males displaying higher levels compared to females. This suggests variations in emotional coping strategies and self-perceptions between genders.

Self-Efficacy Subscales

The study assesses self-efficacy across three domains: academic, social, and emotional. It reveals variations in self-efficacy levels with these domains. Notably, academic self-efficacy stands out, with a majority of children exhibiting high levels.

This reflects the significance of education and its potential role in personal and social transformation, which aligns with Pherali & Turner (2017).

Conclusion

In conclusion, the results of this study shed light on the complex interplay between traumatic life events and self-efficacy among Palestinian refugee children. These findings underscore the resilience of these children in the face of adversity and emphasize the importance of education as a source of empowerment and hope in their lives. However, it is essential to consider the nuanced sociodemographic factors that influence both exposure to trauma and self-efficacy levels among these young individuals.

Limitations

Some of the limitations of this study include:

1. Sampling bias: The study used a purposive sampling method, which may introduce bias in participant selection. It might not represent the entire population of Palestinian refugee children, and the findings may not generalize to all Palestinian refugee communities.
2. Limited demographic variables: The study examined a relatively narrow set of sociodemographic variables (e.g., gender, age, household size, school grade). Other important factors, such as socioeconomic status, parental education, or length of time in the refugee camp, were not explored but could impact the results.
3. Lack of control group: The study did not include a control group of non-refugee children for comparison. This absence makes it challenging to determine whether the observed effects are specific to the refugee population or common among children in similar conflict-affected regions.
4. Long-term effects: The study primarily examined current experiences and self-efficacy. Understanding the long-term effects of trauma and self-efficacy requires longitudinal research.

Implications

The implications of this research are multifaceted and have relevance for various stakeholders, including policymakers, educators, mental health professionals, and humanitarian organizations. Some key implications include:

1. Mental health support for Palestinian refugee children including trauma-informed care and early intervention. The study highlights that a significant number of Palestinian refugee children have experienced traumatic events. This underscores the need for trauma-informed mental health care and support services within refugee communities. Moreover, identifying and addressing trauma-related issues at an early stage is crucial. Schools and community centers can play a vital role in offering counseling and mental health support to affected children.
2. Education as a coping mechanism: Palestinian refugee children place a high value on education. Policymakers should prioritize investments in educational resources, facilities, and programs to support these children in achieving academic success and enhancing their self-efficacy.
3. Gender-specific interventions/approaches: The study identifies gender differences in exposure to traumatic events and self-efficacy levels. Interventions and support programs should be tailored to address the unique needs of boys and girls separately.
4. Family and household dynamics: The correlation between household size and exposure to trauma suggests the importance of family support. Programs that empower parents and caregivers with coping strategies and resources can contribute to children's well-being.
5. Resilience and self-efficacy promotion: The study's findings highlight the resilience of Palestinian refugee children, particularly in developing self-efficacy. Educators and mental health professionals should incorporate resilience-building activities and interventions into their practices.
6. Community and collective well-being: The sense of collective belonging and strength within the community plays a significant role in children's resilience. Encouraging community-based initiatives and support networks can bolster children's emotional well-being.
7. Policy and advocacy: Beyond the scope of this study, the research adds to the body of evidence illustrating the challenges faced by Palestinian refugees. It can serve as a basis for advocacy efforts to address the broader political and humanitarian issues affecting this population.
8. Further research and longitudinal studies: While this research provides valuable insights, further in-depth studies and longitudinal research are needed to explore the long-term effects of trauma and self-efficacy on the well-being and life outcomes of Palestinian refugee children.
9. Cross-cultural application: The findings from this study may have relevance to other conflict-affected and refugee populations. Researchers and practitioners working in similar contexts can draw lessons from this research to inform their work.

References

Alazzeh, S., Galaitsi, S., Bishara, A., Al-Azraq, N., & Durant, J. (2019). Impacts of intermittent water supply on water quality in two Palestinian refugee camps. *Water, 11*(4), 670. https://doi.org/10.3390/w11040670

Alissa, F. (2012). *The effectiveness of EMDR treatment approach in treating the parents or the caregivers and the wives of young martyrs with PTSD and depression symptoms in Bethlehem district* [Unpublished master's thesis]. Al-Quds University.

Al-Khatib, I., & Tabakhna, H. (2006). Housing conditions and health in Jalazone Refugee Camp in Palestine. *EMHJ Eastern Mediterranean Health Journal, 12*(1–2), 144–152.

Al-Khatib, I., Ju'ba, A., Kamal, N., Hamed, N., Hmeidan, N., & Massad, S. (2003). Impact of housing conditions on the health of the people at al-Ama'ri refugee camp in the West Bank of Palestine. *International Journal of Environmental Health Research, 13*(4), 315–326. https://doi.org/10.1080/0960312031000161 6092

Al-Khatib, I., Arafat, R., & Musmar, M. (2005). Housing environment and women's health in a Palestinian refugee camp. *International Journal of Environmental Health Research, 15*(3), 181–191. https://doi.org/10.1080/09603120500105950

Al-Sheikh, N., & Thabet, A. (2017). Post-traumatic stress disorder due to war trauma, social and family support among adolescents in the Gaza Strip. *Journal of Nursing and Health Sciences, 3*(2), 1–12.

Alzaroo, S., & Hunt, G. (2003). Education in the context of conflict and instability: The Palestinian case. *Social Policy and Administration, 37*(2), 165–180. https://doi.org/10.1111/1467-9515.00332

APA. (2014). *The road to resilience*. American Psychological Association. https://uncw.edu/studentaffairs/committees/pdc/documents/the%20road%20to%20resilience.pdf

Asthana, S. (2017). Youth, self, other: A study of Ibdaa's digital media practices in the West Bank, Palestine. *International Journal of Cultural Studies, 20*(1), 100–117. https://doi.org/10.1177/1367877915600546

Badawy, D., Salha, R., Jawabrah, M., Jarada, A., Hawajri, E. L., & A. (2013). Urban planning analyses of refugee camps, Jabalia as case study-Gaza Strip, Palestine. *International Journal of Science and Research, 5*(4), 678–688.

Bandura, A. (1994). Self-efficacy. In V. S. Ramachandran (Ed.), *Encyclopedia of human behavior, Vo. 4*. Academic Press.

Bandura, A. (1999). Social cognitive theory: An agentic perspective. *Asian Journal of Social Psychology, 2*(1), 21–41. https://doi.org/10.1111/1467-839x.00024

Bandura, A., & Adams, N. (1977). Analysis of self-efficacy theory of behavioral change. *Cognitive Therapy and Research, 1*(4), 287–310.

Basak, P. (2012). The impact of ocupation on child health in a Palestinian refugee camp. *Journal of Tropical Pediatrics, 58*(6), 423–428. https://doi.org/10.1093/tropej/fms008

Benight, C., & Bandura, A. (2004). Social cognitive theory of posttraumatic recovery: The role of perceived self-efficacy. *Behaviour Research and Therapy, 42*(10), 1129–1148. https://doi.org/10.1016/j.brat.2003.08.008

Benight, C., Freyaldenhoven, R., Hughes, J., Ruiz, J., Zoschke, T., & Lovallo, W. (2000). Coping self-efficacy and psychological distress following the Oklahoma city bombing. *Journal of Applied Social Psychology, 30*(7), 1331–1344. https://doi.org/10.1111/j.1559-1816.2000.tb02523.x

Benight, C., Harding-Taylor, A., Midboe, A., & Durham, R. (2004). Development and psychometric validation of a domestic violence coping self-efficacy measure (DV-CSE). *Journal of Traumatic Stress, 17*(6), 505–508. https://doi.org/10.1007/s10960-004-5799-3

Bryant, R., Edwards, B., Creamer, M., O'Donnell, M., Forbes, D., & Felmingham, K. (2018). The effect of post-traumatic stress disorder on refugees' parenting and their children's mental health: A cohort study. *The Lancet Public Health, 3*(5), e249–e258. https://doi.org/10.1016/s2468-2667(18)30051-3

Cieslak, R., Benight, C., & Caden Lehman, V. (2008). Coping self-efficacy mediates the effects of negative cognitions on posttraumatic distress. *Behaviour Research and Therapy, 46*(7), 788–798. https://doi.org/10.1016/j.brat.2008.03.007

Erel, D. (2009). The concept of self-efficacy and self-efficiency-performance relationship. *Ankara Üniversitesi SBF Dergisi*, 55–54.

Flatten, G., Walte, D., & Perlitz, V. (2008). Self-efficacy in acutely traumatized patients and the risk of developing a posttraumatic stress syndrome. *GMS Psycho-Social Medicine, 5*, Doc05.

Gangloff, B., & Mazilescu, C. (2017). Normative characteristics of perceived self-efficacy. *Social Sciences, 6*(4), 139. https://doi.org/10.3390/socsci6040139

Gray, M., Litz, B., Hsu, J., & Lombardo, T. (2004). Psychometric properties of the life events checklist. *Assessment, 11*(4), 330–341. https://doi.org/10.1177/1073191104269954

Hjern, A., Angel, B., & Jeppson, O. (1998). Political violence, family stress and mental health of refugee children in exile. *Scandinavian Journal of Social Medicine, 26*(1), 18–25. https://doi.org/10.1177/14034948980260010701

Issa, M., McHenry, M., Issa, A., & Blackwood, R. (2015). Access to safe water and personal hygiene practices in the Kulandia Refugee Camp (Jerusalem). *Infectious Disease Reports, 7*(4). https://doi.org/10.4081/idr.2015.6040

Judge, T., & Bono, J. (2001). Relationship of core self-evaluations traits—self-esteem, generalized self-efficacy, locus of control, and emotional stability—with job satisfaction and job performance: A meta-analysis. *Journal of Applied Psychology, 86*(1), 80–92. https://doi.org/10.1037/0021-9010.86.1.80

Kair, L., Hazena, L., & Alatrash, H. (2007). *Demographic situation and population density in the occupied Palestinian territories*. Institute of Applied Research.

Khoury-Machool, M. (2007). Palestinian youth and political activism: The emerging internet culture and new modes of resistance. *Policy Futures in Education, 5*(1), 17–36. https://doi.org/10.2304/pfie.2007.5.1.17

McKell, C. (2015). *Mental illness in Palestinian refugees living in refugee camps in Jordan: Barriers to access and use of mental health care services and recommendations to overcome such barriers*. Royal College of Psychiatrists. https://www.rcpsych.ac.uk/docs/default-source/members/sigs/volunteering-and-international-vipsig/essay-prize-mckell-mental-illness-in-palestinian-refugees-in-jordan-barriers-toaccess.pdf?sfvrsn=bdae18bb_2

Montgomery, E. (2011). Trauma, exile and mental health in young refugees. *Acta Psychiatrica Scandinavica, 124*, 1–46. https://doi.org/10.1111/j.1600-0447.2011.01740.x

Muris, P. (2001). A brief questionnaire for measuring self-efficacy in youths. *Journal of Psychopathology and Behavioral Assessment, 23*(3), 145–149. https://doi.org/10.1023/A:1010961119608

Najjar, A. (2009). Othering the self: Palestinians narrating the war on Gaza in the social media. *Journal of Middle East Media, 6*, 1–28.

Nguyen-Gillham, V., Giacaman, R., Naser, G., & Boyce, W. (2008). Normalising the abnormal: Palestinian youth and the contradictions of resilience in protracted conflict. *Health & Social Care in the Community, 16*(3), 291–298. https://doi.org/10.1111/j.1365-2524.2008.00767.x

OCHA. (2019). *Humanitarian needs overview*. www.ochaopt.org/sites/files/humanitarian_needs_overview_2019

Pajares, F. (2002). *Overview of social cognitive theory and of self-efficacy*. Western Kentucky University. https://people.wku.edu/richard.miller/banduratheory.pdf

PCBS. (2019). *The international day of refugees 2019*. http://www.pcbs.gov.ps/site/512/default.aspx?lang=en&ItemID=3486

PCBS. (2021). *Annual commemoration of the Palestinian Nakkba 73rd on the numbers of Palestinians Worldwide has doubled about nine times*. http://www.pcbs.gov.ps/post.aspx?lang=en&ItemID=3985

Pherali, T., & Turner, E. (2017). Meanings of education under occupation: The shifting motivations for education in Palestinian refugee camps in the West Bank. *British Journal of Sociology and Education, 39*(4), 567–589. https://doi.org/10.1080/01425692.2017.1375400

Thabet, A., & Vostanis, P. (1999). Visit to the Gaza Community Mental Health Programme: Training in child mental health. *Psychiatric Bulletin, 23*(5), 300–302. https://doi.org/10.1192/pb.23.5.300

Thabet, A. A., Abed, Y., & Vostanis, P. (2001). Effect of trauma on the mental health of Palestinian children and mothers in the Gaza Strip. *EMHJ – Eastern Mediterranean Health Journal, 7*(3), 413–421.

Thabet, A., Abed, Y., & Vostanis, P. (2004). Comorbidity of PTSD and depression among refugee children during war conflict. *Journal of Child Psychology and Psychiatry, 45*(3), 533–542. https://doi.org/10.1111/j.1469-7610.2004.00243.x

Thabet, A., Vostanis, P., & Karim, K. (2005). Group crisis intervention for children during ongoing war conflict. *European Child & Adolescent Psychiatry, 14*(5), 262–269. https://doi.org/10.1007/s00787-005-0466-7

Thabet, A., Thabet, S., & Vostanis, P. (2017). Coping and mental health problems among Palestinian refugee families. *Journal of Psychology and Cognition, 2*(2), 149–156.

Thabet, A. A., Thabet, S. Chih, A., & Wei Huang, W. (2015). Trauma, PTSD, Anxiety, and Resilience in Palestinian Children in the Gaza Strip. *British Journal of Education, Society & Behavioural Science, 11*(1), 1–13. https://doi.org/10.9734/BJESBS/2015/19101

UNRWA. (2011). UNRWA West Bank WASH Program 2011 Emergency Appeal. https://www.unrwa.org/userfiles/2011051512133.pdf

UNRWA. (2015). *Profile: Shu'fat Camp Jerusalem*. https://www.unrwa.org/sites/default/files/shufat_refugee_camp.pdf

UNRWA. (2018). *Condemns the killing of a refugee child during military raid in the Occupied Palestinian Territory*. https://www.unrwa.org/newsroom/official-statements/unrwa-condemns- killing-refugee-child-during-military-raid-occupied

UNRWA. (2019). *Where we work*. https://www.unrwa.org/where-we-work/west-bank

Vostanis, P. (2003). Impact of trauma on Palestinian children's mental health: Lessons from the Gaza studies. Thematic paper – Trauma and the mental health of children. *International Psychiatry, 2*, 5–6.

Violence and Its Associated Psychosocial Factors in Mexican Homeless Females

Susana Castaños-Cervantes

Violence is one of the most widespread, persistent, and devastating human rights violations in our world today. It refers to the situation where an individual suffers intentional physical or psychological harm as a result of actions or omissions of other human beings (United Nations [UN], 2006). It can be physical, psychological, or sexual, and it has been proven to affect the optimal development of individuals (Sadurní et al., 2003). Physical violence includes traumas inflicted upon the person's body, like lacerations, bruises, burns, fractures, or wounds caused by physical punishment (Picornell, 2006). Psychological violence entails forms of chronic verbal hostility such as insults, mockery, contempt, criticism, threats, and emotional negligence (Changa et al., 2008), and sexual violence is unwanted sexual activity, with perpetrators using force, making threats, or taking advantage of victims not able to give consent (American Psychological Association [APA], 2015).

It occurs worldwide, cutting across all generations, nationalities, communities, and spheres of our societies, irrespective of age, ethnicity, disability, or other background, and it is more frequently exerted toward women and girls than men and boys, especially when it comes to sexual violence (Bilginer et al., 2013). One in three females around the world has experienced either physical or sexual violence (World Health Organization [WHO], 2019), and one in twenty cases has needed medical attention (Breiding et al., 2013). In contrast, one in ten men worldwide has suffered sexual violence (Collin-Vézina et al., 2013). Sixty percent of women have been victims of violence in some countries of the Americas (Pan American World Health Organization [PAHO], 2018). In Mexico, 66% of females have suffered from various forms of violence at some point in their lives (Moreno, 2019).

S. Castaños-Cervantes (✉)
Escuela de Psicología, Facultad de Ciencias de la Salud, Universidad Panamericana, Ciudad de México, Mexico
e-mail: scastanos@up.edu.mx

S. Castaños-Cervantes et al. (eds.), *Working with Vulnerable Populations*,
https://doi.org/10.1007/978-3-031-67710-6_12

It is more common in vulnerable groups such as homeless females (da Silva Rosa & Passarella, 2015). The European Federation of National Organizations working with the Homeless (n.d.) revealed that 92% of homeless females have experienced some form of violence throughout their life; 55% have experienced violence as children and during adulthood; 67% have experienced intimate partner violence, 20% of whom by more than one partner; and 46% have experienced sexual abuse during childhood. Globally, homeless females have been victims of domestic violence, school bullying, and social violence at a higher rate than homeless males (Warf et al., 2010) and the rest of the population (Misganaw & Worku, 2013). Such conditions of violence in this group are the leading causes of running away from home (Soriano et al., 2005). Existing information has revealed that homeless female victims of violence display dissociative symptoms (Tyler et al., 2004), mental disorders, depression, and cognitive deficits (Tonmyr et al., 2011). They exhibit poor emotion regulation skills (Kim & Cicchetti, 2010), social incompetence and lack of social abilities, delinquent behavior (Dumain, 2010), prostitution incursion (Helander, 2008), higher victimization (Melander & Tyler, 2010), risky sexual behaviors (Slonim-Nevo & Mukuka, 2007), multiple sexual partners (Lau et al., 2005), suicide ideation and attempt (Capuzzi & Gross, 2008), and substance use and abuse (Douglas et al., 2010). Moreover, they present anxiety (Escribà-Agüir et al., 2010) and can become alcoholic in 45% of the cases (De Rueda, 2007). All of this will eventually exacerbate the effects of violence (Noell et al., 2001). Hence, among the main psychosocial consequences linked to violence in homeless females are the presence of anxiety, depression, and emotion dysregulation, as well as unassertiveness. These outcomes, in turn, negatively impact well-being and lead to several problems (Crawford & Manassis, 2011) when effective and early attention is not provided: devaluated self-concept and self-esteem, decreased perceived self-efficacy, social incompetence, aggression, hostility, frustration, impulsivity and antisocial behavior, health risk behaviors, lack of functional problem solving and coping skills, low school performance and achievement, school dropout, and unemployment. However, particular characteristics of violence and its psychosocial effects on homeless females are partially and superficially known (Williams, 2018), particularly in emerging and developing countries such as Mexico, where the magnitude, dimensions, psychosocial factors, and effects of violence on homeless females are unknown, and well-defined policy actions have not been applied nor developed (Rábago, 2009).

Therefore, this study examined the discrepancies between victims and non-victims of various forms of violence in a group of Mexican homeless females concerning the following psychosocial factors associated with violence (Barman-Adhikari et al., 2016): symptoms of anxiety and depression, emotion dysregulation, low subjective well-being, and unassertiveness. The Ecosystem Model of Belsky (1993), predominantly at the microsystem level, served as the theoretical framework to explain violence and its possible outcomes from the individual ecological level, i.e., assessing the psychosocial functioning of homeless females. Moreover, the individual level of the Social-Ecological Model for Violence Prevention, mainly personal characteristics, behavior, and individual experiences, was taken into account to identify factors that can potentially increase the likelihood of becoming a victim or a perpetrator of violence (Centers for Disease Control and Prevention [CDC], 2019).

It was hypothesized that homeless female victims of violence would experience negative emotions more frequently and with more intensity and would present a higher index of anxiety and depression, unassertiveness, emotion dysregulation, and a lower level of subjective well-being than non-victims. In addition, it was predicted that victims of physical or sexual violence would have a lower level of subjective well-being in comparison to victims of psychological violence.

Materials and Methods

Participants included 240 homeless females ages 6–21 years old ($M[SD]$ = 11.13[3.47]) selected using a purposive sampling method. They were recruited from nine non-governmental organizations in Mexico City that served homeless groups as their primary function. Participants were required to (1) reside within the selected shelter during the data collection period and (2) consent to participate in the study.

Participants were divided into two groups: victims and non-victims of violence. This classification was made considering medical and clinical records, reports to law enforcement, debriefings by social workers, and certified clinical psychologists. Social workers and clinical psychologists worked at the collaborating institutions. Participants with a medical and clinical record of violence or a report to law enforcement concerning violence were classified as victims. Likewise, these participants had to be identified as victims of any form of violence by social workers and certified psychologists. Furthermore, results obtained with a qualitative interview assessing violence were also considered to help differentiate between victims and non-victims of violence.

Measurement. In Mexico, measures for homeless females do not exist. Worldwide, there are significant logistical and measurement issues when assessing homeless children that challenge accurate and thorough assessment of need (Marcal, 2017). All scales were developed during this study using the culturally relevant psychometric validation process proposed by Geisinger (1994) and, specifically for Mexican culture, by Reyes and García (2008). The researcher selected items from various Mexican scales for children and youth that assess anxiety, depression, assertiveness, emotion regulation, and subjective well-being. Items were chosen based upon their relevance for the group under study as they evaluate cognitive (e.g., self-criticism, helplessness, self-devaluation, catastrophic thoughts, self-focused attention), behavioral (e.g., underestimation of the ability to cope and of help available, dependence, withdrawal, failure to resist their peer's influence, aggression reactivity, compliance), emotional (e.g., nervousness, fear, sadness, irritability, anger, guilt), and social (e.g., social interactions, peer approval, peer influence, deviance, risk behaviors) characteristics present in Mexican homeless females according to the results obtained in a previous study (Castaños & Sánchez, 2016). Items of each instrument were rated on a 6-point Likert scale from 1 (Never, 0% of the time) to 6 (Always, More than 80% of the time).

For the psychometric validation process, three pilot studies with differing samples of randomly selected participants were carried out, and psychology experts in the field evaluated the items. The final version of the instrument assessed 240 homeless girls selected using a non-random method and measured self-reported anxiety symptoms, depressive symptoms, assertive skills, emotion regulation, and subjective well-being.

Symptoms of Anxiety Scale: Anxiety was measured using an eight-item scale grouped into two factors that explain 56% of the variance ($\alpha = 0.59$). An example of an anxiety scale item includes the question, "I am worried that something bad will happen to me."

Symptoms of Depression Scale: Depression was measured using an eight-item scale grouped into two factors that explain 50% of the variance ($\alpha = 0.75$). An example of a depression scale item includes the question, "I feel that only bad things happen to me."

Assertiveness Skills Scale: Assertiveness skills were measured using a nine-item scale grouped into two factors that explain 52% of the variance ($\alpha = 0.64$). An example of an assertiveness scale item includes the question, "I can tell someone to stop bothering me when other people are watching."

Emotion Regulation Scale: Emotion regulation was measured using a seven-item scale grouped into two factors that explain 50% of the variance ($\alpha = 0.60$). An example of an emotion regulation scale item includes the question, "I get upset easily." The emotional regulation scale included additional questions to explore strategies individuals use to manage and control their emotions when experiencing anxiety and depression, such as "If you feel worried, what would you do to calm down?"

Subjective Well-Being Scale: Subjective well-being was measured using 32 items grouped into five factors that explain 61% of the variance ($\alpha = 0.85$ to 0.90). An example of a subjective well-being scale item includes the question, "During the last month, I have felt pleased with the support the institutional staff has given me." The subjective well-being scale also evaluated the intensity and frequency of 10 emotions using a 10-point scale from "0 (Never/None)" to "10 (Very often/A lot)."

Data on violence was obtained from debriefs by social workers and certified clinical psychologists of the collaborating institutions. Information was also extracted from medical reports, interviews conducted by certified clinical psychologists involved in the case, reports to law enforcement concerning violence, and results obtained from a qualitative interview about violence. This interview asked specific questions about violence and its various forms, such as "Have you been beaten? If so, by whom? When and where happened?"

Procedure. Because females are more likely to be "hidden" within the homeless population (Timmons et al., 2018), the researcher worked with non-governmental institutions that support homeless children and youth to acquire access to this population. These institutions were informed of the study's purpose and methods and assured that researchers would follow ethical procedures and guidelines specified by the American Psychological Association (APA, 2017), the Mexican General Law of Health, and the Mexican Law of Welfare. The organizations, instead of parental consent, provided permission to conduct the study, as legal authority rested with the institutions to provide consent on the population's behalf. All participants in this study did so voluntarily and provided their fingerprints as written consent. Participants received information about the study's general objectives, use of data, and confidentiality agreement. The researcher took care to answer participants' questions without biasing participation choice. Participants were empowered to refuse to answer any question or to discontinue study participation at any time. This study was reviewed by the Committee of Research and Ethics of the collaborating organizations, who granted permission to conduct this study. This review serves as the Mexican equivalent to an American IRB Review.

The research took place in collaborating institutions' on-site classrooms. Participants were individually interviewed, and responses were recorded on questionnaires by the researcher.

Data Analysis. Statistical analyses were conducted using SPSS version 24. These included differences between victims and non-victims of violence regarding the frequency of emotions displayed using the Chi-square test and concerning various psychosocial characteristics (symptoms of anxiety and depression, emotion regulation strategies, assertiveness, subjective well-being, and intensity of emotions) using the Student's t-test. A discriminant analysis was conducted to identify which psychosocial characteristics previously mentioned accurately differentiate between victims and non-victims of violence. Finally, a multivariate analysis of variance was carried out to examine differences in those psychosocial characteristics concerning age group, type of violence, and time of permanence in a shelter.

Results

Results revealed that 66% of the participants had experienced some form of violence. The most common type of violence was psychological (51%), followed by physical (44%) and sexual (22%). The place in which they most commonly experienced violence was within the family. Homeless females between 10 and 17 years old were the most affected by all forms of violence, followed by girls among 6–9 years old. Additionally, it was found that victims of violence resorted to social isolation, weeping, and self-mutilation behaviors to manage and control their emotions in a higher proportion than non-victims. They also were more prone to exhibiting a lack of self-control and to substance use and abuse.

Findings obtained with the Chi-square test showed that homeless females who had suffered any form of violence displayed negative feelings more than 80% of the time per week than those who had not, $X^2_{(5240)} = 14.97$, $p = 0.010$. Regardless of the type of violence, there were no significant differences between victims and non-victims concerning the frequency of positive emotions presented, $X^2_{(5240)} = 6.24$, $p = 0.284$.

Student's t-test results revealed that homeless female victims of violence significantly use dysfunctional emotion regulation strategies more often, present symptoms of anxiety, depression, and unassertiveness at a higher rate, and experience negative feelings with greater intensity compared to non-victims (Table 1).

Outcomes obtained with the discriminant analysis carried out showed that homeless female victims of physical violence ($n = 105$; function at group centroids = 0.319) were characterized by having low subjective well-being and by presenting a higher emotion dysregulation in comparison to non-victims ($n = 135$; function at group centroids = −0.248). Victims of sexual violence ($n = 59$; function at group centroid = −0.948) were characterized by being older, remaining in a shelter for a shorter time, exhibiting a low level of subjective well-being, and displaying positive emotions more intensely than non-victims ($n = 189$; function at group centroids = 0.256). Finally, victims of psychological violence ($n = 122$; function at group centroids = 0.246) were characterized by presenting a higher index of depression and by expressing positive emotions more intensely than non-victims ($n = 118$; function at group centroids = −0.254) (Table 2).

The overall success rate for predictions of membership of the criterion grouping variable's categories using the discriminant analysis was between 62% and 70%, with sexual violence being the most accurately classified, followed by physical violence and psychological violence being the least accurately classified. Concerning physical violence, 61.7% of initially grouped cases were correctly classified, with victims being the most accurately classified (66.7%) in comparison to non-victims (57.8%). Regarding sexual violence, 69.6% of initially grouped cases were correctly classified, with non-victims being the most accurately classified (70.4%) in comparison to victims (66.7%). Lastly, concerning psychological violence, 62.5% of initially grouped cases were correctly classified, with non-victims being the most accurately classified (66.9%) in comparison to victims (58.2%).

Finally, findings obtained with the multivariate analysis of variance (MANOVA) only indicated significant interaction effects for subjective well-being (sexual violence × time of permanence in a shelter × age group) and for dysfunctional emotion regulation strategies (physical violence × time of permanence in a shelter × age group) (Table 3).

The effects of the significant interactions obtained with MANOVA were analyzed using Bonferroni Correction (Table 4). In the case of subjective well-being, results revealed that older homeless females who did not experience sexual violence and remained for a longer time in a shelter had a higher index of subjective well-being in comparison to those who were younger and had been victims of sexual violence and when their permanence in a shelter was shorter. Regarding dysfunctional emotion regulation strategies, outcomes showed that homeless females who had been victims of physical violence, remained for less than a year in a shelter, and were between 9 and 11 years old were more prone to using dysfunctional emotion regulation strategies than those who have not suffered physical violence.

Table 1 Differences in various psychosocial characteristics among victims and non-victims of violence according to Student's t-test ($N = 240$)

Psychosocial characteristics	*M(SD)*					95% CI		Normality test	
	YES ($n_1 = 157$)	NO ($n_2 = 83$)	*T*	df	*p*	Lower limit	Upper limit	*z* *Kolmogorov-Smirnov*	*p*
Symptoms of anxiety	3.80(0.74)	3.40(0.79)	3.886	238	0.000**	0.19795	0.60489	0.920	0.366
Symptoms of depression	3.08(0.88)	2.71(0.81)	3.179	238	0.002*	0.14020	0.59695	1.104	0.174
Assertiveness	3.54(0.79)	3.77(0.82)	−2.078	238	0.039*	−0.44192	−0.01179	0.833	0.491
Functional emotion regulation strategies	3.86(1.27)	3.75(1.23)	0.657	238	0.516	−0.22523	0.44721	1.279	0.076
Dysfunctional emotion regulation strategies	3.25(1.01)	2.79(1.30)	3.019	238	0.003**	0.15971	0.44448	1.067	0.205
Subjective well-being	4.33(0.75)	4.51(0.65)	−1.841	238	0.067	−0.36936	0.01254	0.822	0.508
Intensity of positive emotions	7.88(2.08)	7.62(2.30)	0.927	238	0.355	−0.30614	0.85074	1.386	0.065
Intensity of negative emotions	5.31(2.62)	4.32(2.60)	2.778	238	0.006*	0.28669	1.68381	1.041	0.228

Note. $^{*}p < 0.05$; $^{**}p < 0.01$

Table 2 Discriminant analysis for victims and non-victims of violence according to various psychosocial characteristics ($N = 240$)

Psychosocial characteristics	Standardized coefficients of the canonical discriminant function	Wilks' lambda	X^2	df	Sig.	Exact F				Eigenvalue	Canonical correlation
						Statistic	df1	df2	*p*		
Physical violence											
Dysfunctional emotion regulation strategies	0.783	0.926	18.213	2	0.000	9.465	2	237.000	0.000	.080[a]	0.272
Subjective well-being	−0.636										
Sexual violence											
Subjective well-being	0.914	0.804	51.625	4	0.000	14.366	4	235.000	0.000	0.245	0.443
Age	−0.460										
Time of permanence in a shelter	0.312										
Positive emotions	−0.384										
Psychological violence											
Depression symptoms	1.097	0.941	14.513	2	0.001	7.483	2	237.000	0.001	0.063	0.244
Positive emotions	0.677										

Note: All results were significant at $p < 0.01$

Table 3 Significant interaction effects of the multivariate analysis of variance ($N = 240$)

Interaction	Dependent variables	gl	*F*	*p*	*Partial* η^2
Sexual violence × time of permanence × age group	Subjective well-being	7	2.323	0.028*	0.094
Physical violence × time of permanence × age group	Dysfunctional emotion regulation strategies	7	2.378	0.025*	0.096
Error		156			
Total		240			

Note: Only significant results were reported. Time of permanence: 1 (1–12 months), 2 (13–36 months), 3 (37–60 months), and 4 (61–204 months). Age Group: 1 (6–8 years old), 2 (9–11 years old), 3 (12–13 years old), and 4 (14–21 years old). Physical violence: victims and non-victims. Sexual violence: victims and non-victims. *$p < 0.05$

Consequently, the first hypothesis was partially supported since it was found that, in comparison to non-victims of violence, homeless female victims of violence experience negative emotions more frequently and with more intensity and present a higher index of anxiety and depression, unassertiveness, and emotion dysregulation. Nonetheless, it was not demonstrated that this group had a lower level of subjective well-being than non-victims. Moreover, the second hypothesis was proven because it was possible to evidence that victims of physical or sexual violence had a lower level of subjective well-being in comparison to victims of psychological violence.

Discussion and Conclusions

Findings showed that Mexican homeless females who had experienced any violence, whether physical, psychological, or sexual, exhibited further psychological impairment compared to those who had not, which is consistent with the microsystem of Belsky's Model and the CDC's Framework. According to previous research in Anglo-Saxon and European countries, homeless females experience physical, sexual, and psychological violence at a higher rate than men (Lepistö et al., 2012; Thompson et al., 2011).

Likewise, it was found that most homeless females have been victims of violence, mainly psychological, followed by physical and sexual, which can be explained as a result of experiencing extreme adverse conditions like harsh parenting, poor parental supervision, sexual violence, exposure to parental intimate partner violence, or aggression in their peer relationships (Belsky, 1993; CDC, 2019; Hipwell et al., 2014).

Furthermore, homeless females exhibited two or more types of violence, and those who suffered more frequently from any form of violence were mostly teenagers. This is consistent with work from other countries where findings show that

Table 4 Significant interaction effects obtained with MANOVA analyzed using Bonferroni Correction ($N = 240$)

Dependent variables	Factors			Statistics		95% CI			
				M(SE)		Lower limit		Upper limit	
Psychosocial characteristics	Type of violence	Time of permanence (months)	Age group (years)	Victims	Non-victims	Victims	Non-victims	Victims	Non-victims
Subjective well-being	Sexual violence	37–60	9–11[a]	3.759(0.382)	4.728(0.206)	3.005	4.321	4.513	5.136
			12–13[b]	3.559(0.317)	4.369(0.234)	2.932	3.907	4.186	4.830
			14–23[c]	3.966(0.441)	5.080(0.312)	3.095	4.465	4.836	5.696
		61–204	9–11[d]	3.477(0.294)	5.031(0.234)	2.897	4.569	4.057	5.493
			12–13[e]	2.000(0.623)	4.409(0.228)	0.769	3.958	3.231	4.859
Dysfunctional emotion regulation strategies	Physical violence	1–12	9–11[f]	4.639(0.400)	2.531(0.329)	3.848	1.881	5.430	3.181

Note: Mean differences are significant at $p < 0.05$. Only significant mean differences were reported

[a] $F_{(1156)} = 4.998$, $p = 0.027$, *partial* $\eta^2 = 0.031$
[b] $F_{(1156)} = 4.214$, $p = 0.042$, *partial* $\eta^2 = 0.026$
[c] $F_{(1156)} = 4.266$, $p = 0.041$, *partial* $\eta^2 = 0.027$
[d] $F_{(1156)} = 17.112$, $p < 0.000$, *partial* $\eta^2 = 0.099$
[e] $F_{(1156)} = 13.170$, $p < 0.000$, *partial* $\eta^2 = 0.078$
[f] $F_{(1156)} = 14.321$, $p < 0.000$, *partial* $\eta^2 = 0.096$

violence in vulnerable people is four times more common during adolescence (De Blake et al., 2014).

In addition, outcomes of this work revealed that homeless females with a history of violence experience more anxiety and depression symptoms, use more dysfunctional emotion regulation strategies (e.g., substance use and abuse, self-mutilating behaviors, social withdrawal) to manage and control their emotions, and have fewer social abilities compared to those without a history of violence. They displayed negative emotions more often and more intensely. Such findings align with literature about violence in children: violence in the short and long term leads to anxiety and depression, difficulties in interpersonal relationships, self-destructive behaviors, substance use and abuse, and a dysfunctional adaptation to society (Rus & Galbeaza, 2013). It also leads to social isolation, chronic stress, suicide ideation and attempts, and post-traumatic stress (Langa-Mlambo & Soma-Pillay, 2014). Hence, homeless female victims of violence have a more impaired psychosocial functioning.

Concerning the types of violence, findings showed that participants who had suffered physical violence had lower subjective well-being and higher emotion dysregulation, unlike those who had not. Similarly, victims of psychological violence exhibited higher symptoms of depression and expressed positive emotions more intensely in comparison to non-victims. These findings concur with previous studies with vulnerable women that have found that physical and psychological violence is associated with depression (Nhi et al., 2019), emotional disorders such as anxiety and somatoform disorders (Savas & Agridag, 2011), and stress (Chandra et al., 2009). Furthermore, victims of sexual violence were older, spent less time in a shelter, exhibited low subjective well-being, and expressed positive emotions more intensely compared to non-victims. Several studies have found that when shelters provide quality services, they can substantially increase the general health of institutionalized children and youth (Lawrence et al., 2006). Thus, facilities serving homeless females can become a protective factor against further victimization or perpetration of violence. Results demonstrated that a longer permanence in a shelter was associated with a higher index of subjective well-being and a lower probability of suffering sexual violence. In contrast, remaining for a brief time in a shelter was related to exhibiting dysfunctional emotion regulation and a higher likelihood of being a victim of physical violence. These outcomes highlight the need to work at a community level with prevention strategies to address these factors and help prevent violence, as stipulated by the CDC's Social Ecological Model (2019).

Finally, both physical and sexual violence were linked with a decreased subjective well-being (i.e., satisfaction with life). These findings agree with previous research that states that physical and psychological violence in children and youth increases the risk of psychiatric disorders (MacMillan et al., 2013), mainly anxiety and depression (Breiding et al., 2013; Calvete, 2014). As a consequence, they display negative emotions more often than individuals without a history of violence. Physical, sexual, or psychological violence lead to poor management and control of emotions, especially negative ones (Zarei et al., 2011). Sexual violence increases depression explicitly (Bilginer et al., 2013; Haileye, 2013; Yüce et al., 2015).

Overall, having been a victim of physical or psychological violence diminishes the psychosocial well-being of individuals and, consequently, the quality and satisfaction with life (Collin-Vézina et al., 2013; Fergusson et al., 2013). As such, violence against women is recognized as a significant impairment to health and social development (Jewkes et al., 2019). These effects can extend to adulthood (United Nations International Children's Fund [UNICEF], 2007).

As seen, violence has severe negative repercussions on the physical, mental, and reproductive health of women and girls (Stewart et al., 2015). When experienced during childhood, as in the case of the participants of this study, it is associated with a greater risk of re-victimization and of presenting anxiety and depression during adulthood (Thoresen et al., 2015). In other words, childhood violence is one of the central causes of emotional, behavioral, and health problems throughout life (Brassard & Fiorvanti, 2015). These effects interfere with healthy physical and psychological development during childhood (Fergusson et al., 2013; Lindauer et al., 2014) and aggravate physical and psychological hassles during adulthood (Bick et al., 2014; Lesmana et al., 2015). According to the Eco-systemic Model (Belsky, 1993) and the CDC (2019) Framework, consequences related to violence negatively impact the cultural microsystem, particularly the individual and his or her family, by increasing family dysfunction and decreasing psychological adjustment of the abused individual.

Early diagnosis, attention, and prevention of violence are crucial to reduce the negative impact on an individual, familial, communal, and social level. Based on early recognition, it is possible to design and carry out effective policy actions and enable treatment and prevention of more adverse conditions in homeless people. It has been shown, for example, that prevention programs aimed at intimate partner violence work when they meet the needs of both homeless youth and those providing services for them (Petering et al., 2014). Interventions should aim to target violence, and service providers should be familiar with how to work with it.

In conclusion, the myriad of psychosocial effects due to violence highlights the extreme inequality suffered by homeless females and their likelihood of presenting cumulative deficits in adulthood. However, due to underreporting, lack of research on this matter, inadequate investigations of violence in homeless females, discrimination, social exclusion, the "hidden nature" of this group, and other factors, not even the exact number of homeless females that have experienced violence are known. The impact of violence on this group has been studied less, and, in Mexico, it has received the least scientific attention. The findings of this study help to identify some psychosocial factors associated with experiencing any form of violence and their impact on each type of violence (i.e., physical, psychological, and sexual). These factors should be addressed to reduce re-victimization, the risk of experiencing violence, and its adverse effects and to promote attitudes, beliefs, and behaviors that foster psychological well-being and resilience and prevent violence. As referred by CDC's framework (2019), specific approaches may include education and life skills training.

This study has some limitations. The results are exploratory rather than confirmatory. The sample size was not large enough, and the relative ethnic homogeneity of the sample reduces the generalizability of the results to homeless females of some regions of Mexico City. Another limitation of this research was the low internal consistency of some of the psychosocial scales used as determined by Cronbach's alpha. Moreover, other factors related to violence in homeless females were not considered in this study, such as sexually transmitted infections, substance use and abuse, parenting styles, and domestic violence. Nonetheless, to the best of the author's knowledge, this study is the first research in Mexico to examine some psychosocial factors associated with violence in homeless females. In addition, it provides a comprehensive description of the current knowledge of violence in homeless females. Further, disparities across types of violence, victims and non-victims of violence, diverse psychosocial factors linked to this violence, age, and time of permanence in a shelter were examined. Since violence against females is recognized as a significant impairment to health and social development (Jewkes et al., 2019), future research should continue assessing violence and its associated psychosocial factors particularly in vulnerable groups like homeless females to enable the design of efficient and sustainable intervention strategies taking into account their needs and characteristics, thus promoting their well-being and improving their quality of life.

References

American Psychological Association. (2017). *Ethical principles of psychologists and code of conduct*. American Psychological Association. Retrieved from: https://www.apa.org/ethics/code/ethics-code-2017.pdf

American Psychological Association (APA). (2015). *APA dictionary of psychology*. American Psychological Association.

Barman-Adhikari, A., Petering, R., Lengnick-Hall, R., Rice, E., Rhoades, H., & McCune, S. (2016). Social context of service use among homeless youth in Los Angeles, California. *Journal of Social Service Research, 42*(4), 501–515. https://doi.org/10.1080/01488376.2016.1153563

Belsky, J. (1993). Etiology of child maltreatment: A developmental-ecological analysis. *Psychological Bulletin, 114*(3), 413–434.

Bick, J., Zajac, K., Ralston, M., & Smith, D. (2014). Convergence and divergence in reports of maternal support following childhood sexual abuse: Prevalence and associations with youth psychosocial adjustment. *Child Abuse and Neglect, 38*(3), 479–487. https://doi.org/10.1016/j.chiabu.2013.11.010

Bilginer, C., Hesapiçioglu, T., & Kandi, S. (2013). Sexual abuse in childhood: A multidimensional look from the view point of victims and perpetrators. *The Journal of Psychiatry and Neurological Sciences, 26*(1), 55–64.

Brassard, M., & Fiorvanti, C. (2015). School-based child abuse prevention programs. *Psychology in the Schools*. https://doi.org/10.1002/pits.21811

Breiding, M., Mercy, J., Gulaid, J., Reza, A., & Hleta-Nkambule, N. (2013). A national survey of childhood physical abuse among females in Swaziland. *Journal of Epidemiology and Global Health, 3*, 73–81.

Calvete, E. (2014). Emotional abuse as a predictor of early maladaptive schemas in adolescents: Contributions to the development of depressive and social anxiety symptoms. *Child Abuse and Neglect, 38*(4), 735–765. https://doi.org/10.1016/j.chiabu.2013.10.014

Capuzzi, D., & Gross, D. (2008). *Youth at risk: A prevention resource for counselors, teachers and parents*. Pearson-Merrill Prentice Hall.

Castaños, S., & Sánchez, J. J. (2016). Hacia una construcción de una concepción psico-sociocultural de niñas y jóvenes mexicanas en situación de calle: Una aproximación cualitativa. *Anales de Psicología / Annals of Psychology, 32*(2), 516–527. https://doi.org/10.6018/analesps.32.2.204721

Centers for Disease Control and Prevention. (2019). *The social-ecological model: A framework for prevention.* Retrieved from: https://www.cdc.gov/violenceprevention/publichealthissue/social-ecologicalmodel.html

Chandra, P., Satyanarayana, V., & Caray, M. (2009). Women reporting intimate partner violence in India: Associations with PTSD and depressive symptoms. *Archives of Women's Mental Health, 12*(4), 203–209.

Changa, J., Theodore, A., Martin, S., & Runyan, D. (2008). Psychological abuse between parents: Associations with child maltreatment from a population-based sample. *Child Abuse & Neglect, 32*(8), 819–829.

Collin-Vézina, D., Daigneault, I., & Hébert, M. (2013). Lessons learned from child sexual abuse research: Prevalence, outcomes, and preventive strategies. *Child and Adolescent Psychiatry and Mental Health, 7*(22), 1–9.

Crawford, M., & Manassis, K. (2011). Anxiety, social skills, friendship quality, and peer victimization: An integrated model. *Journal of Anxiety Disorders, 25*, 924–931.

da Silva Rosa, A., & Passarella, A. (2015). Violence in the lives of homeless women in the city of Sao Paulo, Brazil. *Interface (Botucatu), 19*(53). https://doi.org/10.1590/1807-57622014.0221

De Blake, M., Drezett, J., Vertamatti, M., Adami, F., Valenti, V., Paiva, A., Viana, J., Pedroso, D., & de Abreu, L. (2014). Characteristics of sexual violence against adolescent girls and adult women. *Women's Health, 14*(15). https://doi.org/10.1186/1472-6874-14-15

De Rueda, B. (2007). *La educación de las jóvenes que viven en la calle* (Education of girls who live on the street). United Nations Educational, Cultural and Scientific Organization (UNESCO).

Douglas, K., Chan, G., Gelerneter, J., Arias, A., Anton, R., Weiss, R., Brady, K., Poling, J., Farrer, L., & Kranzler, H. (2010). Adverse childhood events as risk factors for substance dependence: Partial mediation by mood and anxiety disorders. *Addictive Behaviors, 35*, 7–13.

Dumain, K. (2010). *Optimism, hope, problem solving and runaway behavior in adolescents in the dependency system* (Doctoral dissertation). Pepperdine University.

Escribà-Agüir, V., Ruiz-Pérez, I., Montero-Piñar, M., Vives-Cases, C., Plazaola-Castaño, J., & Martín-Baena, D. (2010). Partner violence and psychological well-being: Buffer or indirect effect of social support. *Psychosomatic Medicine, 72*, 383–389.

European Federation of National Organisations working with the Homeless. (n.d.). *The links between violence against women and homelessness.* Retrieved from: https://www.feantsa.org/download/vaw_background_paper_final507550159640577037.pdf

Fergusson, D., McLeod, G., & Horwood, J. (2013). Childhood sexual abuse and adult developmental outcomes: Findings from a 30-year longitudinal study in New Zealand. *Child Abuse and Neglect, 37*, 664–674.

Geisinger, K. (1994). Cross-cultural normative assessment: Translation and adaptation issues influencing the normative interpretation of assessment instruments. *Psychological Assessment, 6*(4), 304–312.

Haileye, A. (2013). Psychopathological correlates of child sexual abuse: The case of female students in Jimma zone, South West Ethiopia. *Ethiopian Journal of Health Sciences, 23*(1), 32–28.

Helander, E. (2008). *Children and violence: The world of the defenseless.* Pallgrave Macmillan.

Hipwell, A., Stepp, S., Xiong, S., Keenan, K., Blokland, A., & Loeber, R. (2014). Parental punishment and peer victimization as developmental precursors to physical dating violence involvement against girls. *Journal of Research on Adolescence, 24*(1), 65–79. https://doi.org/10.1111/jora.12016

Jewkes, R., Corboz, J., & Gibbs, A. (2019). Violence against Afghan women by husbands,mothers-in-law and siblings-in-law/siblings: risk markers and health consequences in an analysis of the baseline of a randomised controlled trial. *PLoS One, 14*(2), e0211361. https://doi.org/10.1371/journal.pone.0211361

Kim, J., & Cicchetti, D. (2010). Longitudinal pathways linking child maltreatment, emotion regulation, peer relations, and psychopathology. *Journal of Child Psychology and Psychiatry, 51*(6), 706–716.

Langa-Mlambo, L., & Soma-Pillay, P. (2014). Violence against women in South Africa. *Obstetrics & Gynaecology Forum, 24*, 17–21.

Lau, J., Kim, J., Tsui, H., Cheung, A., Lau, M., & Yu, A. (2005). The relationship between physical maltreatment and substance use among adolescents. A survey of 95,788 adolescents in Hong Kong. *Journal of Adolescent Health, 37*(2), 110–119.

Lawrence, C., Carlson, E., & Egeland, B. (2006). The impact of foster care on development. *Development and Psychopathology, 18*(1), 57–76. https://doi.org/10.1017/S0954579406060044

Lepistö, S., Joronen, K., Åstedt-Kurki, P., Luukkaala, T., & Paavilainen, E. (2012). Subjective well-being in Finnish adolescents experiencing family violence. *Journal of Family Nursing, 18*(2), 200–233.

Lesmana, C., Suryani, L., & Tiliopoulos, N. (2015). Cultural considerations in the treatment of mental illness among sexually abused children and adolescents: The case of Bali, Indonesia. *New Directions for Child and Adolescent Development, 147*, 109–116. https://doi.org/10.1002/cad.20092

Lindauer, R., Brilleslijper-Kater, S., Diehle, J., Verlinden, E., Teeuw, A., Middeldorp, C., Tuinebreijer, W., Bosschaart, T., van Duin, E., & Verhoeff, A. (2014). The Amsterdam Sexual Abuse Case (ASAC)-study in day care centers: Longitudinal effects of sexual abuse on infants and very young children and their parents, and the consequences of the persistence of abusive images on the internet. *BMC Psychiatry, 14*(1), 295. https://doi.org/10.1186/s12888-014-0295-7

MacMillan, H., Tanaka, M., Duku, E., Vaillancourt, T., & Boyle, M. (2013). Child physical and sexual abuse in a community sample of young adults: Results from the Ontario Child Health Study. *Child Abuse and Neglect, 37*, 14–21.

Marcal, K. (2017). A theory of mental health and optimal service delivery for homeless children. *Child and Adolescent Social Work Journal, 34*, 349–359. https://doi.org/10.1007/s10560-016-0464-2

Melander, L., & Tyler, K. (2010). The effect of early maltreatment, victimization, and partner violence on HIV risk behavior among homeless young adults. *Journal of Adolescent Health, 47*(6), 575–581.

Misganaw, A. C., & Worku, Y. A. (2013). Assessment of sexual violence among street females in Bahir-Dar town, North West Ethiopia: a mixed method study. *BMC Public Health, 13*, 825. https://doi.org/10.1186/1471-2458-13-825

Moreno, T. (2019). *UN: Mexican government must tackle violence against women.* Retrieved from: https://www.eluniversal.com.mx/english/un-mexican-government-must-tackle-violence-against-women

Nhi, T., Hanh, N., Hinh, N., Toan, N., Gammeltoft, T., Rasch, V., & Meyrowitsch, D. (2019). Intimate partner violence among pregnant women and postpartum depression in Vietnam: A longitudinal study. *BioMed Research International*. https://doi.org/10.1155/2019/4717485

Noell, J., Rohde, P., Seeley, J., & Ochs, L. (2001). Childhood sexual abuse, adolescent sexual coercion and sexually transmitted infection acquisition among homeless female adolescents. *Child Abuse & Neglect, 25*(1), 137–148.

Pan American World Health Organization. (2018). *Violence against women affects almost 60% of women in some countries of the Americas.* Retrieved from: https://www.paho.org/hq/index.php?option=com_content&view=article&id=14830:violence-against-women-affects-almost-60-of-women-in-some-countries-of-the-americas&Itemid=1926&lang=en

Petering, R., Wenzel, S., & Winetrobe, H. (2014). Systematic review of current intimate partner violence prevention programs and applicability to homeless youth. *Journal of the Society for Social Work & Research, 5*(1), 107–135. https://doi-org.ucapr.cobimet3.org/10.1086/675851

Picornell, A. (2006). *La infancia en desamparo* (Childhood in distress). Nau Libres.

Rábago-González, M. (2009). Las niñas en situación de calle en la ciudad de México: una visión de género (Homeless girls in Mexico City: A gender perspective). *Revista Iberoamericana sobre Infancia y Juventud en Lucha por sus Derechos, 1*(1), 107–109.
Reyes, I. & García, L. (2008). Procedimiento de validación psicométrica culturalmente relevante: un ejemplo (Psychometric culturally relevant validation procedure: an example). In Asociación Mexicana de Psicología Social [AMEPSO] (Ed.), *La Psicología Social en México XII* (pp. 625–630). AMEPSO.
Rus, M., & Galbeaza, A. (2013). Psychological aspects of child sexual abuse. *Contemporary Readings in Law and Social Justice, 5*(2), 499–510.
Sadurní, M., Rostán, C. & Serrat, E. (2003). *El desarrollo de los niños paso a paso* (Child development step by step). UOC.
Savas, N., & Agridag, A. (2011). The relationship between women's mental health and domestic violence in semirural areas: A study in Turkey. *Asia Pacific Journal Public Health, 23*(3), 399–407.
Slonim-Nevo, V., & Mukuka, L. (2007). Child abuse and AIDS-related knowledge, attitudes and behavior among adolescents in Zambia. *Child Abuse & Neglect, 31*(2), 143–159.
Soriano, A., Ochoa, F. & Jiménez, F. (2005). *Una luz en el sendero de la oscuridad. Experiencia en la enseñanza de valores a adolescentes en situación de calle* (A light in the path of darkness. Experience in the teaching of values to homeless teenagers). Maurilio Olivera, A.C., Instituto de Asistencia e Integración Social (IASIS) y Gobierno del Distrito Federal.
Stewart, D., Aviles, R., Guedes, A., Riazantseva, E., & MacMillan, H. (2015). Latin American and Caribbean countries' baseline clinical and policy guidelines for responding to intimate partner violence and sexual violence against women. *Public Health, 15*(665). https://doi.org/10.1186/s12889-015-1994-9
Thompson, S., Bender, K., & Kim, J. (2011). Family factors as predictors of depression among runaway youth: Do males and females differ? *Child and Adolescent Social Work Journal, 28*, 35–48.
Thoresen, S., Myhre, M., Wentzel-Larsen, T., Aakvaag, H., & Hjemdal, O. (2015). Violence against children, later victimisation, and mental health: A cross-sectional study of the general Norwegian population. *European Journal of Psychotraumatology, 6*, 26259. https://doi.org/10.3402/ejpt.v6.26259
Timmons, V., Coomber-Bendtsen, M. & Zederayko, A. (2018). *Gender-based violence and homelessness: Two sides of the same coin*. Retrieved from: https://www.schoolofpublicpolicy.sk.ca/documents/research/policy-briefs/JSGS-policybriefs-Gender-Based%20Violence%20and%20Homelessness.pdf
Tonmyr, L., Williams, G., Hovdestad, W., & Draca, J. (2011). Anxiety and/or depression in 10-15 years old investigated by child welfare in Canada. *Journal of Adolescent Health, 48*, 493–498.
Tyler, K., Cauce, A., & Whitbeck, L. (2004). Family risk factors and prevalence of dissociative symptoms among homeless and runaway youth. *Child Abuse & Neglect, 28*(3), 355–366.
United Nations. (2006). *La violencia contra niños, niñas y adolescentes. Informe de América Latina en el marco del estudio mundial de las Naciones Unidas* (Violence against boys, girls, and teenagers. Report on Latin America in the framework of the world study of the United Nations). United Nations.
United Nations International Children's Fund. (2007). *La infancia y los objetivos de desarrollo del Milenio* (Childhood and developmental objectives of the Millennium). Retrieved from: https://www.unicef.org/media/92991/file/UNICEF-informe-anual-2007.pdf
Warf, C., Clark, L., Desai, M., Calvo, R., Agahi, G., & Hoffman, J. (2010). Coming of age on the streets; survival sex among homeless adolescent females in Hollywood. *Journal of Adolescent Health, 46*(2), 37–38.
Williams, M. (2018). *Women's hidden homelessness*. Retrieved from: https://www.homeless.org.uk/connect/blogs/2018/feb/27/women%E2%80%99s-hidden-homelessness

World Health Organization. (2019). *Displaced or refugee women are at increased risk of violence. What can WHO do?* Retrieved from: https://www.who.int/reproductivehealth/displaced-refugee-women-violence-risk/en/

Yüce, M., Karabekiroğlu, K., Yildirim, Z., Şahin, S., Sapmaz, D., Babadaği, Z., Turla, A., & Aydin, B. (2015). The psychiatric consequences of child and adolescent sexual abuse. *Noro Psikiyatri Arsivi, 52*(4), 393–399. https://doi.org/10.5152/npa.2015.7472

Zarei, J., Rostami, R., Farhanian, F., Pour, S. G., & Sadeghian, E. (2011). Prevalence of anxiety disorders and its relation to past child abuse and general health in Universities Students of Iran. *Procedia – Social and Behavioral Sciences, 30*, 283–286. https://doi.org/10.1016/j.sbspro.2011.10.056

Part III
Social Vulnerability

Cognitive Abilities in the Learning of Children in Residential Care: Toward the Development of Their Potential

José Anibal Ojeda-Nuñez, Jacqueline Espinosa-Bautista, and Ximena Andrea González-Grandón

Introduction

To optimize the cognitive development of individuals, it is imperative to recognize the role of emotions. Plato's assertion that "all learning has an emotional base" (Porras, 2020, p. 11) underscores the importance of emotions in the learning process. Despite this, little attention has been given to considering emotions as the foundational axis of programs influencing cognitive processes. Elizondo et al. (2018) point out that when fear, sadness, and desolation are prevalent in learning environments, neurotransmitters such as adrenaline, noradrenaline, and cortisol are activated. The prolonged presence of these neurotransmitters can lead to cognitive blocks, negatively impacting memory and attention—critical elements for the learning process.

Conversely, rigorous research findings suggest that activities and environments promoting joy, surprise, tranquility, and calmness yield positive effects at the neuronal level. Such positive effects include increased memory retention, improved reading comprehension, and enhanced reasoning (Pekrun, 2014). Recognizing and leveraging the influence of emotions on cognitive processes can contribute significantly to fostering a conducive and effective learning environment.

Martelo & Arévalo (2017) analyzed attention, memory, language, and executive functions, examining their correlation with literacy and numeracy skills. The study involved 30 participants aged 7–17, chosen based on low academic performance and the absence of neuropsychiatric history. The findings revealed that in the semantic fluency subdomain, 39.6% of participants scored below average, 72.6%

J. A. Ojeda-Nuñez (✉) · X. A. González-Grandón
Universidad Iberoamericana (IBERO), Mexico City, Mexico
e-mail: kanibalin17@gmail.com

J. Espinosa-Bautista
Universidad Nacional Autónoma de México (UNAM), Mexico City, Mexico

S. Castaños-Cervantes et al. (eds.), *Working with Vulnerable Populations*,
https://doi.org/10.1007/978-3-031-67710-6_13

exhibited very low scores in working memory, and 42.9% were classified as extremely low in calculation skills. The authors highlighted that attention disorders are interconnected with other cognitive abilities and emotional processes, as they share interacting brain structures. This underscores the intricate relationship between attention, cognition, and emotions in the context of academic performance.

In the given context, Novoa et al. (2021) highlight that reading comprehension involves a range of cognitive-linguistic skills. These skills encompass decoding, utilizing prior knowledge, understanding vocabulary, recognizing textual structures, and applying mental frameworks to enhance comprehension. Additionally, cognitive skills such as self-reflection, self-regulation, and the capacity to employ various strategies when interpreting a text are also activated. The mention of these cognitive-linguistic and metacognitive processes underscores the multifaceted nature of reading comprehension and the diverse cognitive skills that contribute to it.

In Mexico, the outcomes of the 2018 national assessment for sixth-grade primary education students revealed that 49% performed at Level I, indicating insufficient performance. Students at this level demonstrated limited comprehension skills to identify explicit information in texts. Conversely, only 3% reached Level IV, representing outstanding proficiency (INEE, 2018). In the realm of mathematics, which involves cultivating critical-scientific thinking such as interpreting, explaining, and predicting, assessments like PISA and PLANEA indicate that Mexico ranks fifth among countries with the lowest mathematical performance statistics (OECD, 2018). These findings underscore the challenges and disparities in academic achievement faced by students in Mexico, particularly in the areas of reading comprehension and mathematical proficiency.

According to UNESCO (2015), the goal by 2030 is to ensure that children and adolescents receive an inclusive, intercultural, and equitable education that defends and protects their rights with a focus on social justice. This education is envisioned to be rooted in learning opportunities and encompass skills such as creativity, problem-solving, teamwork, communication, and resilience. A foundational principle of Mexican basic education is to promote inclusive and equitable education that revolves around rights, interculturality, and human dignity. This involves providing access to education for the entire population without any form of distinction. As a result, childhood centers are expected to adhere to the stipulations set forth by international and national organizations to support the integral well-being of society (SEP, 2019).

The synergy between inclusion and intercultural approaches can be most effectively established by emphasizing intercultural competence, encompassing cognitive, affective, sociocultural, and behavioral skills that facilitate adept and meaningful interactions in diverse cultural settings. The cornerstone of cognitive competency is cultural self-awareness, while curiosity serves as the pivotal affective competency, and empathy is the fundamental behavioral competency. This chapter meticulously explores each of these competencies before delving into the future practical application of intercultural concepts and models. The objective is to construct a cohesive bridge that seamlessly connects diversity, inclusion, and global diversity perspectives in institutionalized educational contexts.

This prompts the question: How can this be achieved without leaving any children and young people without these opportunities?

Characteristics of Vulnerable Child Population

Meta-analyses conducted by Elegbeleye (2013) and Tagurum et al. (2015) focusing on children living in vulnerable conditions and orphanages reveal that exposure to traumatic experiences often results in a lack of access to education and deficiencies in other essential services, such as:

- *Nutrition Services*: Malnutrition can lead to illnesses and fatalities due to a lack of proper nourishment.
- *Clothing and Access to Personal Hygiene Items*: Inadequate housing conditions contribute to neglect, impacting the overall well-being of children from a biopsychosociocultural perspective.
- *Stigma and Social Abandonment*: These children often encounter additional challenges related to the lack of protection of their rights, leading to stigma and social abandonment.
- *Primary Health Care*: Deficient healthcare can affect the overall integrity of these children, including issues related to the lack of application and follow-up of vaccination schedules.
- *Psychosocial Support and Extracurricular Activities*: Respecting these rights fosters teamwork, empathy, and communication skills. The absence of these experiences can result in delays in their overall development.
- *Continued Education and Vocational Opportunities*: Constant changes in educational institutions, high absenteeism, dropping out of school cycles, and limited support for higher education tuition perpetuate inequality and hinder social integration. These challenges make it difficult for affected children to access continued education and vocational opportunities, perpetuating disparities in their long-term prospects.

Other research supports the observation that children in residential care often experience educational lag, with potential consequences such as social exclusion and marginalization. Consequently, institutions must prioritize successful academic learning within their plans and programs. Obtaining information about educational backgrounds, attitudes, and motivations within the classroom is crucial for understanding and advocating for better education. Early identification of individuals who may require specific support for improved learning is essential and can be easily accessible (Olsen & De Montgomery, 2018; Rodríguez & Pérez, 2022). This emphasis on recognizing and addressing educational challenges early on is key to mitigating the potential negative outcomes associated with educational lag among children in residential care or institutionalized education.

From the perspective of healthcare professionals, the review by Fernández et al. (2021) highlights that children and adolescents in residential care often display little or no interest in interaction, minimal motivation to cooperate, difficulties in their social life, and a tendency to disregard established norms and limits. Consequently, they may exhibit violent behaviors toward objects, peers, adults, and the various professionals supporting them. Reasons for seeking psychological and psychiatric consultations typically include attention deficit hyperactivity disorder (ADHD), oppositional defiant disorder (caused by anger and irritability), anxious and depressive behaviors, as well as self-harming behaviors such as suicidal ideation and attempts. It is noteworthy that caregivers predominantly report these reasons, as children and adolescents in residential care are often reluctant to express their experiences and emotional challenges directly. This underscores the importance of a comprehensive approach involving both caregivers and healthcare professionals to address the mental health and behavioral issues faced by this population.

A study conducted with 111 institutionalized children found statistically significant differences, using the Capacities and Difficulties Questionnaire (SDQ), in emotionally problematic behaviors reported by teachers, caregivers, and family members compared to a control group. Participants in residential care showed lower scores, with areas of major concern being emotional difficulties, behavioral problems, hyperactivity, and conflicts with peers (Fernández-Daza & Fernández-Parra, 2017).

Another study by Sölva et al. (2020), involving 147 children from foster care institutions in Lower Austria, demonstrated a relationship between post-traumatic stress and various types of abuse they are exposed to. This is in addition to the diverse issues resulting from high levels of neglect and lack of protection. Constant abuse was associated with increased severity of post-traumatic stress disorder. Children under abuse also showed high indicators of anxiety, often comorbid with depression and other affective disorders. These data correlate with poor performance in intellectual skills and tasks, which may be connected to cognitive deficits and impairments (Deambrosio et al., 2018). Robledo (2017) mentions that most institutionalized children in foster homes in Mexico City harbor resentment and anger toward their initial caregivers because they have often experienced violence, perpetuating a negative environment for their psychosocial development.

In the social interaction of peers who spend significant time together and face emotional difficulties and learning problems, another important characteristic to consider is the manifestation of bullying. According to Balluerka et al. (2023), bullying represents a serious psychosocial challenge with detrimental effects, serving as a major risk factor for the onset of psychological disorders and psychopathological manifestations during childhood and adolescence. If not resolved, these effects can persist into adulthood. Oppong et al. (2015) highlight a connection between substance use, suicidal ideation, and perceived resilience with emotional problems. Predictive factors encompass violent behavior, stigma, and a lack of social support. In their study, resilience, as the primary indicator, offered insights into individuals' perceived ability to cope and recover from challenges. Suicidal ideation and substance abuse explored critical dimensions of mental health that can significantly impact development and emotional well-being. Recognizing and addressing bullying within the context of emotional difficulties and learning problems is crucial for mitigating long-term psychosocial consequences for these individuals.

Justification

As of the present date in Mexico, the personal strengths and cognitive and socio-emotional capacities of institutionalized children remain unknown. This information is crucial for the complete restoration of their rights, unlocking their potential, reducing and eventually overcoming their conditions of vulnerability, and facilitating their successful social integration, inclusion, and adaptation. Existing studies on this matter have primarily focused on the learning difficulties of the institutionalized population (Deambrosio et al., 2018; Tagurum et al., 2015), their psychiatric disorders (Elegbeleye, 2013; Fernández & Fernández, 2017; Oppong et al., 2015), and the detrimental effects of institutionalization (Rodríguez, 2016). The absence of comprehensive data on the personal strengths and capacities of institutionalized children highlights the need for research in this area to inform targeted interventions and support mechanisms for their holistic development and well-being.

Indeed, in our country, interventions have predominantly focused on cognitive rehabilitation and psychiatric care, often overlooking the stipulations outlined in Mexican regulations. According to the General Health Law, the General Education Law, the General Victims Law, and the General Law for the Rights of Girls, Boys, and Adolescents, institutionalized children have the right to comprehensive intervention aimed at ensuring their complete reintegration into society. This intervention should be integral to their life plan, to enhance their overall well-being, improve their quality of life, and to overcome their conditions of vulnerability. Recognizing and addressing the diverse needs and capacities of institutionalized children, beyond cognitive and psychiatric aspects, aligns with the principles of these laws and regulations, emphasizing a more holistic and inclusive approach to their development and successful integration into society.

The ascent of the inclusive education movement accentuates its reliance on pathologizing paradigms deeply entrenched in the foundations of traditional special or institutionalized education. Over its recent history, the application of a positivist research and practice approach for neurodivergent students or children experiencing prolonged institutionalization, whether in segregated or integrated mainstream classrooms, has perpetuated a disability-fixing ideology. In contrast, the neurodiversity, inclusive, and intercultural framework takes an integrative stance, encompassing psychosocial, sociocultural, and political elements to disrupt the systematic categorization of diverse neurological and cognitive embodiments and expressions as threatening "learning disorders." Traditionally, such conditions are addressed through cures, training, masking, or behavioral interventions within the classroom or institution (Acevedo & Nusbaum, 2020).

By centering on the personal lived experiences and perspectives of neurotypical, neurodiverse, and institutionalized children, an emancipatory lens emerges. This lens serves as a platform for representing and embodying neurological, socioemotional, or economic differences outside the deficit-based discourses and practices of traditional special or institutionalized education. The emphasis on socioemotional learning and the promotion of cultural agency effectively challenges universalizing assumptions about whose students are deemed "educable" and under what auspices concepts such as agency, care, self-awareness, and social consciousness are constructed and incorporated into general education curricula.

An increasing number of children from institutionalized educational backgrounds are entering academic environments without the essential skills for success. In this chapter, our concern extends beyond cognitive abilities to encompass the social and emotional skill deficits that we find particularly problematic. We examine the recognition of family and community risk factors, such as affective deprivation and educational neglect associated with prolonged institutionalization. We explore strategies to address these issues within educational spaces, emphasizing socioemotional learning as a crucial component that can be fostered in both institutionalized and non-institutionalized settings.

Our focus is on providing the foundation for the development of social-emotional skills, shedding light on various programs that educators and policymakers should be aware of. These initiatives are essential for supporting children at risk of academic underperformance due to deficits in social and emotional skills. By understanding the impact of institutionalization on socioemotional development and implementing effective programs, we aim to contribute to the creation of educational environments that foster holistic skill development in children.

Social and Emotional Learning (SEL) represents a strengths-based, developmental process that initiates from birth and continues to evolve across the entire lifespan (Weissberg et al., 2015). This comprehensive process involves the acquisition of skills by children, adolescents, and adults to foster healthy development and well-being within relationships. Key components of SEL include emotion regulation, self-awareness, and social consciousness. Through SEL, individuals cultivate the necessary tools to navigate and contribute positively to their emotional landscape, fostering meaningful connections and promoting overall emotional and social well-being.

Intercultural education focuses on cultural diversity as opposed to merely addressing those who are culturally different. It rejects romanticized notions of diversity and stresses the importance of cultivating the ability to live together creatively in today's global context. Intercultural education aims to go beyond traditional boundaries, viewing diversity—such as races, ethnic groups, or environments marked by affective deprivation—as a valuable force for mutual enrichment rather than a weakness to overcome. The approach involves promoting optimal development, fostering intercultural relations, eliminating prejudice, and providing quality education for all, with the ultimate goal of contributing to a more just and united society. Implementation involves shaping the curriculum to develop intercultural skills, including cultural self-awareness, enhanced communication, and positive attitudes toward diverse cultures (Schmelkes, 2013).

This study was conducted from an inclusive and intercultural perspective to explore the strengths, cognitive abilities, and socioemotional capacities of a group of institutionalized children aged between 8 and 12 years. The primary objective is to formulate an intervention proposal grounded in Neuroeducation and Socioemotional Education, aiming to facilitate the complete restoration of their rights, foster social integration, promote inclusion in a socio-familial system, and reduce their conditions of vulnerability. Masten's (2011) Risk and Resilience Model served as the theoretical framework, guiding the development and implementation of this study. The utilization of this model reflects a comprehensive approach that considers both the challenges and protective factors influencing the development of institutionalized children, contributing to the formulation of targeted and effective interventions.

Methodology

A non-experimental, cross-sectional, quantitative study with descriptive and correlational scope was conducted.

Participants

A total of 34 male children in residential care participated, ranging in age from 9–13 years (mean age = 10.5, standard deviation (SD) = 1.13). They were intentionally and non-probabilistically selected from a publicly funded social assistance house that serves children in vulnerable conditions. The institutional authorities determined the feasibility, relevance, and ethics of the study. Once approved, the general purpose of the study was explained to the participants. Every child participated voluntarily with informed consent. Descriptive, correlation and mean difference analyses were performed using Jamovi software version 2.3.28.0, depending on the measurement level of the variables.

Instruments

- *Intelligence Assessment*: Based on theory of fluid and crystallized intelligence (Cattell, 1963), Colored Progressive Matrices Test (Raven et al., 1998) was applied to assess non-verbal reasoning. An incomplete figure is presented, and the child must choose from 6 possible answers, with one point awarded for each correct answer, and a maximum score of 36. To evaluate verbal reasoning, the

Verbal Analogies Test (Ramírez-Benítez et al., 2016) was used. An incomplete sentence is presented in the format "A is to B as C is to D" with 4 possible answers (D, E, F, G). One point is awarded for each correct answer, with a maximum score of 16.

- *Words and Pseudowords Reading Task*: This test evaluates the use of phonological and lexical reading strategies. Stimuli were presented one by one on a computer, and each child had to read as quickly as possible. Reading speed was recorded via a microphone, and accuracy was indicated on the keyboard. The variables recorded include reading speed for words and pseudowords, as well as reading efficiency for both routes. The variant by Reigosa (2019) was utilized.
- *Oral Reading and Comprehension Test*: A text was presented on the screen (Reigosa-Crespo et al., 2020), which each child had to read aloud. Subsequently, they were asked a series of 10 true or false questions to assess reading comprehension. The reading time of the text and reading efficiency were also recorded. Reading efficiency is calculated by dividing the reading speed of texts by the comprehension score.
- *Mental arithmetic*: The consolidation of the direct route of mental calculation was assessed (Reigosa-Crespo et al., 2011). Two sets of 15 additions, 15 subtractions, and 15 multiplications were presented, and each child had to solve them. The motor reaction time was calibrated beforehand as an individual measure for each participant. Each numerical operation was presented in the form "3+2," and two possible answers were shown, for example, 5 and 6. Each child selected the correct answer on the keyboard.

Procedure

Each child was individually assessed on a laptop, where each test was presented. There was no time limit during the application. Researchers administered each test, controlling the lighting of the room and ensuring it was quiet and peaceful. Only two children were unable to take the mental calculation test as they had not acquired the necessary arithmetic procedures for this test.

Results

Descriptive Analysis of Cognitive Variables

Table 1 displays the percentage of children with typical and atypical development in each variable. To assign the atypical label, it is analyzed whether the child falls below 2 standard deviations compared to the theoretical mean of each variable. More than half of the evaluated population (55.9%) exhibited difficulties in verbal

Table 1 Descriptive analysis of variables

Variables	Mean	SD	Minimum	Maximum	Outliers	Percentage of outliers	Typical	Percentage of typical
Verbal analogies	10.294	3.850	2	16	19	55.9%	15	44.1%
Matrix sequences	25.147	5.361	13	34	2	5.9%	32	94.1%
Speed of word reading	2213.662	836.706	1242.500	4672.00	6	17.6%	28	82.4%
Efficiency of word reading	5588.587	12333.49	617.5	58776.5	8	23.5%	26	76.5%
Speed of pseudoword reading	2535.235	1003.464	0.01	4750.0	4	11.8%	30	82.2%
Efficiency of pseudoword reading	12101.092	24204.517	843.857	91949.0	14	41.2%	20	58.8%
Reading speed	12009.147	10559.258	5625	66921	3	8.8%	31	91.2%
Reading efficiency	96.772	196.826	24.316	1195.02	6	17.6%	28	82.4%
Comprehension index	0.765	0.155	0.400	1.0	4	11.8%	30	88.2%
Efficiency in exact calculation	5306.353	1866.885	2925.333	9428.57	24	75%	8	25%
Efficiency in addition	5534.839	2465.329	2967.742	14344.0	19	59.4%	13	40.6%
Efficiency in subtraction	5833.417	2771.109	2883.2	14769.23	16	50%	16	50%
Efficiency in multiplication	4950.546	1914.223	2677.677	10579.2	26	76.5%	8	23.5%

SD Standard deviation

reasoning. This test relies on previously learned knowledge and the influence of cultural aspects, making its content a good indicator of vocabulary development. On the other hand, only 5.9% of the children reached an atypical label in the matrix reasoning test, where problem-solving with visual content through inductive-deductive reasoning is not appropriate.

In reading, 82.4% of the population demonstrated an adequate word reading speed with 76.5% accuracy. For the use of the phonological route, 82.2% read pseudowords with 58.8% accuracy, which is lower compared to the lexical route. Depending on the phonological route is slower for children with difficulties or those in the process of acquiring reading skills. About 91.2% of the population has a normal text reading speed, with 88.2% capable of understanding to some extent. This results in lower reading efficiency, making reading activities faster. Around 82.4% of the population scores lower in this variable, as it is inversely proportional, indicating that a lower value allows the child to read and comprehend the text without difficulties.

However, in the area of mathematics, there are more areas of opportunity. The direct route of mental calculation has not yet consolidated, with only 25% of the sample able to solve different mathematical operations (addition, subtraction, and multiplication) without any additional assistance, such as counting on fingers. Efficiency in accurate calculation increases. Multiplication operations pose the primary challenge for children, leading to significantly greater cognitive fatigue and longer response times compared to addition (59.4% atypical development) and subtraction (50% atypical development) mathematical operations.

Correlations of Reading and Arithmetic Variables

Table 2 shows that word reading speed scores significantly correlated with word reading efficiency ($r = 0.733$, $p < 0.001$), pseudoword reading efficiency ($r = 0.871$, $p < 0.001$), reading speed ($r = 0.414$, $p < 0.05$), and reading efficiency ($r = 0.521$, $p < 0.01$). Word reading efficiency only correlated with pseudoword reading efficiency ($r = 0.888$, $p < 0.001$). Regarding reading and comprehension, it is essential to note that text reading speed significantly correlated with reading efficiency ($r = 0.943$, $p < 0.001$) but did not correlate with comprehension ($r = -0.322$, $p > 0.05$), although the latter showed a negative correlation with the measure of reading efficiency ($r = -0.437$, $p < 0.01$).

In Table 3, it is shown that efficiency in exact calculation positively correlates with efficiency in addition ($r = 0.764$, $p < 0.001$), efficiency in subtraction ($r = 0.844$, $p < 0.001$), and efficiency in multiplication (0.586, $p < 0.001$). Efficiency in addition significantly correlates with efficiency in subtraction ($r = 0.498$, $p < 0.01$) but not with efficiency in multiplication ($r = 0.340$, $p > 0.05$). Additionally, efficiency in subtraction correlates with efficiency in multiplication ($r = 0.408$, $p < 0.05$).

Table 2 Correlation matrix of reading variables

	Word reading speed	Word reading efficiency	Pseudoword reading speed	Pseudoword reading efficiency	Reading speed	Reading efficiency	Comprehension index
Word reading speed	—						
Word reading efficiency	0.733***	—					
Pseudoword reading speed	0.296	−0.131	—				
Pseudoword reading efficiency	0.871***	0.888***	0.086	—			
Reading speed	0.414*	0.216	0.408*	0.391*	—		
Reading efficiency	0.521**	0.328	0.350*	0.506**	0.943***	—	
Comprehension index	−0.229	−0.205	−0.038	−0.292	−0.322	−0.437**	—

Note. $*p < .05$, $**p < .01$, $***p < .001$

Table 3 Correlation matrix of arithmetic calculation variables

	Efficiency in exact calculation	Efficiency in addition	Efficiency in subtraction	Efficiency in multiplication
Efficiency in exact calculation	—			
Efficiency in addition	0.764***	—		
Efficiency in subtraction	0.844***	0.498**	—	
Efficiency in multiplication	0.586***	0.340	0.408*	—

Note. $^{*}p < .05$, $^{**}p < .01$, $^{***}p < .001$

Discussion

The significance of this study is pioneering in Mexico, as it identifies and characterizes the cognitive learning abilities of a group of institutionalized children.

Crystalized intelligence, which involves culturally learned knowledge, underscores the importance of speech development and vocabulary acquisition in cognitive and academic development. Verbal reasoning plays a crucial role in influencing reading skills, and children with poor performance in this task may encounter difficulties in more intricate reading tasks, such as comprehension and silent reading (Ramírez-Benítez et al., 2016). This research contributes to filling a gap in understanding the cognitive capacities of institutionalized children, shedding light on crucial aspects that can impact their academic development and overall well-being.

The acquisition of reading represents a pivotal milestone in social and cognitive development during the early years of schooling. The primary aim of early education is for each child to adeptly name symbolic stimuli, such as letters and numbers, through the retrieval of long-term memory until mastering both reading routes. This initiates with the phonological route in the early years of schooling, gradually evolving into a stage where expert readers predominantly rely on the lexical route (Mosquera et al., 2016; Sanabria et al., 2009). Understanding and facilitating this progression is essential for educators and caregivers to support children's effective development as readers.

The relationship between reading efficiency, reading comprehension, and text reading speed is interconnected. Reading efficiency, defined by the ability to read accurately and quickly, is closely linked to reading speed, with faster reading often associated with improved performance in comprehension tasks. However, the relationship between speed and comprehension is intricate, as excessively fast reading can negatively impact comprehension by overlooking crucial details. Reading comprehension relies not only on speed but also on the reader's capacity to analyze and relate information in the text (Jiang et al., 2012). Striking a balance between speed and comprehension is essential for effective reading skills.

The study identified several areas of opportunity in the processes of solving arithmetic operations. According to the functional neuroanatomical model of

Dehaene and Cohen (1995), a direct route for solving arithmetic problems is mentioned, manifested in the memory of numerical facts and verbal sequences for overlearned mathematical operations. The research indicates that the direct route of mental calculation has not yet fully consolidated in most children. This is attributed to the need to strengthen the memory of numerical facts, comprehend the abstract concept of arithmetic operations, and apply procedures correctly.

Furthermore, Yang et al. (2017) suggest the existence of different neural networks for addition and subtraction operations. Subtraction is considered more challenging than addition due to the involvement of phonological and visual processes in the mental representation of numerosity. Understanding these cognitive processes is crucial for developing targeted interventions to enhance arithmetic skills in children.

The consolidation of the memory of numerical facts is a time-consuming process that demands slow and complex cognitive strategies to arrive at the correct result (Estévez et al., 2019). To tackle these challenges, it is essential to implement teaching methods that foster a conceptual understanding of multiplication. Strategies such as problem-based learning and linking multiplications to real-world situations can render the process more meaningful. Additionally, regular practice and the integration of educational games can enhance the learning experience, making it more engaging and motivating. This approach facilitates the assimilation of multiplications through the use of concrete materials and calculation practices in the classroom (Lampert, 1986). Implementing diverse and interactive teaching methods can contribute to a more comprehensive and effective learning experience for students.

Incorporating playful activities into the learning process ensures an emotionally stable environment, fostering feelings of optimism, satisfaction, tranquility, calmness, and achievement, as suggested by Pekrun (2014). On the contrary, constant exposure to situations of high stress, often stemming from vulnerability and violence, can lead to emotions such as sadness, disappointment, discouragement, rejection, and boredom. These emotional experiences trigger detrimental neurocognitive changes in crucial brain structures like the amygdala, hippocampus, and thalamus, which are fundamental for learning. Unfortunately, the consequences of such exposure are more pronounced when experienced at a younger age, influencing future behaviors and learning outcomes (Glejzer et al., 2019). Creating a positive and engaging learning environment through playful activities becomes particularly crucial in mitigating the impact of stress and promoting healthy cognitive development in children.

Proposal for a Neuroeducational and Socioemotional Model

Based on the obtained results and drawing from Masten's Risk and Resilience Model (2011) and in alignment with Mexican regulations, a proposal for psychopedagogical intervention centered on Neuroeducation and Socioemotional Education was crafted to facilitate the development of institutionalized children's potentials and help them overcome their conditions of vulnerability. The implementation of a neuroeducation program is deemed necessary as a targeted intervention strategy for neurocognitive development. According to Reigosa-Crespo et al. (2020), this strategy should be grounded in the following assumptions:

1. *Closed cycle among alerts, neurocognitive profile, intervention, and monitoring*: Identify early signs of alerts in the school population, assess the learning profile of children, intervene, and provide necessary follow-up throughout the school cycle.
2. *Take advantage of ICTs*: Use evidence-based technological tools to diagnose, intervene, and provide corresponding follow-up by teachers and primary caregivers.
3. *Train teachers and caregivers*: Rely on the foundations of school neurocognition so that teachers can produce timely and well-directed interventions for the target population.
4. *Ecological approach*: Utilize tools and knowledge provided by neuroscience and school psychology in the classroom. This would be the primary place for neurocognitive intervention.

The analyzed data exemplify the need to look at and address the cognitive abilities of the population in residential care. The reviewed references provide insights into vulnerabilities and other elements in childhood, but they are limited to such characteristics. Therefore, it is urgent to focus on the potentials instead of solely concentrating on deficiencies in order to impact holistic development and facilitate social, institutional, group, and individual processes and expenditures that arise from the habit of fixing what is damaged instead of addressing crucial aspects. In this regard, the systemic solution-focused model applied to the school population, as proposed by Herrero & Beyebach (2018), seeks to influence well-being through the following premises:

1. Recognize each child as the protagonist of infinite personal resources to improve solutions within their context.
2. Pay attention to particular possibilities to address cases through specific interactional behaviors instead of focusing on labels and limitations.
3. Consider childhood and adolescent issues as products of social factors rather than individual pathologies.

Similarly, the appreciative intervention proposed by Varona (2007) suggests an approach centered on strengths to bring about changes in private and/or government institutions working with diverse populations. This model aims to achieve objectives through equal collaboration, cooperation, commitment, and self-motivation. In line with this, Tagurum et al. (2015) emphasize the urgency of addressing current difficulties to resolve long-term vulnerability needs and point out that emotional skills should take precedence.

Resilience models suggest the possibility of reducing certain influences or vulnerability factors by strengthening protective influences. In this regard, risk-oriented interventions seek to reduce and prevent exposure to conditions that could threaten human development, such as preventing homelessness and ending armed conflicts. On the other hand, interventions aimed at potentials seek to increase protective factors such as providing food, medical care, housing, income, schools, books, recreational centers, neighborhood safety, and effective caregivers. It is anticipated that the incorporation of such assets will contribute to good adaptation in the majority of children and young people (Masten, 2011).

In conclusion, this research lays the groundwork for working with institutionalized male children from an intercultural, inclusive perspective that guarantees rights, aiming at promoting their cognitive and socioemotional well-being for their full integration into society. It is essential to consider that to enhance cognitive skills in all learning, it is important to promote emotional states such as enjoyment, calmness, and pride to increase autonomy, independence, motivation, and, of course, emotional regulation, coping, and resilience strategies throughout childhood, i.e., starting from a neuroeducation model. The results obtained show the need to generate evidence-based intervention strategies, allowing the acquisition of reading and numerical learning processes to develop according to the age and grade level of the assessed children, intending to improve their cognitive and emotional well-being and, therefore, the full restitution of their rights.

Regarding the limitations of this research, it is necessary to include a female sample in future studies, allowing for comparisons based on participants' gender. Similarly, it is important to assess general mastery skills, such as attention, executive functions, vocabulary, and the socioemotional profile of the participants.

References

Acevedo, S. M., & Nusbaum, E. A. (2020). Autism, neurodiversity, and inclusive education. In *Oxford research encyclopedia of education*. Oxford University Press.

Balluerka, N., Aliri, J., Goñi-Balentziaga, O., & Gorostiaga, A. (2023). Association between bullying victimization, anxiety and depression in childhood and adolescence: The mediating effect of self-esteem. *Revista de Psicodidáctica, 28*(1), 26–34. https://doi.org/10.1016/j.psicoe.2022.11.001

Cattell, R. B. (1963). Theory of fluid and crystallized intelligence: A critical experiment. *Journal of Educational Psychology, 54*(1), 1. https://doi.org/10.1037/h0046743

Deambrosio, M., Vázquez, M., Arán-Filippetti, V., & Román, F. (2018). Efectos del maltrato en la neurocognición. Un estudio en niños maltratados institucionalizados y no institucionalizados. *Revista Latinoamericana de Ciencias Sociales, Niñez y Juventud, 16*(1), 239–253. https://doi.org/10.11600/1692715x.16114

Dehaene, S., & Cohen, L. (1995). Towards an anatomical and functional model of number processing. *Mathematical Cognition, 1*(1), 83–120. https://doi.org/10.1155/2014/461647

Elegbeleye, A. (2013). Predictors of the mental health of orphans and vulnerable children in Nigeria. *IFE PsychologIA, 21*(2), 170–180.

Elizondo, A., Rodríguez, J. V., & Rodríguez, I. (2018). La importancia de la emoción en el aprendizaje: Propuestas para mejorar la motivación de los estudiantes. *Revista de Didácticas Específicas, 19*, 37–42.

Estévez-Pérez, N., Castro-Cañizares, D., Martínez-Montes, E., & Reigosa-Crespo, V. (2019). Numerical processing profiles in children with varying degrees of arithmetical achievement. *Acta Psychologica, 198*, 102849. https://doi.org/10.1016/j.actpsy.2019.05.001

Fernández, O. M., Irarrázaval, M., Ortega, B., Carrasco, P., Martínez, P., Rojas, G., & Mundt, A. P. (2021). Salud mental primaria para niños, niñas y adolescentes institucionalizados: perspectiva de equipos de salud. *Revista Latinoamericana de Ciencias Sociales, Niñez y Juventud, 19*(2), 1–19. https://doi.org/10.11600/rlcsnj.19.2.4175

Fernández-Daza, M., & Fernández-Parra, A. (2017). Problemas de comportamiento, problemas emocionales y de atención en niños y adolescentes que viven en acogimiento residencial. *Psychologia, 11*(1), 57–70.

Glejzer, C., Ciccarelli, A., & Ricci, A. (2019). The incidence of emotions on learning processes in children and youth in contexts of social vulnerability. *Educación socioemocional: implicaciones teóricas y evidencias científicas*, 2448–6248.

Herrero, M., & Beyebach, M. (2018). *Intervención escolar centrada en soluciones. Conversaciones para el cambio en la escuela*. Herder.

Instituto Nacional para la Evaluación de la Educación [INEE]. (2018). *Planea. Resultados Nacionales 2018.* http://planea.sep.gob.mx/content/general/docs/2018/RESULTADOS_NACIONALES_PLANEA2018_INEE.pdf

Jiang, X., Sawaki, Y., & Sabatini, J. (2012). Word reading efficiency, text reading fluency, and reading comprehension among Chinese learners of English. *Reading Psychology, 33*(4), 323–349. https://doi.org/10.1080/02702711.2010.526051

Lampert, M. (1986). Knowing, doing, and teaching multiplication. *Cognition and Instruction, 3*(4), 305–342.

Martelo, O. M., & Arévalo, J. M. (2017). Funcionamiento cognitivo y estados emocionales de un grupo de niños y adolescentes con bajo rendimiento académico. *Revista Neuropsicología Latinoamericana, 9*(3), 13–22.

Masten, A. S. (2011). Resilience in children threatened by extreme adversity: Frameworks for research, practice, and translational synergy. *Development and Psychopathology, 23*(2), 493–506. https://doi.org/10.1017/S0954579411000198

Mosquera-Suárez, R., Torres, R., Reigosa-Crespo, V., González, E., & Valdés-Sosa, M. (2016). Written word processing as predictor of Spanish reading proficiency: A longitudinal study. *International Journal of Psychophysiology, 100*(108), 169. https://doi.org/10.1016/j.ijpsycho.2016.07.484

Novoa, P. F., Uribe, Y. C., Garro, L. L., & Cancino, R. F. (2021). Estrategias metacognitivas en entornos digitales para estudiantes con baja comprensión lectora. *Revista Electrónica de Investigación Educativa*, 1–34. https://doi.org/10.24320/redie.2021.23.e28.3953

Olsen, R., & De Montgomery, C. (2018). Revisiting out-of-home placed children's poor educational outcomes – Is school change part of the explanation? *Children and Youth Services Review, 88*, 103–113. https://doi.org/10.1016/j.childyouth.2018.03.005

Oppong, K., Meyer-Weitz, A., & Petersen, I. (2015). Correlates of psychological functioning of homeless youth in Accra, Ghana: A cross-sectional study. *International. Journal of Mental Health Systems, 9*(1). https://doi.org/10.1186/1752-4458-9-1

Organización de las Naciones Unidas para la Educación, la Ciencia y la Cultura (UNESCO). (2015). *Educación 2030. Declaración de Incheon y marco de acción para la realización del objetivo de desarrollo sostenible 4.* UNESCO https://unesdoc.unesco.org/ark:/48223/pf0000245656_spa

Organización para la Cooperación y el Desarrollo Económico [OCDE]. (2018). *Rendimiento matemático.* https://www.oecd.org/espanol/estadisticas/pisa-matematicas.htm

Pekrun, R. (2014). *Emotions and learning.* International Academy of Education. Educational Practices Series. UNESCO. http://www.ibe.unesco.org/

Porras, R. (2020). *Inteligencia emocional y relaciones interpersonales en estudiantes de V ciclo.* [Tesis de maestría, Universidad César Vallejo].

Ramírez-Benítez, Y., Torres-Diaz, R., & Amor-Diaz, V. (2016). Contribución única de la inteligencia fluida y cristalizada en el rendimiento académico. *Revista Chilena de Neuropsicología, 11*(2), 1–5. https://doi.org/10.5839/rcnp.2016.11.02.01

Raven, J., Raven, J., & Court, J. (1998). *Manual for Raven's progressive matrices and vocabulary scales. Part 2. Coloured progressive matrices*. Oxford Psychologist Press Ltd.

Reigosa-Crespo, V. (2019). *Education 2030 agenda's targets: Implementing neuroscience findings. Prospects*. (in press).

Reigosa-Crespo, V., Valdes-Sosa, M., Butterworth, B., Estévez, N., Rodríguez, M., Santos, E., Torres, P., Suarez, R., & Lage, A. (2011). Basic numerical capacities and prevalence of developmental dyscalculia: The Havana survey. *Developmental Psychology, 48*(1), 123–135. https://doi.org/10.1037/a0025356

Reigosa-Crespo, V., Valdes-Sosa, M., BuReigosa-Crespo, V., Castro-Cañizares, D., Estévez-Pérez, N., Santos, E., Torres, R., Mosquera, R., et al. (2020). Numerical skills and dyscalculia. From basic research to practice in Cuba (Habilidades numéricas y discalculia. De la investigación básica a la práctica en Cuba). *Studies in Psychology, 41*(2), 373–403. https://doi.org/10.1080/02109395.2020.1749502

Robledo, C. L. (2017). *Desarrollo emocional en niños y adolescentes de una casa hogar del DIF* [Tesis de licenciatura, Universidad Nacional Autónoma de México]. http://132.248.9.195/ptd2019/junio/0790499/Index.html

Rodríguez Juárez, G. (2016). Situación de los niños, niñas y adolescentes privados de cuidados parentales en México. *Entretextos, 8*(22), 1–14. https://doi.org/10.59057/iberoleon.20075316.201622393

Rodríguez, D., & Pérez, H. (2022). Revisión sobre el desarrollo educativo de los menores en acogimiento residencial. Una comparación internacional. *Perfiles Educativos, 44*(177), 183–198. https://doi.org/10.22201/iisue.24486167e.2022.177.60077

Sanabria Díaz, G., del Rosario Torres, M., Del, R., Iglesias, J., Mosquera, R., Reigosa, V., Santos, E., et al. (2009). Changes in reading strategies in school-age children. *The Spanish Journal of Psychology, 12*(2), 441–453. https://doi.org/10.1017/s1138741600001827

Schmelkes, S. (2013). Educación para un México intercultural. *Sinéctica, 40*, 01–12.

Secretaría de Educación Pública. SEP. (2019). *Rediseño del marco curricular común de la educación media superior 2019–2022*. Subsecretaría de Educación Media Superior.

Sölva, K., Haselgruber, A., & Lueger-Schuster, B. (2020). Latent classes of childhood maltreatment in children and adolescents in foster care: associations with ICD-11 PTSD and complex PTSD. *European Journal of Psychotraumatology, 11*(1) https://doi-org.pbidi.unam.mx:2443/10.1080/20008198.2020.1832757

Tagurum, Y., Chirdan, O., Bello, D., Afolaranmi, T., Hassan, Z., Iyaji, A., & Idoko, L. (2015). Situational analysis of orphans and vulnerable children in urban and rural communities of Plateau State. *Annals of African Medicine, 14*(1), 18–24. https://doi.org/10.4103/1596-3519.148714

Varona, F. (2007). La intervención apreciativa: Una nueva manera de descubrir, crear, compartir e implementar conocimiento para el cambio en instituciones gubernamentales o privadas. *Investigación & Desarrollo, 15*(2), 394–419.

Weissberg, R. P., Durlak, J. A., Domitrovich, C. E., & Gullotta, T. P. (2015). *Social and emotional learning: Past, present, and future.*

Yang, Y., Zhong, N., Friston, K., Imamura, K., Lu, S., Li, M., Zhou, H., Wang, H., Li, K. and Hu, B. (2017). The functional architectures of addition and subtraction: Network discovery using fMRI and DCM. *Human Brain Mapping, 38*(6), 3210–3225. https://doi.org/10.1002/hbm.23585

Ethnic Identity, Conflict, and Discrimination Among Ancient Nahuatl-Speaking Peoples

Jaime Echeverría-García

Introduction

Social exclusion and ethnic discrimination are not a product of the modern world; they have represented constant aspects of the interactions between different human groups through the ages. In the process of development of an ethnic identity, the boundaries define themselves for the group who sustains that identity. It brings about discrimination: members take their place within a group, differentiating themselves and distancing themselves from others. Otherwise, the boundaries of the ethnic identity would be diluted to the point of not being able to keep their members. It is clear that this primary meaning of discrimination points more to the differentiation between groups than to the systematic practices of harassment and segregation that one group inflicts on another due to their ethnic origin.

The purpose of this article is to outline the relationships that existed between ethnic identity, conflict, and discrimination between the populations that inhabited the Valley of Mexico on the eve of the Spanish Conquest. This geographical region was originally an endorheic basin made up of five lakes: to the north, the Zumpango and Xaltocan lakes; Lake Texcoco, in the central area; and to the south, the lakes of Xochimilco and Chalco. Today, the Valley of Mexico encompasses Mexico City and parts of the State of Mexico. It was inhabited mainly by Nahuatl-speaking populations, the Mexica or Aztecs being the best-known and dominant group in the region. Other non-Nahuatl-speaking ethnic groups that also inhabited the Valley were the Otomíes and, in smaller numbers, the Matlatzincas and Mazahuas. The Nahua populations were concentrated in the lake areas and the other ethnic groups in the mountains.

J. Echeverría-García (✉)
Humanities and Social Sciences Department, La Salle University Mexico, Mexico City, Mexico
e-mail: jaime.echeverria@lasalle.mx

S. Castaños-Cervantes et al. (eds.), *Working with Vulnerable Populations*, https://doi.org/10.1007/978-3-031-67710-6_14

Returning to our topic, the interest here lies in demonstrating that, in the particular case of Mexico, ethnic discrimination was present prior to colonial imposition. However, under no circumstance can we consider that the discrimination and racism that are experienced in the country today have their antecedents in pre-Hispanic times, since the historical relationships that were forged at that time were nothing like the relationships of inequality and oppression that ethnic groups have been experiencing since colonial times to the present day. Therefore, the importance of knowing about ethnic discrimination in pre-Hispanic times has two purposes: (1) to account for the universality of the phenomenon of discrimination over time and (2) not tend to idealize the forms of social relationship between ancient and current non-Western populations, thinking that the different indigenous groups, before the conquest, lived in a state of harmony. This helps us to measure the historical depth of discrimination and racism in Mexico and its complications in eradicating these phenomena, but it forces us to think about more suitable strategies to do so.

One way to approach the study of the relationships between the elements mentioned above is to identify the conflicts in the intergroup relations. While it has been demonstrated that simple interaction between groups promotes categories and stereotypes between groups and that the reference group is valued positively to the detriment of the other groups (Tajfel, 1984), it has also become apparent that conflicts in intergroup relations activate ethnic elements of identity and intensify them in such a way that the exaltation of the group itself and the stereotypes toward the other group become more evident (see Dijk, 2000; Sandstrom, 2008; Terraciano, 2013). A second approach is to take into account the worldview of the study groups to explain the way in which they processed intergroup relations. If we do not know the ideology of the peoples, we would fall into very superficial explanations and interpretations that would not result in any knowledge generation.

Intergroup interactions between the ancient Nahuas should be conceived as relationships between native, Nahuas themselves, and foreign groups, as Nahuatl-speaking peoples of different cities as non-Nahuatl-speaking peoples like Otomí and Huastec peoples, among other ethnic groups, which were largely concentrated around conflicts, such as the individual presence of strangers in the neighborhoods, the arrival of migratory groups looking for land to settle, the invasion of territorial borders, the competition for natural resources, and the separatist tendencies. Because shared history and place—in addition to kinship—were determining criteria in the building of ethnic identity, any situation that compromised the privacy or autonomy of cities and neighborhoods was seen as an attack on ethnic identity and, therefore, was against the moral and ethical values of a people. As access to land determined ethnic identity, foreigners living in the neighborhoods in which they did not own their own land created a differential situation that could border on exclusion (see Berdan, 2008; Chance, 2008; Escalante, 2004; Lockhart, 2013; Stark, & Chance, 2008).

The work material to be used are the published historical sources that were elaborated mainly during the 16th and 17th centuries and that refer to the history and culture of the Nahua peoples who inhabited not only the Valley of Mexico but also the Central Highlands.[1]

Additionally, I will have at my disposal the studies, carried out by specialists, that were conducted on these groups and that mainly talk about issues of identity and intergroup relations.

The article is divided into two parts. The first one provides information about the *altepetl*—a concept in the Nahuatl language that refers to the city-state: the elements that constituted it, its origins, and its role in shaping the identity of its members—and an overview of inter-ethnic relations between Nahua groups. The second part offers two historical examples in which the relationships between ethnic identity, conflict, and discrimination were connected.

Altepetl and Ethnic Identity

The Nahua *altepetl* was the independent political entity similar to the city-state. The concept alludes to two essential elements: the sacred hill, the residence of the tutelary deity, and the source of water, which indicated the physical and agricultural subsistence of its inhabitants. These elements show how the notion of *altepetl* linked the social, natural, and supernatural realms (Navarrete, 2011a; see Reyes, 1996). This political entity then had a defined territory and a sacred center (Navarrete, 2011a; Lockhart, 2013; Horn, 1997). Other elements inherent to the *altepetl* were the ruler's palace and the market (Horn, 1997; Lockhart, 2013). In a concise way, María Castaneda (2013, p. 71) defines it as "a sovereign territory inhabited by a multi-ethnic population." Each *altepetl* built an ethnic identity linked to political power and territory.

The constituent parts of the *altepetl* were called *calpulli* or *tlaxilacalli*. The *calpulli* arose both from a process of division of a previous unit of people and from a process of addition in which the *altepetl* welcomed foreigners who were settled in well-differentiated *calpulli*, either as refugees or as part of a systematic administrative measure of inserting peoples in different *altepetls* (Gibson, 2000; Berdan, 2008; Lockhart, 2013). As Charles Gibson (2000: 26) well points out, "the result was the formation of enclaves, not mixtures, of populations." This is reflected in the names of the *calpulli* that made up the *altepetl*, which in most cases referred to geographic features or ethnic affiliation (Lockhart, 2013). So, we have, for example, two *calpulli* in Tulancingo that were called Colhuacan and Mexicatzinco, which would surely be populated by Colhuas and Mexicas (Carrasco, 1963), and Chimalhuacan included a *calpulli* also called Colhuacan, possibly inhabited by Colhuas (Gibson, 2000). So, "...while the *altepetl* was often multi-ethnic, the small *calpulli* more often exhibited a unique ethnic composition" (Berdan, 2008, p. 109).

[1]This region includes the Basin of Mexico in the center, the Morelos Valley in the south, the Puebla-Tlaxcala Valley in the east, and the Toluca Valley in the west.

The multi-ethnicity that characterized the Postclassic city-states (900/1000–1521 AD) was the product of the great demographic mobility caused by the climate of political instability and adverse environmental conditions. Therefore, successive waves of various ethnic groups who migrated together (see Kirchhoff, 2002/1962) came to settle in certain areas of the Mesoamerican territory. This trait had its first manifestations in the transitional Epiclassic period (650/800–900/1000 AD) (López Austin & López Luján, 1997).

According to indigenous historical traditions, the origins of the human groups, or at least of those who considered themselves Chichimecs,[2] were found in cavernous places. Chicomoztoc, the place of the seven caves, was one of the most common. The different groups waited separately in each of the caves, and they came out at different historical moments, each with its patron deity, from whom they received their language, particular customs, divine image, sacred bundle, and profession (López Austin & López Luján, 1999).

During the migration, the human groups went on a pilgrimage in various subgroups of different ethnic affiliations or came to differentiate themselves along the way. In the times of Chichimec Xólotl, the Acolhuas arrived in the Anahuac region divided into three "biases"—the Tepanecas, the Otomí, and the Acolhuas themselves—and "each of them had a different language, each bringing its chief and lord" (Alva Ixtlilxóchitl, 1997, Volume II, Chapter V, p. 17). While the Mexicas, Tarascos, and Malinalcas formed a single migratory group of the same language and guided by the same deity, because of dissensions inland, the original group split along the way, in such a way that the Tarascos and the Malinalcas lived in different geographical areas, and they even, in the case of the first ones, changed their language, according to the information gathered by Friar Diego Durán (2002, Volume I, Book I, Chapter III).

Once the Nahua groups had reached their final destination, the takeover of the territory would provide legitimacy vis-à-vis their neighbors. That was carried out through various means: through a long migration, through the conquest of neighboring towns, or through the transfer of land achieved by merits (Boone, 1998; Oudijk, 2002). The legitimacy of the territory also implied a political legitimacy, in such a way that the relationship by kinship with ancient peoples and the fusion of ethnic identities were equally necessary actions. According to Federico Navarrete (2011a, b), in the formation of the *altepetl* of the Valley of Mexico came about a transfer of cultural assets between peoples of different culture and identity, the Chichimecs and the Toltecs, which led to the construction of a new common Toltec-Chichimec identity. Some authors have emphasized that the Nahua ethnic identity was conceived in terms of place and history. The members of the *calpulli* shared a common history because their ancestors came from a particular place and came to settle after a long migratory period; while identifying with the *altepetl* invoked the idea of a common residence and participation in a political order. The ethnic logic was expressed, then,

[2]The different Nahua groups as well as the Purepecha, the Otomí and other peoples of the Sierra of Toluca, called themselves Chichimecs, because they had wandered through the northern lands and returned from there (Sahagún, 2002, Volume II, Book X, Chapter XXIX, pp. 978–979).

as follows: "all who belonged were from the same people, not because they were descendants of the same ancestors [...] but because they lived together in the same place and therefore shared a common history and common interests" (Chance, 2008, p. 136; see Brumfiel, 1994; Stark and Chance, 2008; Berdan, 2008).

History and territory, as well as kinship, were fundamental aspects that were found at the core of the construction of ethnic identity and that, at the same time, helped label the status of foreigners. The interrelation of these aspects is well reflected in the naming. Some of the personal names showed that the origin of the person or of their parents was found outside the community, that is, they highlighted the absence of kinship and friendship ties and, therefore, the absence of a shared history. Among the names used as nicknames recorded in the Cuernavaca censuses in the mid-sixteenth century were Don Pablo Campa huitz, "Where does he come from?"; Juan Quenitoloctzin, "What's his name?"; Juan Atonemac, "Not our inheritance (he is not ours)"; or Pedro Achane, "Homeless" (Lockhart, 2013, pp. 173–174, 178, table IV.2, 179, Table IV.3).

The territory, in particular, is a fundamental criterion to be able to conceptualize the outsider among the Nahuas and understand the interactions between natives and foreigners. This also explains that in conflicts over land and resources in pre-Hispanic and colonial times, ethnicity and ethnic stereotypes invariably came to light, as can be seen in some sources of indigenous tradition (see *Anales de Cuauhtitlán*, 1945; Sousa and Terraciano, 2003).

The *altepetl* provided its members the point of ethnic reference from which they positioned themselves with respect to the other groups and differentiated themselves from them. In the sixteenth-century Nahuatl documents, speaking of themselves or of their rivals, the Nahuas attached greater importance to the ethnicity of the local *altepetl* and *calpulli* than to the broader ethnic categories (Lockhart, 2013). Rebecca Horn (1997) also points out that, in the sixteenth century, the people of Coyoacan were aware of their Tepanecan identity, but instead of using this term in documents in Nahuatl, they invariably identified themselves as belonging to a particular *altepetl*.

From a strongly ethnocentric perspective supported by the *altepetl*, the inhabitants of central Mexico created a dichotomous vision of the various groups, where "we" corresponded to the *altepetl* itself and "they" to the rest of the *altepetl*. From his study of book XII of the *Florentine Codex*, James Lockhart (1993, pp. 14, 21) arrived at the conclusion that "any one *altepetl* has its friends and its enemies among the rest; from the point of view of each *altepetl*, all the others are outsiders." In the same way, Federico Navarrete (2004, pp. 40–41) affirms that "indigenous societies [of the Postclassic period] held very specific ethnic identities, which they defended with all the political and military means at their disposal, and that differentiated them and made their neighbors be their enemies."[3] Lockhart (2013, p. 36) also

[3] "... but" -continues the scholar- "they also had broader cultural identities, which allowed them to trade, dialogue and exchange ideas and people with their neighbors" (Navarrete, 2004, p. 41).

implies that the ethnic identity of the large political units motivated constant "rivalries and feelings of independence and superiority."

The pronounced ethnicity of the *altepetl* was also observed at *calpulli* level; in fact, Frances Berdan (2008) points out that at this level ethnicity surely acquired its greatest meaning. The *calpulli* exhibited a strong sense of micro-patriotism, which could sometimes be accentuated by ethnic differences. And under the right conditions, separatist tendencies could easily emerge among the *calpulli* in the *altepetl* (Horn, 1997).

In line with the above, Rudolf van Zantwijk (1973) states that there was no general trend toward fraternization within ethnic groups or even toward equality of rights between them but that there was also no general trend toward strong ethnic discrimination, persecution of minority groups, or destruction of different ethnic groups. As a rule, such discriminatory trends were clearly frowned upon. This interethnic "tolerance" was closely linked to the principles of social and cosmic organization. Each ethnic group played a role in the system at a certain time: one group was in charge of military functions; another, of the priests; while another one of agricultural or artisanal activities.[4] Likewise, each ethnic group was associated with a certain deity, various dates in the calendar, certain direction, and cosmic designation.

The management model of the ethnic groups was based on myth, among other elements. From there, social relations, political alliances, kinship networks, and friendship between the patron deities were created and justified, which favored the proximity between two villages (López Austin, 1994). Similarly, two deities distanced one from another led to their peoples not recognizing each other and not entering into a relationship of equality. A clear example is found in the document called the *Anales de Cuauhtitlán* (1945, p. 46). When the inhabitants of Cuauhtitlan requested an alliance with the Acolhuas, "they pleaded because they were known for their ancestry and for the arrow and for their god named Mixcohuatl." And they added "that the Tepanecs, whose weapon was the sling, were not their neighbors and that they did not recognize them, because their god was the so called Cuecuex, and that they were not their equals."

Under a situation of political and social stability, the assignment to an ethnic group of a social and cosmic function and order in the great cultural mosaic of the Central Highlands could effectively serve as a way to contain the violent actions of the states against their neighbors. However, in a turbulent Postclassic context, the dominant note was conflict rather than stability. The constant dynamic resided in struggles between the *altepetl* in order to get political control and resources not available in the territory itself. It is precisely in the context of domination or competition that ethnic identity becomes important, both at the level of self-recognition

[4]The idea of performance of social activities based on ethnic criteria was previously pointed out by Paul Kirchhoff (2002/1962, p. 81) and Pedro Carrasco (1971, p. 462).

and of recognition by others (Stark, 2008; Sandstrom, 2008; Terraciano, 2013).[5] So, as Berdan (2008) points out, ethnic interests in central Mexico were rarely active during daily life.

However, recognition of ethnic differences and aggressive actions directed against them may not have necessarily been conditioned by conflict but may have been motivated by the ethnic minority status of some groups. Although the *altepetl* of Coyoacan was predominantly Tepanec, in the mid-sixteenth century the Mexica and Otomí minorities were present and were living in different neighborhoods in mountain environments. In the 1553 inspection, for example, many residents complained that the nobleman of Coyoacan, Don Luis Quauhnochtli, harassed "all the neighborhoods that are next to the mount that belong to them Otomíes and to them Mexicans" (Carrasco & Monjarás-Ruiz, 1976, Volume I, p. 112, see Horn, 1997). Although this information dates from the Colony, I think it can refer us to a practice from earlier times.

The trend toward the separation of the *altepetl*, so characteristic of the pre-Hispanic era, continued to a certain extent during the colonial period, despite the implementation of the congregation process. This consisted of the reduction in number of Indian villages and of their settling in a different place. The demographic dispersion in a vast conquered territory hindered the work of evangelization, the political control of the population, the use of natural resources, and the possibility of using that population as a source of manpower. This panorama caused the state to authorize the resettlement of the population (Torre Villar, 1995), which resulted sometimes in new associations of peoples of different ethnic affiliation (Gibson, 2000; Horn, 1997).

This process was not uniformly successful. In the seventeenth century, populations in many cities resisted being displaced by alleging long-standing hostility between them. And in the case of the populations already settled in the congregation, this argument was good enough for them to be relocated. Other reasons given to avoid resettlement were the permanence near ancestral lands and their agricultural quality, the good climate of their territory, and the maintenance of ties of kinship and friendship, since their relocation to a different territory would make them foreigners (Haskett, 1991; Gibson, 2000). A good example is of the Indians who lived in the villages of Santa Ana and San Ildefonso and of the carpenters of Tlalpujahua, who resisted their congregation in the early seventeenth century: as they are all "of a Mazahua nation and language," "if they were taken to Ucareo [...] they would not have peace and quiet because they were from different nations," as there lived the Otomíes (Torre Villar, 1995, pp. 227–228).

[5] Inter-ethnic relations, Navarrete points out (2004, p. 31), "are always social relations of power, that is to say [...] they are relations of political domination, social control and economic exploitation."

Ethnic Identity, Conflict, and Discrimination Among Pre-Hispanic Nahuas

I am going to present two pre-Hispanic examples narrated by historical sources that tell us about the devaluation of the ethnic identity of the antagonistic group in conflict. In the two examples, a Nahuatl language group and a different language group are confronted. This is the first element of importance that we must consider in order to understand the relationship of feud between them, since language was a fundamental criterion of ethnic differentiation and a marking element of otherness. A different language led to an equally different cultural model: different deities, contrasting ways of treating the body, and contrasting customs and social practices, among other aspects.

The first example focuses on a prolonged conflict between the Chichimecs of Cuauhtitlan and the inhabitants of the city of Xaltocan, where the former spoke the Nahuatl language and the latter was of Otomí descent. Although Nahuas and Otomíes established continuous commercial exchanges during the Postclassic period (Escalante, 2004, p. 202), the relationship between them kept on being marked by criticism, blame, and contempt, which the Nahuas expressed toward its neighbors settled in the peripheral mountain areas of the Valley of Mexico. The Nahuas despised the Otomíes, among other things, for not respecting social differences, for dressing and adorning themselves excessively, and for their immoderate sexual practices and alcohol consumption (Echeverría, 2009; Escalante, 2002, 2004).

According to the *Anales de Cuauhtitlán*, it all started with the conflict that existed between the Mexicas and the Xaltocamecs when, during their pilgrimage, the first one settled in Chapultepec. Due to the friendship that Mexicas had with the Chichimecs of Cuauhtitlan, they inherited the feud with the Xaltocamecs (*Anales de Cuauhtitlán*, 2011).

The ruler Quinatzin of Cuauhtitlan ordered all the Chichimec nobles to no longer be friends with the Xaltocamecs; that "they were never to be friends; and they should never come to their side again." And so it was, as sometimes the Xaltocamecs went to the mount; there, they were attacked by the Chichimecs. In addition, they insulted them by calling them *tlilhuipilleque*, "the owners of black *huipiles*," as well as Nonohualcas and Cozcatecas (*Anales de Cuauhtitlán*, 1945, p. 19).

The hatred for the Xaltocamecs was passed on to the next generations of Cuauhtitlan. Over time, a Chichimec group settled in Tlalcozpan. While there, each time the Xaltocamecs went to hunt quails up the Zoltepetl hill, they harassed them. The people of Cuauhtitlan wondered who the Xaltocamecs were, to which they replied: "We persecute those who will continue to harass us, because they are not good, but evil; they are the ones who made war on the *Mexitins*. And our *tlatoani* has ordered us to never be friends with the Xaltocamecs" (*Anales de Cuauhtitlán*, 2011, pp. 95). So, they attacked them.

During the reigns of Quinatzin and Tezcatlteuctli, the Chichimecs were harassing the Xaltocamecs, since their former rulers had made them known that they were their enemies. During the times under the ruling of Huactzin, the ultimate war against Xaltocan started. The Chichimecs began to fight them from various villages and forced them to move to different places (*Anales de Cuauhtitlán*, 1945, pp. 24–25). According to the historical document, the Xaltocamecs "no longer dared to rebel, because they feared the Chichimecs of Cuauhtitlan" (*Anales de Cuauhtitlán*, 2011, p. 97).

The war between these two people lasted one hundred years. After being defeated at Tecaman, they asked the people of Metztitlan and Tlaxcallan to settle in their domain. When questioned about their decision, the Xaltocamecs replied that "our enemies, the Chichimecs of Cuauhtitlan, are afflicting us and we are about to fall into their hands; they have been fighting us for a long time, since the war began in the days of our parents" (*Anales de Cuauhtitlán*, 2011, p. 99).

This story is one of the many displacements that the Otomíes were subjected to by Nahua peoples. To a large extent, the siege actions that the Nahuatl-speaking groups took against the Otomíes were determined and justified by the representations that had been made out of them based on their cultural difference. In the description above, we not only see exposed an inherited conflict but also the continuous harassment that people with ethnic affiliation different to that of their neighbors could suffer. One of these actions that gets attention are the insults that the Cuauhtitlans uttered to the Xaltocamecs, materialized in nicknames: *Tlilhuipilleque* and *Nonohualca*. Both are concepts in Nahuatl that respectively refer to women and foreigners of different languages.

A very common insult among the Nahua peoples—and other Mesoamerican groups—was the comparison of the defeated warrior with women in the context of war, as eluded in the nickname *Tlilhuipilleque*, which literally means "the owners of black *huipiles*." And on top of that, to confront him even more, they forced him to wear women's clothes (Alvarado Tezozomoc, 1944, Chapter XIII; Durán, 2002, Volume I, Book I, Chapter X; Acosta 2006, Book VI, Chapter XIV). That way, the feminization of the enemy symbolized their defeat and submission, that is, a state of passivity that was attributed to women.

The other insult, *Nonohualca*, referred to the status of foreigner that the Xaltocamecs had for those from Cuauhtitlan. As the Nahuatl language is the main criterion that defined the model of civilization exalted by the Nahua societies, any group that spoke a different language was put in a dimension that was on the edge of culture and morality, always defined from the ethnocentric vision of the Nahuas. Referring to the alien status of a group in derogatory terms denoted the contempt felt against them. It must also be said that the concept of *Otomitl*, which is the name given by the Nahuas to the speakers of the Otomí language, served as an insult within the Nahua society. So, the person who was incapable was affronted by the imputation of said name (Sahagún, 2002, Volume II, Book X, Chapter XXIX).

From the previous example, we can see how ethnic aspects played a role in relationships between adversaries, but when asked how far the enemy can be defined by its ethnicity, Frances Berdan (2008, p. 111) considers that it played a minor role in the military governments of central Mexico in the Late Postclassic period. Rather, "economic gain, strategic advantage, and maintenance of political legitimacy prevailed." Similarly, she affirms that ethnic considerations do not seem to have had a role in the elections or treatment of adversaries between the Mexicas and their allies.

This information should be taken with certain reservations. Although there are not many examples in historical sources that point to discrimination and harassment toward a group based on their ethnic identity, I consider that the above information is paradigmatic of a type of inter-ethnic relations that took place in Mesoamerica. And as proof of this, the second example I provide refers directly to such relationships.

One of the main criticisms that the Mexicas made to the Cuextecs (Huastecs) was about them piercing the septum to insert an ornament (Sahagún, 2002, Volume II, Book X, Chapter XXIX), as instead of reserving this practice for the noble or heroic warriors, as it was customary in Nahua societies, it was used without distinction of social class. And the aversion of the Mexicas to this custom was so great that when the empire defeated the Cuextecs under the rule of Ahuitzotl, they were taken to Tenochtitlan, pulled by cords that went through the holes they had in their noses, and thus they marched in a row, strung together (Durán, 2002, Volume I, Book I, Chapter, XLII; Alvarado Tezozomoc, 1944, Chapter LXV). This Huastec practice on the body was so striking that the Mexicas, and the various Nahua groups in general, made this feature the core of the Huastecs' ethnic identity. And it was reflected as such in the codices of Nahua tradition, where the Cuextecs are always represented in a grotesque way with a large perforation in the nose (Echeverría, 2009).

Conclusions

The study of inter-ethnic relations in pre-Hispanic Mexico shows us the social, psychological, and ideological elements that played a role during its development. They reflect the attitudes and behaviors that the ancient Nahua populations had toward the outsider and their culture and how they determined and justified the way they behaved toward it.

From a strongly ethnocentric view, the development of prejudices and stereotypes among the ancient Nahuas was highly encouraged, as it helped to clearly define ethnic borders between peoples. But although stereotypes fulfill a cultural function, discriminatory attitudes among peoples are based on these stereotypes. The examples from the past that refer to identity and discrimination should shed some light on the situation of ethnic discrimination that we experience in our country. Although we cannot look at discrimination in Mexico as having its antecedents in pre-Hispanic times, the information presented should make us reflect on the historical density of ethnic discrimination and its materialization in stereotypes, its process of development, the favorable contexts for such discrimination to happen, and the elements that played a part in it. This will be a first step in the arduous process of dismantling the prejudices and stereotypes that mestizo society has built on ethnic minorities and that has largely determined their condition of vulnerability.

I will end with a current example, but one whose duration is long-standing. Since pre-Hispanic times, the Nahuas conceived of the Otomíes as impulsive, unskillful, and excessive people in their way of dressing, among other aspects (Sahagún, 2002; Echeverría, 2009). When the Nahuas confronted their culture with that of the Otomíes, they judged the differences from an ethnocentric point of view, in such a way that any Otomí custom that clashed with the Nahua value system was harshly criticized and triggered the construction of negative representations about the Otomíes. Now, these representations have accompanied the Otomíes from pre-Columbian times to the present day, in such a way that, for example, the Nahuas of the municipality of Pahuatlán, in the Sierra Norte of the state of Puebla, who have the Otomíes of the town of San Pablito as neighbors, continue to reproduce them and have added others, such as being dangerous (Echeverría, 2019). This shows us the great strength these representations have had in the system of Nahua representations and their high functionality in the contexts of interethnic interaction. These types of representations, which take the form of ethnic stereotypes, have not gone unnoticed by the mestizo population of Pahuatlán, as they have assimilated them when hearing them from the Nahuas. This assimilation of stereotypes about the Otomíes ends up influencing the relationship that mestizos have with them, which has led, on a certain scale, to unequal treatment because they are perceived as untreatable and dangerous and which can lead to the Otomíes suffering discrimination. Here, we have a clear example of how the history of interethnic relations between pre-Hispanic peoples can shed light on understanding certain discriminatory practices against indigenous people today, as a first step in the eradication of this problem.

References

Alvarado Tezozomoc, H. (1944). Crónica Mexicana, escrita hacia el año de 1598 [Mexican Chronicle, Written Around the Year 1598]. Orozco y Berra, M. (Ed.) Editorial Leyenda.

Anales de Cuauhtitlán [Annals of Cuauhtitlan] (1945). In P. F. Velázquez (Ed.), *Códice Chimalpopoca. Anales de Cuauhtitlán y Leyenda de los Soles* (pp. 3–68). Universidad Nacional Autónoma de México, Instituto de Historia, Imprenta Universitaria.

Anales de Cuauhtitlán [Annals of Cuauhtitlan] (2011). In R. Tena (Ed.). Consejo Nacional para la Cultura y las Artes.

Berdan, F. (2008). Concepts of ethnicity and class in Aztec-Period Mexico. In F. Berdan et al. (Eds.), *Ethnic identity in Nahua Mesoamerica: The view from archaeology, art history, Ethnohistory, and contemporary ethnography* (pp. 105–132). The University of Utah Press.

Boone, E. (1998). Cartografía azteca: Presentaciones de geografía, historia y comunidad [Aztec Cartography: Presentations of geography, history and community]. *Estudios de Cultura Náhuatl, 28*, 17–38.

Brumfiel, E. (1994). Ethnic groups and political development in ancient Mexico. In E. M. Brumfiel & J. W. Fox (Eds.), *Factional competition and political development in the New World* (pp. 89–102). Cambridge University Press.

Carrasco, P. (1963). Los caciques chichimecas de Tulancingo [Chichimec Caciques of Tulancingo]. *Estudios de Cultura Náhuatl, 4*, 86–91.

Carrasco, P. (1971). The peoples of Central Mexico and their historical traditions. In G. Ekholm & I. Bernal (Eds.), *Archaeology of Northern Mesoamerica* (Vol. 11, Part II, pp. 459–473). In R. Wauchope (General Ed.), *Handbook of Middle American Indians*). University of Texas Press.

Carrasco, P. & Monjarás-Ruiz, J. (1976). Colección de documentos sobre Coyoacán (Visita del oidor Gómez de Santillán y su sujeto Tacubaya en el año de 1553) [Collection of Documents on Coyoacán (Visit of the Judge Gómez de Santillán and His Subject Tacubaya in the Year 1553)] (Vol. 1). Instituto Nacional de Antropología e Historia, Centro de Investigaciones Superiores.

Chance, J. (2008). Indigenous ethnicity in Colonial Central Mexico. In F. Berdan et al. (Eds.), *Ethnic identity in Nahua Mesoamerica: The view from archaeology, art history, Ethnohistory, and contemporary ethnography* (pp. 133–149). The University of Utah Press.

de Alva Ixtlilxóchitl, F. (1997). Historia de la nación chichimeca [History of Chichimec Nation]. In E. O'Gorman (Ed.), *Obras Históricas* (Vol. 1–2). Universidad Nacional Autónoma de México, Instituto de Investigaciones Históricas, Instituto Mexiquense de Cultura.

de la Castañeda Paz, M. (2013). *Conflictos y alianzas en tiempos de cambio: Azcapotzalco, Tlacopan, Tenochtitlan y Tlatelolco (siglos XII-XVI).* [Conflicts and Alliances in Changing Times: Azcapotzalco, Tlacopan, Tenochtitlan and Tlatelolco (12th through 16th Centuries)]. Universidad Nacional Autónoma de México, Instituto de Investigaciones Antropológicas.

de Sahagún, B. (2002). *Historia general de las cosas de la Nueva España* [General history of the things of New Spain]. In A. L. Austin & J. G. Quintana (Eds.), (Vol. 1–3). Consejo Nacional para la Cultura y las Artes, Cien de México.

Dijk van, T. A. (Trans.). (2000). *Ideología. Una aproximación multidisciplinaria.* [Ideology: A Multidisciplinary Approach]. Gedisa.

Durán, D. (2002). *Historia de las Indias de Nueva España e islas de tierra firme* [History of Indies of New Spain and Mainland Islands]. In R. Camelo & J. R. Romero (Eds.), (Vol. 1–2). Consejo Nacional para la Cultura y las Artes, Cien de México.

Echeverría. (2019). Representaciones nahuas sobre los 'otros' indígenas en el Municipio de Pahuatlán de Valle, Sierra Norte de Puebla [Nahua representations about the indigenous 'others' in the Municipality of Pahuatlán de Valle, Sierra Norte de Puebla]. *Dimensión Antropológica, 26*(77), 93–130.

Echeverría García, J. (2009). *Representación y miedo al otro entre los antiguos nahuas* [Representation and Fear to the Other among Ancient Nahuas]. Unpublished master 's thesis. Universidad Nacional Autónoma de México.

Escalante Gonzalbo, P. (2002). Primer espejo [First Mirror]. In E. Florescano (Coord.) (Ed.), *Espejo mexicano* (pp. 48–71). Consejo Nacional para la Cultura y las Artes, Fundación Miguel Alemán, A. C., Fondo de Cultura Económica.

Gibson, Ch. (Trans.). (2000). *Los aztecas bajo el dominio español 1519-1810.* [The Aztecs under Spanish Rule]. Siglo XXI.

Haskett, R. (1991). Indigenous Rulers. An Ethnohistory of Town Government in Colonial Cuernavaca. University of New Mexico Press.

Horn, R. (1997). *Postconquest Coyoacan. Nahua-Spanish relations in Central Mexico, 1519-1650.* Stanford University Press.

Kirchhoff, P. (2002/1962). Dos tipos de relaciones entre pueblos en el México antiguo [Two Types of Relationships among Peoples of Ancient Mexico]. In C. García Mora, L. Manzanilla, & J. Monjaráz-Ruiz (Eds.), *Paul Kirchhoff. Escritos selectos. Estudios mesoamericanos, Volumen 1 Aspectos Generales* (pp. 79–82). UNAM, Instituto de Investigaciones Antropológicas.

Lockhart, J. (1993). Introduction. In J. Lockhart (Ed.), *We people here: Nahuatl accounts of the Conquest of Mexico* (Vol. 1, pp. 1–46). University of California Press.

Lockhart, J. (2013). *Los nahuas después de la Conquista. Historia social y cultural de los indios del México central, del siglo XVI al XVIII.* [The Nahuas After the Conquest. A Social and Cultural History of the Indians of Central Mexico, Sixteenth Through Eighteenth Centuries]. Fondo de Cultura Económica.

López Austin, A. (1994). *Tamoanchan y Tlalocan.* [Tamoanchan and Tlalocan]. Fondo de Cultura Económica.

López Austin, A., & López Luján, L. (1997). *El pasado indígena.* [Indigenous Past]. Fondo de Cultura Económica, El Colegio de México.

López Austin, A., & López Luján, L. (1999). Mito y realidad de Zuyuá. Serpiente Emplumada y las transformaciones mesoamericanas del Clásico al Posclásico [Myth and Reality of Zuyuá. Feathered Serpent and the Mesoamerican Transformations from the Classic to Postclassic]. Colegio de México, Fideicomiso Historia de las Américas, Fondo de Cultura Económica.

Navarrete, F. (2011a). *Los orígenes de los pueblos indígenas del valle de México. Los altépetl y sus historias* [The Origins of Indigenous Peoples of Mexico's Valley. The *Altepetl* and its histories]. Universidad Nacional Autónoma de México, Instituto de Investigaciones Históricas.

Navarrete, F. (2011b). Chichimecas y toltecas en el valle de México [Chichimecs and Toltecs in Mexico's Valley]. *Estudios de Cultura Náhuatl, 42*, 19–50.

Navarrete, F. (2004). *Las relaciones interétnicas en México.* [Interethnic Relations in Mexico]. Universidad Nacional Autónoma de México, Dirección General de Publicaciones y Fomento Editorial.

Oudijk, M. (2002). La toma de posesión: un tema mesoamericano para la legitimación del poder [Taking of possession: A Mesoamerican theme for the legitimation of power]. *Relaciones, XXIII*(91), 95–131.

Escalante, P. (Coord.). (2004). La ciudad, la gente y las costumbres [City, People and Customs]. In *Mesoamérica y los ámbitos indígenas de la Nueva España* (Vol. I, pp. 199–230). In P. Gonzalbo Aizpuru (Dir.), *Historia de la vida cotidiana en México*). Fondo de Cultura Económica, El Colegio de México.

Reyes, L. (1996). El término calpulli en documentos del siglo XVI [The Term Calpulli in Documents of the 16th Century]. In Luis Reyes García et al. (Authors), Documentos nauas de la ciudad de México del siglo XVI (pp. 21–68). CIESAS, Archivo General de la Nación.

Sandstrom, A. R. (2008). Blood sacrifice, curing, and ethnic identity among contemporary Nahua of Northern Veracruz, Mexico. In F. Berdan et al. (Eds.), *Ethnic identity in Nahua Mesoamerica: The view from archaeology, art history, Ethnohistory, and contemporary ethnography* (pp. 150–182). The University of Utah Press.

Sousa, L., & Terraciano, K. (2003). The "Original Conquest" of Oaxaca: Nahua and Mixtec accounts of the Spanish Conquest. *Ethnohistory, 50*(2), 349–400.

Stark, B. (2008). Archaeology and Ethnicity in Postclassic Mesoamérica. In F. Berdan et al. (Eds.), Ethnic identity in Nahua Mesoamerica: The view from archaeology, art history, Ethnohistory, and contemporary ethnography (pp. 38–63). The University of Utah Press.

Stark, B., & Chance, J. (2008). Diachronic and multidisciplinary perspectives on Mesoamerican ethnicity. In F. Berdan et al. (Eds.), *Ethnic identity in Nahua Mesoamerica: The view from archaeology, art history, Ethnohistory, and contemporary ethnography* (pp. 1–37). The University of Utah Press.

Tajfel, H. (Trans.). (1984). *Grupos humanos y categorías sociales.* [Human Groups and Social Categories]. Herder.

Terraciano, K. (Trans.). (2013). *Los mixtecos de la Oaxaca colonial. La historia ñudzahui del siglo XVI al XVIII.* [The Mixtecs of Colonial Oaxaca. Ñudzahui History, Sixteenth trough Eigtheenth Centuries]. Fondo de Cultura Económica.

Torre Villar, E. (1995). Las congregaciones de los pueblos de indios. Fase terminal: aprobaciones y rectificaciones [Congregations of the Indian Peoples. Final Phase: Approvals and Rectifications]. Universidad Nacional Autónoma de México, Instituto de Investigaciones Históricas.

van Zantwijk, R. (1973). Politics and ethnicity in a Prehispanic Mexican state between the 13th and 15th centuries. *Plural Societies, 4*(2), 23–52.

The Role of Higher Education in Prison Settings

Cristina L. Reitz-Krueger, Morgan McConnell, and Julie Wilson

The United States has the highest incarceration rate in the world (Walmsley, 2010). At the end of 2016, 2.16 million Americans were incarcerated in state prisons, federal prisons, and jails (Kaeble & Cowhig, 2018). The incarceration rate skyrocketed in the 1980s and the 1990s during the War on Drugs, when drug use was disproportionately criminalized in Black communities (Alexander, 2012; Vesely-Flad, 2017). This situation compounded racial bias already existing in the US carceral system and in the culture at large to criminalize Black men (Alexander, 2012; Vesely-Flad, 2017).

The incarceration rate leveled off in the 2000s and, over the past decade, has begun to decline. However, Black people are still six times more likely to be incarcerated than White people (Gramlich, 2019). Furthermore, while the overall incarceration rate is declining, the rate of incarceration for women is rising, including for drug offenses, "fighting back against domestic violence," and sex work (Equal Justice Initiative, 2018). Currently, women comprise 7% of the overall incarcerated population in the United States.

Regardless of race, ethnicity, or gender, poverty exacerbates one's chances of being incarcerated, with people who are incarcerated earning 41% less than non-incarcerated peers just prior to their incarceration (Rabuy & Kopf, 2015). Incarceration increases socioeconomic vulnerability, as prison time carries "collateral consequences" beyond time served. Formerly incarcerated people face challenges to obtaining employment, education, housing, public benefits, and voting rights, with specific barriers varying by state and locale (Alexander, 2012; Vesely-Flad, 2017).

C. L. Reitz-Krueger (✉)
Department of Psychology, Warren Wilson College, Asheville, NC, USA
e-mail: creitz-krueger@warren-wilson.edu

M. McConnell · J. Wilson
Warren Wilson College, Asheville, NC, USA

S. Castaños-Cervantes et al. (eds.), *Working with Vulnerable Populations*,
https://doi.org/10.1007/978-3-031-67710-6_15

For many, then, incarceration may be viewed as the culmination of various vulnerabilities that predated their time in prison or jail. However, all incarcerated individuals share the particular vulnerabilities associated with their current loss of freedom and the constraints imposed by the penal system of which they are currently a part. An awareness of the pre-existing and current risks, challenges, and vulnerabilities faced by incarcerated individuals is necessary for effective work with this population. In this chapter, we consider the role of higher education inside detention centers. In particular, we address challenges and ethical concerns involved in teaching and conducting research with incarcerated individuals.

We would also like to note that, for the sake of ease, we use the term "prison" and "detention center" interchangeably to refer generally to any of the various facilities used to house those who are either awaiting trial or incarcerated as a result of a criminal conviction. Similarly, "prisoner" is sometimes used exclusively to refer to those held in a prison; when it is employed here, it refers to anyone who is currently incarcerated.

Post-Secondary Education in Prison

Access to college education in prison can change the culture of prison and also enhance opportunities for those leaving prison (Davis, 2018; Meyer et al., 2010). Currently, educators in the United States are seeking to differentiate "higher education in prison" from "correctional education" (Castro & Gould, 2018). Correctional education includes a broad swath of programs within a rehabilitative framework, based on the premise that people in prison can change their circumstances through participation in educational programming. By contrast, the movement toward higher education in prison asks colleges and universities to step up to our nation's problem of mass incarceration by providing equitable opportunities to incarcerated students (Castro & Gould, 2018).

In 2018, an estimated 202 colleges and universities offered credit-bearing courses in prisons (Castro et al., 2018). Even more college-in-prison programs existed prior to 1994, when Congress rescinded incarcerated students' access to Pell Grants through the Violent Crime Control and Law Enforcement Act (Oakford et al., 2019). The Second Chance Pell Act of 2016 has restored some higher education programs to prisons, yet many prisoners still lack access to higher education. This is unfortunate; postsecondary opportunities in prison reduce recidivism rates and lead to better-paying jobs for students post-release (Meyer et al., 2010). Others argue that colleges and prisons shouldn't limit their goals for incarcerated students to post-release outcomes but rather set the same expansive learning outcomes on the inside as on the outside (Castro & Gould, 2018).

Pedagogical Challenges

Prison as an educational setting presents a unique set of barriers between students and teachers. Historically, education in prison was approached using the "banking model" wherein students were treated as receptacles to be filled with the teacher's knowledge and wisdom, and learning was a passive experience (Bidhan, 2018). These teaching methods often invite "second-order speech," meaning dialogue that is only welcomed when students are called upon by the teacher and the content of which is a reiteration of what has already been taught. These methods raised questions about the ethicality of education in prison, where the teacher is an authority figure much like the guards, and students are meant to consume and reiterate any information given. This led to the idea, largely adapted from Paolo Freire's concept of critical pedagogy (Freire, 1970) that the classroom should be tailored in ways specific to the demographic composition of prison, namely, that written text should be avoided when possible due to high illiteracy rates, texts should be used by demographically representative authors, and the structure and dynamic of the classroom should be constantly molded by the students' needs, to combat issues with the student-teacher power dynamic (Bidhan, 2018).

The dialogical approach, which was adapted largely from Freire's (1970) approach to critical pedagogy, was put forth as a strategy for building a productive educational setting within prison, one that is dialogue-based and is meant to be tailored to varying demographics, education levels, and general life experiences (Bidhan, 2018). Many teachers report challenges surrounding lack of prior formal education among students, linguistic differences between students and teachers, as well as the presence of trauma and PTSD creating disempowerment in the classroom (Flores, 2012; Golden, 2018). The dialogical approach seeks to create an egalitarian space that is inclusive of students with these educational barriers.

Students without much prior formal education often benefit from being able to influence the structure of the course and being able to connect the content to their own life experiences. In an effort to create autonomy within incarcerated students for their own learning experiences, Allred (2009) solicited feedback from students about specific course features that were found to be most helpful in a class that combined both incarcerated and non-incarcerated students. Students rated the structure of a class as the most important aspect, stating that icebreakers were important for acclimating to the classroom setting and integrating incarcerated students with non-incarcerated students. This research also found that students strongly emphasized small group discussions over large class discussions. Involvement of the larger group was more welcome during low-stakes activities, such as brainstorming. Students appreciated readings that had connections to their own experience, as this allowed them to relay knowledge acquired without formal education. McCarthy (2006) provides a good example of this when talking about how, in their history class, they began a unit on the civil rights movement before realizing that they had a former Black Panther and a former freedom fighter in the class. This was an opportunity to allow students to be experts in their own education and use learning that is not purely academic.

In some prisons, as many as one-third of the prisoners are suffering from some form of PTSD (Flatt et al., 2017). Trauma symptoms are so prevalent that the history of physical abuse in women's prison is often referred to as "the sexual abuse to prison pipeline" (Golden, 2018). Working with a population where PTSD is so prevalent calls for trauma-informed pedagogy by teachers working in prison. In a class conducted by Bidhan (2018), it was clear that disempowerment was one of the biggest hurdles to an effective classroom. This was further perpetuated by the nature of prison, where writing is subject to censorship by the prison guards. Because of this, it is important to be able to ensure that class can be kept confidential or to make it abundantly clear when it cannot. Despite issues with censorship, Golden (2018) emphasizes writing prompts that invite the difficult or disturbing, though never pushing this and modeling a level of self-disclosure. This can be especially important because trauma can affect one's understanding of appropriate levels of disclosure. In terms of lesson plans, she found five general components most effective for working with a traumatized population. It is important to create a safe space through encouragement and confidentiality, to leave space for laughter, to use materials that have specificity and familiarity, to use visuals when possible, and to allow for imitation of text during writing exercises.

In many ways, the dialogical approach is an attitude for teaching in prison rather than a specific methodology. This attitude requires teachers to constantly question and edit the structure of the classroom to meet the needs of the students. This is particularly important in prison settings where there is a larger power differential in the learning process and students often have unique challenges such as educational gaps, linguistic differences, and learning barriers created by the high prevalence of PTSD (Flores, 2012; Golden, 2018). The strategies mentioned for these emphasize allowing students to be experts in their own learning, engaging with their own thoughts and experiences using a platform that respects their unique learning styles and needs.

The Role of Writing Centers

Writing is the most common learning outcome across colleges and universities (Hart, 2015) and therefore needs to be a priority of college in prison programs. Yet, resources that support writing are limited in carceral settings. Many college writing assignments are research-based, but most prisons lack access to academic journals and books (Jones, 2016; McAleese, 2016). Castro and Gould (2018) note that most incarcerated students lack access to writing courses, writing centers, and individualized support with writing.

Writing centers are a common feature in "free-world" colleges and universities today. According to Salem (2014), 90% of US colleges and universities offer some type of individualized writing support; 52% have a stand-alone writing center, and

25% include writing support within larger centers that offer support with various academic skills and content. In a carceral setting, writing centers can meet the needs of writers from a diverse range of academic backgrounds by offering individualized feedback and providing foundational resources.

Writing centers offer a pedagogical approach that makes them the better fit for carceral settings over a more generalized academic support model. For incarcerated tutors and tutees, the writing center offers a space for writing to be honed as a tool of critical thinking. Even when students also need support with grammatical correctness and formatting to be successful in their academic courses, writing centers prioritize higher-level writing skills of argumentation, evidentiary support, and analysis, as well as exposure to writing as a process of meaning-making (Fitzgerald & Ianetta, 2016). The opportunity to use writing as a tool to further critical thinking is a necessary opportunity in the restrictive and dehumanizing setting of the prison (Davis, 2018; Jones, 2016). Furthermore, writing center pedagogy centers the student as the decision-maker over their written work (Fitzgerald & Ianetta, 2016), an approach aligned with trauma-informed pedagogy.

We are also now seeing some institutions able to offer writing center tutor training courses inside penal settings, creating an opportunity for advanced undergraduates and alumni to become writing center tutors while in prison. As tutors, these students and alumni can experience a higher academic challenge and an opportunity to mentor students coming after them (Moore, 2019; VanBerkum, 2017). Such opportunity further enhances the important role writing centers can play in academic life in carceral settings.

Research in Correctional Settings

Another opportunity for the intersection of higher education and the penal system is in the realm of academic research. Research in correctional settings is haunted by two contradictory concerns: overuse and underuse of incarcerated individuals as research participants.

Historically, prisoners have been treated with little consideration for their welfare. Hornblum's concise history of research conducted in American correctional facilities paints a grim portrait of medical experimentation up to the middle of the twentieth century, with some prisons "[becoming] supermarkets of investigatory opportunity" for studies of little value to anyone other than the (often for-profit) industries that sponsored them (Hornblum, 1997, pp. 1440). During the mid-1970s, for example, some 90% of drug trials in the United States were conducted on prisoners (Pont, 2008).

By the late 1970s, and largely due to the abuses of the earlier part of the century, medical research in prisons significantly declined (Hornblum, 1997). And while forgoing the use of prisoners as research subjects altogether is one sure way to ensure a reduction in ethical violations, it also prevents individuals who might benefit from clinical trials and other experimental interventions from having an opportunity to reap any potential benefits. The second concern, then, is that an ever-growing segment of the population may be denied access to experimental treatments that could substantially improve or even save their lives (Cislo & Trestman, 2013; Pont, 2008; Trestman, 2014).

This issue of denied access is particularly concerning given that health disparities abound within the American penal system. As of 2012, incarcerated individuals were more likely than the general population to have had a chronic health condition, or infectious disease such as tuberculosis, hepatitis B or C, or an STI (Maruschak et al., 2015). Forty percent of incarcerated individuals reported currently having a chronic health condition, and nearly three-quarters were overweight, obese, or morbidly obese (Maruschak et al., 2015). Mental health is no better. Compared with 5% in the general population, between 14 and 32% of incarcerated people (depending on gender and type of facility) met the threshold for serious psychological distress in the past 30 days (Bronson & Berzofsky, 2017).

Of course, medical research is only one area that may be appropriate for a prison setting. There are many questions specific to the penal system that are addressable by social scientists as well. Questions related to reentry programs, for instance, could benefit both incarcerated individuals as well as the communities into which they're released. For researchers who are funded by the Department of Health and Human Services (DHHS), 45 C.F.R. Part 46, Subpart C regulates the types of research permissible with prisoners, limiting it to questions specifically related to incarceration and prisons as institutions or on conditions particularly affecting prisoners and ways in which to alleviate those conditions (45 C.F.R. Subpart C). In 2006, recommendations were made to extend these limitations to all research within the United States, not just those funded by the government (Committee on the Ethical Considerations for Revisions to DHSS Regulations for Protection of Prisoners Involved in Research, 2007).

Others note the importance of research on the potential ethical issues of prison-based research itself. Studies on topics such as prisoners' competence to consent to research, the presence of coercion, misconceptions about potential benefits, and IRBs' standards of rigor are all needed to inform and improve the current landscape of research within correctional facilities (Christopher et al., 2011). Of course, as Christopher et al. note, even researching the ethics of research can be ethically challenging! However, there are several resources to at least guide us in that aspiration.

The Nuremberg Code, created in response to horrific human experimentation by the Nazis during WWII, laid out a series of requirements for ethical research with human participants, chief among those being the ability to voluntarily consent ("Trials of War Criminals before the Nuremberg Military Tribunals," 1949). In addition to voluntary participation, there must also be a consideration of the risk/reward ratio, i.e., the potential risks to individuals in the study must not outweigh the potential benefits to society. The Belmont Report reiterates many of the tenets found in the Nuremberg Code in its three "Basic Ethical Principles:" (1) respect for persons, (2) beneficence, and (3) justice (National Commission for the Protection of Human Subjects of Biomedical and Behavioral Research, 1979). Respect for persons encompasses consent, beneficence demands that we do no harm, and justice speaks to the need to spread the burdens as well as the benefits of research participation among various groups of people. Ironically, justice, as it pertains to research among incarcerated populations, was a particular violation in the earlier part of the twentieth century due to the great burden placed upon prisoners, yet it persists today in the opposite form.

While there are several ethical standards in place to help ensure that research with prisoners proceeds without a repeat of a deeply regrettable past, meeting these standards is not always straightforward. For example, ensuring that the IRBs in our respective institutions are set up with knowledgeable members and adequate prisoner representation is a legitimate challenge for many institutions (Christopher et al., 2011). We must also ask ourselves how consent obtained from the average community member differs from that within the walls of a prison due the inherent imbalance of power (e.g., see Moser et al., 2004).

The use of Participatory Action Research (PAR) may be one avenue for reducing power asymmetries by engaging prisoners as part of the research team (Resnik & Kennedy, 2011). For example, using Participatory Action Research, Penrod and colleagues worked with both staff and prisoners to identify concerns and help facilitate system changes surrounding end-of-life care within the prison community (Penrod et al., 2016). Creative research methodologies, such as PAR, may facilitate the ethical collection of data while providing empowering opportunities for prisoners to affect changes from within.

While prisoners may have once been used as test subjects simply because "they were cheap and available" (Hornblum, 1997), today, scientists are in a position to do a great deal of good in the realms of biomedical, mental, and socioemotional health inside correctional facilities. However, each researcher has a responsibility to think deeply about how beneficence and justice apply to this particular class of vulnerable participants.

Conclusions

Teaching and research are two common ways that those working in higher education might interact with incarcerated populations. Both these endeavors have the potential to positively impact the lives of prisoners, the penal system more broadly, and, we would argue, students and educators who are on the outside of the prison walls. In order to do this work well, we must also consider the particular ethical and pedagogical challenges that accompany such work. This is a challenge, but a worthy one. Locked away with the experiences and knowledge of millions of Americans, there are clues to some of society's most pressing questions—clues that those in higher education have a responsibility to explore.

References

Alexander, M. (2012). *The new Jim Crow: Mass incarceration in the age of colorblindness*. The New Press.
Allred, S. L. (2009). The inside-out prison exchange program: The impact of structure, content, and readings. *The Journal of Correctional Education, 60*(3), 240–259.
Bidhan, C. R. (2018). Words uncaged: A dialogical approach to empowering voices. In J. Lockard & S. Rankins-Robertson (Eds.), *Prison Pedagogies* (pp. 32–48).
Bronson, J., & Berzofsky, M. (2017). *Indicators of Mental Health Problems Reported by Prisoners and Jail Inmates, 2011–12*. (U.S. Department of Justice Special Report: NCJ 250612). Retrieved from https://www.bjs.gov/content/pub/pdf/imhprpji1112.pdf
Castro, E. L., & Gould, M. R. (2018). What is higher education in prison? Introduction to radical departures: Ruminations on the purposes of higher education in prison. *Critical Education, 9*(10), 1–16. Retrieved from https://ices.library.ubc.ca/index.php/criticaled/article/view/186439/185511
Castro, E. L., Hunter, R. K., Hardison, T., & Johnson-Ojeda, V. (2018). The landscape of postsecondary education in prison and the influence of Second Chance Pell: An analysis of transferability, credit-bearing status, and accreditation. *The Prison Journal, 98*(4), 405–426.
Christopher, P. P., Candilis, P. J., Rich, J. D., & Lidz, C. W. (2011). An empirical ethics agenda for psychiatric research involving prisoners. *AJOB Primary Research, 2*(4), 18–25. https://doi.org/10.1080/21507716.2011.627082
Cislo, A. M., & Trestman, R. (2013). Challenges and solutions for conducting research in correctional settings: The U.S. experience. *International Journal of Law and Psychiatry, 36*(3–4), 304–310. https://doi.org/10.1016/j.ijlp.2013.04.002
Committee on the Ethical Considerations for Revisions to DHSS Regulations for Protection of Prisoners Involved in Research. (2007). *Ethical Considerations for Research Involving Prisoners*. https://doi.org/10.17226/11692
Davis, J. (2018). Caught somewhere between. *Critical Education, 9*(15), 1–12. Retrieved from https://ices.library.ubc.ca/index.php/criticaled/article/view/186355
Equal Justice Initiative. (2018). *Incarceration of women is growing twice as fast as that of men*. Retrieved from https://eji.org/news/female-incarceration-growing-twice-as-fast-as-male-incarceration
Fitzgerald, L., & Ianetta, M. (2016). *The Oxford guide for writing tutors: Practice and research*. Oxford University Press.
Flatt, J., Williams, B., Barnes, D., Goldenson, J., & Ahalt, C. (2017). Post-traumatic stress disorder symptoms and associated health and vulnerabilities in older jail inmates. *Aging & Mental Health, 21*(10), 1106–1112.
Flores, J. (2012). Jail pedagogy: Liberatory education inside a California juvenile detention Facility. *Social Work Publications, 154*, 1–44.
Freire, P. (1970). *Pedagogy of the oppressed*. The Continuum International Publishing Group Ltd.
Golden, T. (2018). Writing with incarcerated teen women: Trauma-informed pedagogy, health, and gender equity. In J. Lockard & S. Rankins-Robertson (Eds.), *Prison Pedagogies* (pp. 127–147).
Gramlich, J. (2019). *The gap between the number of blacks and whites in prison is shrinking*. Pew Research Center. Retrieved from https://www.pewresearch.org/fact-tank/2019/04/30/shrinking-gap-between-number-of-blacks-and-whites-in-prison/
Hart Research Associates. (2015). *Recent trends in general education design, learning outcomes, and teaching approaches*. Association of American Colleges & Universities. Retrieved from https://www.aacu.org/sites/default/files/files/LEAP/2015_Survey_Report2_GEtrends.pdf
Hornblum, A. M. (1997). They were cheap and available: Prisoners as research subjects in twentieth century America. *British Medical Journal, 315*(7120), 1437–1441. Retrieved from https://www.ncbi.nlm.nih.gov/pmc/articles/PMC2127868/

Jones, M. (2016). Incarcerated scholars, qualitative inquiry, and subjugated knowledge: The value of incarcerated and post-incarcerated scholars in the age of mass incarceration. *Journal of Prisoners on Prison, 25*(2), 98–111. Retrieved from http://www.jpp.org/documents/back%20 issues/JPP%2025-2.pdf

Kaeble, D., & Cowhig, M. (2018). *Correctional populations in the United States, 2016* (No. NCJ 251211). Bureau of Justice Statistics, US Department of Justice. Retrieved from https://www.bjs.gov/content/pub/pdf/cpus16.pdf.

Maruschak, L. M., Berzofsky, M., & Unangst, J. (2015). *Medical problems of state and federal prisoners and jail inmates, 2011–12.* (U.S. Department of Justice Special Report: NCJ 248491). Retrieved from https://www.bjs.gov/content/pub/pdf/mpsfpji1112.pdf

McAleese, S. (2016). Looking back on learning inside the walls: A review of previous JPP special issues on prison education. *Journal of Prisoners on Prisons, 25*(2), 112–130.

McCarty, H. (2006). Educating felons: Reflections on higher education in prisons. *Radical History Review, 96*, 87–94.

Meyer, S. J., Fredericks, L., Borden, C. M., & Richardson, P. L. (2010). Implementing postsecondary academic programs in state prisons: Challenges and opportunities. *Journal of Correctional Education, 61*(2), 148–184.

Moore, S. (2019). Collaborative learning in a prison context. *Praxis: A Writing Center Journal.* Blogpost. Retrieved from http://www.praxisuwc.com/praxis-blog/2019/6/3/collaborative-learning-in-a-prison-context?rq=prison

Moser, D. J., Arndt, S., Kanz, J. E., Benjamin, M. L., Bayless, J. D., Reese, R. L., et al. (2004). Coercion and informed consent in research involving prisoners. *Comprehensive Psychiatry; New York, 45*(1), 1–9. https://doi.org/10.1016/j.comppsych.2003.09.009

National Commission for the Protection of Human Subjects of Biomedical and Behavioral Research. (1979). *The Belmont report: Ethical principles and guidelines for the protection of human subjects of research.* Retrieved from https://www.hhs.gov/ohrp/regulations-and-policy/belmont-report/read-the-belmont-report/index.html

Oakford, P., Brumfield, C., Goldvale, C., Tatum, L., diZerega, M., & Patrick, F. (2019). *Investing in futures: Economic and fiscal benefits of postsecondary education in prison.* Vera Institute of Justice. Retrieved from https://storage.googleapis.com/vera-web-assets/downloads/Publications/investing-in-futures-education-in-prison/legacy_downloads/investing-in-futures.pdf

Penrod, J., Loeb, S. J., Ladonne, R. A., & Martin, L. M. (2016). Empowering change agents in hierarchical organizations: Participatory action research in prisons. *Research in Nursing and Health, 39*, 142–153.

Pont, J. (2008). Ethics in research involving prisoners. *International Journal of Prisoner Health; Bingley, 4*(4), 184–197. https://doi.org/10.1080/17449200802473107

Rabuy, B., & Kopf, D. (2015). *Prisons of poverty: Uncovering the pre-incarceration incomes of the imprisoned.* Prison Policy Initiative. Retrieved 21 June 2019, from https://www.prisonpolicy.org/reports/income.html

Resnik, D. B., & Kennedy, C. E. (2011). Balancing scientific and community interests in community-based participatory research. *Account Research, 17*, 198–210. https://doi.org/10.1080/08989621.2010.493095

Salem, L. (2014). Opportunity and transformation: How writing centers are positioned in the political landscape of higher education in the United States. *The Writing Center Journal, 34*(1), 15–43.

Trestman, R. L. (2014). Ethics, the law, and prisoners: Protecting society, changing human behavior, and protecting human rights. *Journal of Bioethical Inquiry, 11*(3), 311–318. https://doi.org/10.1007/s11673-014-9560-1

Trials of War Criminals before the Nuremberg Military Tribunals under Control Council Law No. 10. (1949). (Vol. 2, pp. 181–182). U.S. Government Printing Office. Retrieved from https://history.nih.gov/research/downloads/nuremberg.pdf

VanBerkum, M. (2017). Writing centers partner with educational facility. *The Irish Rover*. Retrived from https://irishrover.net/2017/10/writing-center-partners-with-correctional-facility/

Vesely-Flad, R. L. (2017). *Racial purity and dangerous bodies: Moral pollution, Black lives, and the struggle for justice*. Fortress Press.

Walmsley, R. (2010). *World prison population list*. Institute for Criminal Policy Research World Prison Brief. Retrieved from https://www.prisonstudies.org/sites/default/files/resources/downloads/world_prison_population_list_11th_edition_0.pdf

Understudied Populations Within the Sexual Assault Literature

Cristina L. Reitz-Krueger, Lucy A. Guarnera, and Susana Castaños-Cervantes

Sexual violence impacts millions of people worldwide, is considered a human rights violation, and is often associated with a host of negative consequences for survivors including physical injuries, STIs, and psychological consequences such as posttraumatic stress disorder (World Health Organization, 2002). Given this global impact, sexual assault has received a great deal of attention from the scientific community; a quick search with Google Scholar elicits around 1.25 million articles on the subject. This research attention is unsurprising given the scope and severity of the issue, and the many facets of sexual assault that merit empirical investigation. However, within the broader domain of sexual violence, there are several subgroups that remain underexplored.

This chapter highlights just three understudied populations affected by sexual violence that have thus far received less attention from the scientific community: women who conceive in rape, homeless youth, and male college students. While this list is by no means exhaustive, available research on these three groups illustrates how a nuanced, fine-grained investigation of circumscribed populations can reveal unique patterns and outcomes of sexual violence that require different kinds of services and policy solutions to intervene effectively.

C. L. Reitz-Krueger (✉)
Department of Psychology, Warren Wilson College, Asheville, NC, USA
e-mail: creitz-krueger@warren-wilson.edu

L. A. Guarnera
Institute of Law, Psychiatry, and Public Policy, University of Virginia, Charlottesville, VA, USA

S. Castaños-Cervantes
Escuela de Psicologia, Facultad de Ciencias de la Salud, Universidad Panamericana, Ciudad de México, Mexico

S. Castaños-Cervantes et al. (eds.), *Working with Vulnerable Populations*,
https://doi.org/10.1007/978-3-031-67710-6_16

Women Who Conceive in Rape

Women who conceive in rape experience multiple risks and needs in addition to those shared by sexual assault survivors generally. Although rape-related pregnancy occurs around the world, the most recent, most rigorous research hails from the United States and estimates that 2.4% of all US women, or 2.9 million American women total, have experienced rape-related pregnancy (Basile et al., 2018). Incidence and prevalence rates likely vary widely from locality to locality[1] depending on local rates of sexual assault, contraception usage, and other contextual factors. Notably, rates of rape-related pregnancy can increase dramatically in the context of wartime rape—e.g., in Bosnia-Herzegovina during the Yugoslav wars of the 1990s (Erjavec & Volčič, 2010) or during the Rwandan Civil War (1990–1994; Mukangendo, 2007)—since combatants often intentionally impregnate victims in order to infiltrate their bloodlines as a means of genocide. Research suggests that one-fifth to one-half of women who conceive in rape raise their rape-conceived children themselves, again with estimates varying by study locality, time period, and methodology (de Haas et al., 2012; Gil et al., 2001; Holmes et al., 1996; Londoño et al., 2000; Reardon et al., 2000). Although relatively little is known about this understudied population, some recent research has begun to shed more light on the unique vulnerabilities of this subgroup. Several of these special considerations are outlined below.

First, both pregnancy and the acute post-rape period are times of heightened risk for physical and mental health problems, so women experiencing both states simultaneously may be at super-elevated risk. Recent research in the USA indicates that close to one in seven women experience physical injury as a result of sexual assault (Black et al., 2011), and this figure may be much higher in contexts such as war rape. In addition to potential injuries from the sexual assault itself, pregnancy is a time of increased physical vulnerability for women (particularly in low-income nations), ranging from more common impairments such as fatigue, nausea, and back pain to rarer and more serious conditions such as hypertension, infection, fistula, hemorrhage, kidney failure, cardiac arrest, and even death (Koblinsky et al., 2012). Although global maternal morbidity and mortality have fallen steadily over the past decades, maternal conditions still account for 12% of deaths of women of childbearing age worldwide (Ribeiro et al., 2008). Along these lines, both the perinatal period and acute post-rape period are times of elevated mental health concerns, including posttraumatic stress disorder, depression, substance abuse, and suicide (Campbell, 2008; Oates, 2003; Söderquist et al., 2009). Overlapping mental health risk may result in interactive effects among women experiencing rape-related pregnancy.

Second, recent research within the USA suggests that rape-related pregnancy occurs predominantly within the context of intimate partner violence, with 77.3% of

[1] See, e.g., de Haas et al. (2012), who estimated that 1% of all Dutch women have experienced a rape-related pregnancy.

women reporting a current or former intimate partner as the perpetrator (Basile et al., 2018). The same study found that over one-quarter of intimate partner rape victims became pregnant from assault (26.2%), as compared to only 5.2% of women raped by an acquaintance and 6.9% of victims raped by a stranger (Basile et al., 2018). At least in the USA, rape-related pregnancy appears to occur most commonly in the context of an ongoing sexually violent relationship in which the woman is raped many times over a period of months or years, which creates an increased opportunity for rape conception to occur. Further, within the context of intimate partner violence, rape-related pregnancy seems to exist on the spectrum of reproductive coercion, a collection of behaviors intended to maintain power and control over a romantic partner by interfering with reproductive decision-making (e.g., sabotaging contraceptive methods or coercing a partner into having unprotected sex; Basile et al., 2018; Miller et al., 2010, 2014). Pregnancy resulting from an intimate partner rape may render the female partner more physically vulnerable and financially dependent on the abusive male partner, as well as creating an enduring legal tie if the pregnancy results in the birth of a child, all of which may make it more difficult for the woman to escape the abusive relationship.

Third, women who give birth to their rape-conceived children may face numerous legal obstacles related to custody, visitation, child support, government assistance, adoption, stepparent adoption, and related issues. For example, in most jurisdictions, a man who fathers a child via rape has the same parental rights as any other father, unless his parental rights are specifically terminated as the result of a rape conviction or civil proceeding—both of which are rare and may be difficult or impossible for a woman to achieve (Bitar, 2011; Prewitt, 2009; Stevens, 2014). This enduring legal tie may force interaction between a woman and the perpetrator for years, inviting continued manipulation and abuse, creating an opportunity for the perpetrator to blackmail the victim into dropping criminal charges (see, e.g., Sheehan, 2004), and subjecting her to the financial loss and emotional toll of lengthy custody battles.

Finally, along these lines, sexual assault has already been identified as a source of serious and continuing financial loss, with an estimated lifetime cost $122,461 per rape survivor in the USA (Peterson et al., 2017). In addition to the financial burdens common to all rape victims, rape-related pregnancy can impose additional economic loss by way of costs related to pregnancy, perinatal health concerns, abortion, custody proceedings, stepparent adoption, and, of course, potentially raising a child. Rape-related pregnancy can also impose more indirect financial costs, because at least in the USA, a single parent applying for government assistance (such as Temporary Assistance for Needy Families) may be required to pursue the absent parent for child support, and individuals who refuse to cooperate with the child support requirement may face a reduction or denial of benefits (Nusbaum, 2013). Because a woman raising a child conceived in rape may not want to pursue the perpetrator for child support—correctly perceiving that this kind of contact may prompt continuing interference or retaliation from the perpetrator—she may not be eligible for government benefits sorely needed by a single parent (Nusbaum, 2013).

In sum, women who conceive in rape face numerous additional medical, legal, and financial vulnerabilities over and above the risks common to all sexual assault survivors. Particularly for women raising their rape-conceived children, these vulnerabilities may continue for many years after the assault itself and require improved responses from medical, legal, and cultural institutions to begin to be adequately addressed.

Homeless Female Youth

Homeless female youth experience a complex web of vulnerabilities that make them particularly susceptible to sexual violence and its consequences. To begin, research suggests that close to 50% of homeless females experienced childhood sexual abuse, and this sexual violence is often a key factor leading them to abandon their homes in the first place (Pojomovsky, 2008).

Once on the streets, homeless youth experience numerous risks and deficits that may set the stage for sexual victimization. Research suggests that homeless youth exhibit cognitive deficits (Tonmyr et al., 2011), poor emotion regulation skills (Kim & Cicchetti, 2010), limited social abilities, delinquent behavior (Dumain, 2010), substance use problems (Douglas et al., 2010), physical violence (Melander & Tyler, 2010), and suicidal ideation and suicide attempts (Capuzzi & Gross, 2008). Homeless girls and young women are also more likely to engage in risky sexual behaviors that are associated with increased risk for sexual violence (Slonim-Nevo & Mukuka, 2007), including having multiple sexual partners (Lau et al., 2005) and engaging in sex work (Helander, 2008).

Unsurprisingly then, homeless youth suffer sexual violence at an extremely high rate compared with non-homeless populations (Feitel et al., 1992; Timmons et al., 2018). Homeless girls and young women experience many short and long-term consequences of sexual violence (Barman-Adhikari et al., 2016). In addition to acute psychological trauma and injuries, homeless youth may face other ongoing health issues including unintended pregnancy, mental health problems, and sexually transmitted infections, including HIV. Homeless sexual violence survivors may face stigma and rejection, making it more difficult to return to their families and communities and thus making them vulnerable to further sexual violence (World Health Organization, 2019). Compounding these problems, in many settings the health services that respond to survivors of sexual violence are inadequately prepared to meet the special needs (i.e., homelessness, social stigma, discrimination, lack of resources, abandonment, lack of social resources, presence of internalizing and externalizing behaviors, health risk behaviors, substance use and abuse, affiliation to organized crime) of the homeless population, meaning that many homeless survivors never receive care.

Despite this multifaceted vulnerability, the particular characteristics of sexual violence and its psychosocial effects on homeless girls and homeless young women are only superficially understood because research has been insufficient (Williams, 2018). This lack of empirical knowledge hinders the design and implementation of effective intervention strategies that may decrease the likelihood of running away from home and buffer the effects associated with sexual violence (García-Moreno & Watts, 2011). This lack of research is particularly troubling in localities with a large homeless population, such as Mexico City (Rábago-González, 2009).

To try to address this lack of research, in 2018, Castaños and Vélez interviewed over 200 homeless girls and young women in Mexico City between 11 and 20 years old. Results revealed that more than half of the participants were victims of intra-familial sexual abuse before the age of 11, which was the primary reason for leaving home. Once homeless, females suffered further sexual abuse by other homeless youth and adults, as well as other adults they encountered on the streets, such as police officers. Moreover, many participants described joining semi-organized groups of other homeless individuals in order to receive support, protection, and provision of basic needs; however, joining a homeless group led to sexual victimization by all male members of the group. Furthermore, in approximately 50% of cases, participants were forced into prostitution or became victims of human trafficking. Other participants chose to engage in sex work in exchange for food, shelter, or protection.

Interviews suggested that homeless women and girls continued to face disadvantages if they sought help for the consequences of sexual violence, including sexually transmitted infections and pregnancy. At least 10% of the participants reported facing discrimination in institutional health centers in Mexico City due to their homeless status (e.g., being denied care). Homeless youth who did receive care frequently reported sexual harassment or assault by healthcare providers (e.g., "The doctor who treated me told me that he would cure me if I gave him oral sex"; "When they treated me, the doctor put his hand inside my vagina without gloves"). Such brazen sexual perpetration within health centers may be explained by the low social status of homeless females, whose homelessness renders them invisible to law enforcement.

This research with homeless women and girls in Mexico City suggests both the multifaceted ways that homeless youth become victims of sexual violence and the complex influences of victimization on their life courses. Findings suggest the urgent need to study factors that increase the likelihood of sexual victimization among homeless females, as well as how these factors can be addressed to reduce the risk of sexual violence. For example, targeted prevention programming, such as education and life skills training, has the potential to promote attitudes, beliefs, and behaviors that prevent sexual violence among homeless individuals (Centers for Disease Control and Prevention, 2019). Future research should continue assessing sexual violence and its psychosocial consequences in this population to enable the design of efficient and sustainable intervention strategies that consider the special needs and characteristics of the homeless population.

Male College Students

Research stretching back to the 1980s has identified high rates of sexual assault against women on US college campuses (e.g., Koss & Dinero, 1989). College-age women are four times as likely to be sexually assaulted as women in other age groups (Moreno, 2015), and in some colleges, more than a quarter of the female seniors reported experiencing some form of unwanted sexual contact during their tenure (Cantor et al., 2015). And although research typically finds that women are more likely to experience sexual assault than men (e.g., Banyard et al., 2007; Elliott et al., 2004), rates among male US college students are still troubling. In terms of prevalence, estimates vary widely from around 3% (Hines et al., 2012) to 7–8% (Banyard et al., 2007; Reitz-Krueger et al., 2017), up to 22% (Tewksbury & Mustaine, 2001).

This wide range of prevalence estimates is likely related, at least in part, to differences in how sexual assault is defined by the various researchers. Sexual assault as a construct can encompass a wide range of behaviors, from unwanted kissing to forced penetration, and is measured differently in different studies. In practice, researchers often collapse distinct types of forced or unwanted sexual acts into a single overall prevalence score (e.g., Banyard et al., 2007; Elliott et al., 2004). Doing so, however, may obscure more nuanced comparisons between men and women (Abbey et al., 2005; Reitz-Krueger et al., 2017). When sexual assault is broken down into distinct acts, more complicated patterns emerge. For instance, while college women are overwhelmingly more likely to experience unwanted sexual acts *in general,* several studies have found that college men are equally likely to experience rape or attempted rape (Hines, 2007; Hines et al., 2012; Reitz-Krueger et al., 2017). The similar rate of rape and attempted rape among college men and women is in contrast to community-wide samples, which find higher rates of all types of sexual assault, including rape, among women (Weiss, 2010). This suggests qualitative differences between the sexual assaults men experience on college campuses as compared to those occurring elsewhere.

Like their female counterparts, males are also at risk of negative physical and psychological outcomes following a sexual assault (Choudhary et al., 2010; Davies, 2002; Davies et al., 2010; Frazier, 1993). Men, however, are less likely to seek help or report the incident (Weiss, 2010). There are many reasons why victims of sexual assault may choose not to disclose their experience, and both college men and women report that common barriers to reporting included shame, embarrassment, and a fear of not being believed (Sable et al., 2006). For men, however, another barrier to reporting is that sexual assault may undermine a sense of heteronormative masculinity that underpins traditional gender roles (Javaid, 2016; Weiss, 2010).

One way these kinds of gender norms are propagated is via rape myths—beliefs about rape that tend to blame the victim or justify sexual violence. Although rape myths were initially conceptualized with female victims in mind (Burt, 1980), researchers have recently begun to describe rape myths specifically for male victims—for example, beliefs that all men want sex (particularly with women) or that they should be strong enough to fight off a sexual offense. Ironically, men themselves are most likely to endorse these types of myths about male victims (Reitz-Krueger et al., 2017), and when they are victimized, many men are forced to renegotiate their self-conceptions of gender and sexuality (Weiss, 2010).

Unfortunately, the smaller proportion of male victims who do seek help are often met with some skepticism from service-providing agencies, perhaps due to the widespread acceptance of male rape myths even among service providers (Javaid, 2016). Javaid (2016) argues that, because many agencies dedicated to intimate partner violence and sexual assault were designed with female victims in mind, service providers may not be equipped to effectively and empathetically handle male clients. Ironically, then, these agencies, which are often grounded in feminist thinking, may inadvertently reinforce the same package of male gender norms that are linked with violence against women.

While male college students have typically not been considered a population that is vulnerable to sexual assault, they are understudied compared with their female counterparts, and available research suggests a unique pattern of risk and barriers to help-seeking. Unlike community samples, samples of college students reveal that men appear to be about as likely to suffer rape or attempted rape as women. This flies in the face of conventional wisdom and highlights the importance of studying sexual assault in a more fine-grained way, beyond overall prevalence rates. Further, men are less likely to seek help than women and face gender-specific challenges that many agencies may not be prepared to handle. More research is needed to identify how colleges and universities can best support *all* victims of sexual assault regardless of gender.

Conclusions

The global problem of sexual violence has received widespread concern, policy action, and research over the past several decades, allowing the scientific community to begin turn its attention to smaller sub-populations with special patterns and consequences of victimization. Women who conceive in rape face a myriad of additional emotional, physical, and potentially legal challenges in the wake of their assaults. Youth who flee sexual violence within their families of origin are often met with further victimization in their new life on the streets. And college men experiencing sexual assault may be overlooked by service providers that have traditionally focused on female victims. Although such understudied groups represent a relatively small percentage of the overall number of sexual assault victims, further research and specialized interventions are required to address their unique challenges.

References

Abbey, A., Parkhill, M. R., & Koss, M. P. (2005). The effects of frame of reference on responses to questions about sexual assault victimization and perpetration. *Psychology of Women Quarterly, 29*(4), 364–373. https://doi.org/10.1111/j.1471-6402.2005.00236.x

Banyard, V. L., Ward, S., Cohn, E. S., Plante, E. G., Moorhead, C., & Walsh, W. (2007). Unwanted sexual contact on campus: A comparison of women's and men's experiences. *Violence and Victims, 22*, 52–70.

Barman-Adhikari, A., Petering, R., Lengnick-Hall, R., Rice, E., Rhoades, H., & McCune, S. (2016). Social context of service use among homeless youth in Los Angeles, California. *Journal of Social Service Research, 42*(4), 501–515. https://doi.org/10.1080/01488376.2016.1153563

Basile, K. C., Smith, S. G., Liu, Y., Kresnow, M., Fasula, A. M., Gilbert, L., & Chen, J. (2018). Rape-related pregnancy and association with reproductive coercion in the U.S. *American Journal of Preventive Medicine, 55*(6), 770–776. https://doi.org/10.1016/j.amepre.2018.07.028

Bitar, K. N. (2011). The parental rights of rapists. *Duke Journal of Gender Law & Policy, 19*, 275–302.

Black, M. C., Basile, K. C., Breiding, M. J., Smith, S. G., Walters, M. L., Merrick, M. T., & Stevens, M. R. (2011). *The National Intimate Partner and Sexual Violence Survey (NISVS): 2010 Summary Report*. National Center for Injury Prevention and Control, Centers for Disease Control and Prevention.

Burt, M. R. (1980). Cultural myths and supports for rape. *Journal of Personality and Social Psychology, 38*(2), 217–230. https://doi.org/10.1037/0022-3514.38.2.217

Campbell, R. (2008). The psychological impact of rape victims' experiences with the legal, medical, and mental health systems. *American Psychologist, 63*(8), 702–717. https://doi.org/10.1037/0003-066X.63.8.702

Cantor, D., Fisher, B., Chibnall, S., Townsend, R., Lee, H., Carol, B., & Thomas, G. (2015). *Report on the AAU Campus Climate Survey on sexual assault and sexual misconduct* (pp. 1–302). University of Virginia.

Capuzzi, D., & Gross, D. (2008). *Youth at risk: A prevention resource for counselors, teachers and parents*. Pearson-Merrill Prentice Hall.

Centers for Disease Control and Prevention. (2019). *The Social-Ecological Model: A framework for prevention*. Retrieved from: https://www.cdc.gov/violenceprevention/publichealthissue/social-ecologicalmodel.html

Choudhary, E., Coben, J., & Bossarte, R. M. (2010). Adverse Health Outcomes, Perpetrator Characteristics, and Sexual Violence Victimization Among U.S. Adult Males. *Journal of Interpersonal Violence, 25*(8), 1523–1541. https://doi.org/10.1177/0886260509346063

Davies, M. (2002). Male sexual assault victims: A selective review of the literature and implications for support services. *Aggression and Violent Behavior, 7*, 203–214.

Davies, M., Walker, J., Archer, J., & Pollard, P. (2010). A comparative study of long-term psychological functioning in male survivors of stranger and acquaintance rape. *Journal of Aggression, Conflict and Peace Research, 2*(4), 25–33.

de Haas, S., van Berlo, W., Bakker, F., & Vanwesenbeeck, I. (2012). Prevalence and characteristics of sexual violence in The Netherlands, the risk of revictimization and pregnancy: Results from a national population survey. *Violence and Victims, 27*(4), 592–608. https://doi.org/10.1891/0886-6708.27.4.592

Douglas, K., Chan, G., Gelerneter, J., Arias, A., Anton, R., Weiss, R., Brady, K., Poling, J., Farrer, L., & Kranzler, H. (2010). Adverse childhood events as risk factors for substance dependence: Partial mediation by mood and anxiety disorders. *Addictive Behaviors, 35*, 7–13.

Dumain, K. (2010). *Optimism, hope, problem solving and runaway behavior in adolescents in the dependency system* (Unpublished doctoral dissertation). Pepperdine University, Culver City, CA, USA.

Elliott, D. M., Mok, S. M., & Briere, J. (2004). Adult sexual assault: Prevalence, symptomatology, and sex differences in the general population. *Journal of Traumatic Stress, 17*(3), 203–211.

Erjavec, K., & Volčič, Z. (2010). Living with the sins of their fathers: An analysis of self-representation of adolescents born of war rape. *Journal of Adolescent Research, 25*(3), 359–386. https://doi.org/10.1177/0743558410361373

Feitel, B., Margetson, N., Chamas, J., & Lipman, C. (1992). Psychosocial background and behavioral and emotional disorders of homeless and runaway youth. *Hospital & Community Psychiatry, 43*(2), 155–159.

Frazier, P. A. (1993). A comparative study of male and female rape victims seen at a hospital based rape crisis program. *Journal of Interpersonal Violence, 8*(1), 64–76.

García-Moreno, C., & Watts, C. (2011). Violence against women: An urgent public health priority. *Bulletin of the World Health Organization, 89*, 2–2. https://doi.org/10.2471/BLT.10.085217

Gil, M., Ortiz, B., & Jaramillo, A. M. (2001). Pregnancy resulting from rape: Breaking the silence of multiple crises. In A. Gomez & D. Meacham (Eds.), *Women's Health Collection (Reflections of inequality: Women and mental health)* (Vol. 6, pp. 109–113). Latin American and Caribbean Women's Health Network.

Helander, E. (2008). *Children and Adolescence: The World of the Fefenseless*. Palgrave Macmillan.

Hines, D. A. (2007). Predictors of sexual coercion against women and men: A multilevel, multinational study of university students. *Archives of Sexual Behavior, 36*(3), 403–422.

Hines, D. A., Armstrong, J. L., Reed, K. P., & Cameron, A. Y. (2012). Gender differences in sexual assault victimization among college students. *Violence and Victims, 27*(6), 922–940.

Holmes, M. M., Resnick, H. S., Kilpatrick, D. G., & Best, C. L. (1996). Rape-related pregnancy: Estimates and descriptive characteristics from a national sample of women. *American Journal of Obstetrics and Gynecology, 175*(2), 320–325. https://doi.org/10.1016/S0002-9378(96)70141-2

Javaid, A. (2016). Voluntary agencies' responses to, and attitudes toward male rape: Issues and concerns. *Sexuality and Culture, 20*(3), 731–748.

Kim, J., & Cicchetti, D. (2010). Longitudinal pathways linking child maltreatment, emotion regulation, peer relations, and psychopathology. *Journal of Child Psychology and Psychiatry, 51*(6), 706–716.

Koblinsky, M., Chowdhury, M. E., Moran, A., & Ronsmans, C. (2012). Maternal morbidity and disability and their consequences: Neglected agenda in maternal health. *Journal of Health, Population, and Nutrition, 30*(2), 124–130.

Koss, M. P., & Dinero, T. E. (1989). Discriminant analysis of risk factors for sexual victimization among a national sample of college women. *Journal of Consulting and Clinical Psychology, 57*, 242–250.

Lau, J., Kim, J., Tsui, H., Cheung, A., Lau, M., & Yu, A. (2005). The relationship between physical maltreatment and substance use among adolescents. A survey of 95,788 adolescents in Hong Kong. *Journal of Adolescent Health, 37*(2), 110–119.

Londoño, L., Ortiz, B., Gil, A., Jaramillo, A., Castro, R., & Pineda, N. (2000). *Embarazo por violación. La crisis múltiple [Rape pregnancy: Multiple crises]*. Colciencias [Administrative Department of Science, Technology, and Innovation].

Melander, L., & Tyler, K. (2010). The effect of early maltreatment, victimization, and partner violence on HIV risk behavior among homeless young adults. *Journal of Adolescent Health, 47*(6), 575–581.

Miller, E., Jordan, B., Levenson, R., & Silverman, J. G. (2010). Reproductive coercion: Connecting the dots between partner violence and unintended pregnancy. *Contraception, 81*(6), 457–459. https://doi.org/10.1016/j.contraception.2010.02.023

Miller, E., McCauley, H. L., Tancredi, D. J., Decker, M. R., Anderson, H., & Silverman, J. G. (2014). Recent reproductive coercion and unintended pregnancy among female family planning clients. *Contraception, 89*(2), 122–128. https://doi.org/10.1016/j.contraception.2013.10.011

Moreno, M. A. (2015). Sexual assault and rape among college students. *JAMA Pediatrics, 169*(12), 1184. http://jamanetwork.com/journals/jamapediatrics/fullarticle/2474665

Mukangendo, M. C. (2007). Caring for children born of rape in Rwanda. In R. C. Carpenter (Ed.), *Born of war: Protecting children of sexual violence survivors in conflict zones* (pp. 40–52). Kumarian Press.

Nusbaum, A. (2013). The high cost of child support in rape cases: Finding an evidentiary standard to protect mother and child from welfare's cooperation requirement. *Fordham Law Review, 82*, 1331–1365.
Oates, M. (2003). Perinatal psychiatric disorders: A leading cause of maternal morbidity and mortality. *British Medical Bulletin, 67*(1), 219–229. https://doi.org/10.1093/bmb/ldg011
Peterson, C., DeGue, S., Florence, C., & Lokey, C. N. (2017). Lifetime economic burden of rape among US adults. *American Journal of Preventive Medicine, 52*(6), 691–701. https://doi.org/10.1016/j.amepre.2016.11.014
Pojomovsky, J. (2008). *Cruzar la calle. Niñez y adolescencia en las calles de la ciudad [Crossing the street. Homeless childhood and adolescence in the city]*. Espacio Editorial. First Volume.
Prewitt, S. R. (2009). Giving birth to a rapist's child: A discussion and analysis of the limited legal protections afforded to women who become mothers through rape. *The Georgetown Law Journal, 98*, 827–862.
Rábago-González, M. (2009). Las niñas en situación de calle en la ciudad de México: una visión de género [Homeless girls in Mexico City: A gender perspective]. *Revista Iberoamericana sobre Infancia y Juventud en Lucha por sus Derechos, 1*(1), 107–109.
Reardon, D., Makimaa, J., & Sobie, A. (Eds.). (2000). *Victims and victors: Speaking out about their pregnancies, abortions and children resulting from sexual assault*. Acorn Books.
Reitz-Krueger, C. L., Mummert, S. J., & Troupe, S. M. (2017). Real men can't get raped: An examination of gendered rape myths and sexual assault among undergraduates. *Journal of Aggression, Conflict, and Peace Research, 9*(4), 314–323.
Ribeiro, P. S., Jacobsen, K. H., Mathers, C. D., & Garcia-Moreno, C. (2008). Priorities for women's health from the Global Burden of Disease study. *International Journal of Gynaecology and Obstetrics: The Official Organ of the International Federation of Gynaecology and Obstetrics, 102*(1), 82–90. https://doi.org/10.1016/j.ijgo.2008.01.025
Sable, M. R., Danis, F., Mauzy, D. L., & Gallagher, S. K. (2006). Barriers to reporting sexual assault for women and men: Perspectives of college students. *Journal of American College Health, 55*(3), 157–162.
Sheehan, R. (2004, September 6). Rapists lose facet of power. *Raleigh News & Observer*. Retrieved from http://www.go2gbo.com/forums/round-the-'ole-pot-bellied-stove/rapists-lose-facet-of-power/
Slonim-Nevo, V., & Mukuka, L. (2007). Child abuse and AIDS-related knowledge, attitudes and behavior among adolescents in Zambia. *Child Abuse & Neglect, 31*(2), 143–159.
Söderquist, J., Wijma, B., Thorbert, G., & Wijma, K. (2009). Risk factors in pregnancy for post-traumatic stress and depression after childbirth. *BJOG: An International Journal of Obstetrics & Gynaecology, 116*(5), 672–680. https://doi.org/10.1111/j.1471-0528.2008.02083.x
Stevens, M. E. H. (2014). Rape-related pregnancies: The need to create stronger protections for the victim-mother and child. *Hastings Law Journal, 65*(3), 865–898.
Tewksbury, R., & Mustaine, E. E. (2001). Lifestyle factors associated with the sexual assault of men: A routine activity theory analysis. *The Journal of Men's Studies, 9*, 153–182.
Timmons, V., Coomber-Bendtsen, M., & Zederayko, A. (2018). *Gender-based violence and homelessness: Two sides of the same coin*. Retrieved from: https://www.schoolofpublicpolicy.sk.ca/documents/research/policy-briefs/JSGS-policybriefs-Gender-Based%20Violence%20and%20Homelessness.pdf
Tonmyr, L., Williams, G., Hovdestad, W., & Draca, J. (2011). Anxiety and/or depression in 10-15 years old investigated by Child Welfare in Canada. *Journal of Adolescent Health, 48*, 493–498.
Weiss, K. G. (2010). Male sexual victimization: Examining men's experiences of rape and sexual assault. *Men & Masculinities, 12*(3), 275–298.
Williams, M. (2018). *Women's hidden homelessness*. Retrieved from: https://www.homeless.org.uk/connect/blogs/2018/feb/27/women%E2%80%99s-hidden-homelessness
World Health Organization. (2002). *World report on violence and health*. Retrieved from https://www.who.int/violence_injury_prevention/violence/world_report/en/introduction.pdf
World Health Organization. (2019). *Displaced or refugee women are at increased risk of violence. What can WHO do?* Retrieved from: https://www.who.int/reproductivehealth/displaced-refugee-women-violence-risk/en/

The Vulnerability of Women as a Subject and Contemporary Theological Action: A Review of the Genesis and Evolution of Feminist Theology

Ricardo Alberto Rodríguez Villanueva

From the Theological Blush

This work aims to create a space for readers to reflect on the challenges and significance of Feminist Theology (FT). It also seeks to engage with concrete issues that require a deeper commitment to this theological perspective. To begin, I would like to share some data that reflects the current context in Mexico, which is similar to other Latin American countries like Brazil, Honduras, Argentina, and Colombia (Galván, 2019).

According to the UN, nine women are killed every day in Mexico. Since 2015, there have been 3200 femicides nationwide. From January to June 2019 alone, 470 cases were reported, based on figures from the Executive Secretariat of the National Public Security System (SESNSP). Mexico City has recorded 206 femicides over the past five years, with 18 occurring in the first half of 2019. Veracruz is currently the most dangerous state for women, with 104 femicide victims from January to June this year, followed by the State of Mexico with 42 cases during the same period (SESNSP).

From January to August of this year, 292 women were victims of sexual abuse in Mexico City; four of these cases involved gang rape, according to the capital's Open Data Portal (Agencia Digital de Innovación Pública, 2019). From 2013 to 2018, the perception of insecurity among women rose from 74.7% to 82.1%, as reported by the National Survey of Victimization and Perception of Public Security (Envipe) 2018 (El Instituto Nacional de Estadística y Geografía, 2018).

The same data shows that women feel more insecure than men in both public and private places: ATMs on public streets (87.4%), public transport (74.2%), streets (72.9%), highways (69.5%), markets (65.5%), parks (62.1%), cars (48.9%), schools (39.2%), workplaces (36.2%), and homes (26.7%). Women are the primary victims

R. A. Rodríguez Villanueva (✉)
UMG- Universidad Marista de Guadalajara, Guadalajara, Jalisco, Mexico

S. Castaños-Cervantes et al. (eds.), *Working with Vulnerable Populations*,
https://doi.org/10.1007/978-3-031-67710-6_17

of sexual crimes; in 2017, the crime rate was 2733 per 100,000 women, up from 1764 in 2016 (INEGI).

Given this harsh reality, I wish to highlight points that connect the reader with the theological reflection and the topic of Feminist Theology. First, I am presenting data that centralizes the discussion on the disadvantages faced by women in countries like Mexico. Next, I will discuss the work of James Alison, who introduces the concept of doing theology from a place of "blush"—a state of vulnerability that can be a starting point for developing theological ideas. With this in mind, I will outline the genesis and evolution of Feminist Theology to explore its contributions toward creating a world with greater justice and solidarity for women, who are a significant voice of God's revelation in contemporary times.

At this juncture, I would like to revisit some aspects that James Alison deems fundamental in locating the theological space. He places the prophet Elijah, after his conflict with the prophets of Baal, in a cave where he experiences a "crisis of confidence." In this moment, Elijah encounters different divine manifestations, which bring him closer to his own understanding of the transcendent. These revelations ultimately lead him to discover God's true presence in the simple—like a gentle breeze. Alison (2000) suggests that this realization involves "an authentic revolution that devastates personal structures and transforms how we speak of God" (Alison, 2000, p. 5).

Alison draws a parallel to Paul's experience in Jerusalem, B.o (1999), where Paul's conversion reveals that the truth he sought was not found in violence and persecution but in the peace offered by the Lord. These moments, as Alison illustrates, entail a new vision and a redefinition of the concept and following of God. I identify this phase of the theological space as a "blush"—a place of feeling ashamed or vulnerable.

This "blush" now allows for a discourse on the vulnerability of women within the theological field. This work aims to examine the origins and evolution of Feminist Theology, alongside various theoretical contributions that help position the discourse and practice of faith from a feminine perspective. Feminist Theology emerged from Liberation Theology and later evolved by critiquing and sometimes diverging from it. Feminist Theology has faced numerous challenges in giving voice to the voiceless, fighting for credibility, and developing its own theological methods.

This is why I mentioned earlier that this theological "blush" guides this work. As a Mexican man, I find the inequality and vulnerability that women experience simply for being women to be both outrageous and concerning. Engaging with the theological principles and methods of Feminist Theology provides a pathway to a new understanding of masculinity that acknowledges and respects the femininity inherent in God, which deserves to be heard, valued, and expressed in a manner that fosters a more supportive, just, and fraternal world for all.

By addressing Feminist Theology, I also seek a new way of understanding and interpreting the world. This highlights the importance of using a new theological method that generates new pathways for approaching the divine, from the perspective of women, while also shedding light on the Mexican context and the multifaceted violence it perpetuates against women.

Feminist Theology or theology by women (Velez, 2001, pp. 549–564) can be traced through various stages of development. From the 1960s, it began to formally critique patriarchal society, its norms, traditions, and practices that perpetuate the oppression and repression of women. Feminist Theology also draws from the methods of Liberation Theology, employing the "see-judge-act" approach: observing the reality of women's lives, judging it through the lens of God's word, and acting to transform women's reality. The objective of any new theological response is to propose a system of analysis that addresses and resolves reality by offering new hope from a transcendent perspective.

To achieve this, the feminist approach has undergone various evolutionary stages or trends, which I will detail further (Velez, 2001, pp. 547–549).

Waves of Feminist Theology

First Wave

- *Focus*: Challenges the foundational authority of the entire Judeo-Christian tradition, which, by tradition, could be considered patriarchal.
- *Approach*: Moves away from classical sources of theology, including Sacred Scripture, Tradition, and the Magisterium.
- *Key Figure*: Mary Daly.

Second Wave

- *Focus*: Questions the overarching structures of theology while maintaining the basic framework. This wave is considered reformist, introducing a new hermeneutical approach.
- *Approach*: Advocates for the renewal of biblical scholarship and the discovery of new elements within the biblical message.
- *Key Figure*: Elizabeth Schüssler Fiorenza.

Contemporary Waves

- *Focus*: Encompasses a diverse range of feminist theological perspectives, including:
- Feminist Theology.
- Feminist Liberation Theology.
- Womanist Theology.
- African-American Feminist Theology.
- Latin American Feminist Liberation Theology.
- Latin American Ecofeminist Theology.
- *Approach*: Reflects the varied struggles, expressions, and realities of women. It represents the evolution of theology from a feminine perspective.
- *Key Figures*: Various female authors and theologians contribute to this wave.

Methodological Foundations

This feminist theological framework is inspired by the methodological approach of the Second Vatican Council, emphasizing inductive reasoning over deductive. It values the experiences of women, transforming these experiences into theological reflections that support, guide, and reformulate the feminine experience. This process has been gradual, with numerous modifications, additions, and even internal disagreements along the way.

Elizabeth Schüssler Fiorenza (1996) proposes a model of feminist liberation interpretation, focusing on antihierarchy, which opposes the traditional model that is steeped in experiences of oppression and is deeply influenced by patriarchal traditions. She also critiques the androcentric interpretation and hermeneutics of the Bible, which have historically centered on male perspectives.

Elements of Feminist Hermeneutics

Velez (2001) provides a systematic outline of the main elements characterizing Elisabeth Schüssler Fiorenza's (1996) model, which I find helpful in understanding the feminist theological approach.

Review of Women's Representation in Scripture It is essential to carefully examine the information provided in the Scripture about women. We must recover and highlight the contributions women have made at various times and consider the multiple traditions—both biblical and extra-biblical—that have influenced the Church's teachings. Traditionally, these have often been viewed from an androcentric perspective, leading to the neglect of women's roles in the process of salvation. For instance, consider the enduring image of Mary Magdalene in Catholic tradition, where she is often depicted as a woman possessed by demons or traditionally mischaracterized as a prostitute (Ristine, 2018).

Critique of Patriarchal Interpretations It is important to recognize that biblical texts have often been interpreted in a way that reflects patriarchal cultural norms. We need to identify other traditions that support the liberation of women, moving away from traditional interpretations that prioritize an androcentric view. This shift allows for a more dignified understanding of women's roles.

Reimagining Women's Roles We must start envisioning women's presence and actions in biblical stories or historical moments where they have been overlooked due to an androcentric perspective. Employing a "hermeneutics of suspicion" is crucial to avoid falling back into traditional, biased portrayals of women. It is also essential to demystify the notion that women cannot be authors or interpreters of Sacred Scripture. We should return women to history and history to women and work toward developing sociopolitical and religious cultural models that place women at the center of the struggles and history of early Christianity. This approach ensures that women are recognized for their contributions and are no longer marginalized in the construction of the collective Christian imagination.

Critical Model of Feminist Interpretation of Liberation

To discuss this model, it's important to clarify its commitment to creating a different approach to developing theology. Unlike traditional hermeneutics, which aim to explore the meaning of texts, this feminist model focuses on the elements that shaped the construction of the text itself. It delves into the symbols each society used while writing the texts and examines the moral norms that influenced the biblical texts' characteristics. This approach involves reading, reconstructing, and practicing theology in a way that resists androcentrism and aims to transform gender relations.

Feminist Theology is dedicated to reclaiming the place of women in theology, a role that has been historically denied. This method seeks to revisit and emphasize the often-forgotten importance of women throughout history. Therefore, its author suggests that a dance serves as an ideal analogy for this interpretative method. Unlike classical hermeneutics with its linear and structured approach, this method allows movement between moments in a rhythmic and dynamic way, adapting as needed.

The dance metaphor highlights the fluidity and adaptability of this method, contrasting with the rigid steps of traditional hermeneutics, which adhere to a dogmatic structure often steeped in social, political, and religious contradictions that obscure the feminine perspective. This rhetoric involves the following steps:

(1) *Ideological Suspicion (Hermeneutics of Suspicion)*:

- This step involves examining texts with a focus on patriarchal, androcentric elements and the interpretations they have produced. By acknowledging that these texts may reflect such biases, we can develop a new perspective and approach to the text.

(2) *Historical Reconstruction (Hermeneutics of Proclamation)*:

- Imagine the experiences, feelings, and proclamations of women from the early Christian era. Recognize their participation and influence in various historical moments and even in the formation of the Church.

(3) *Theoretical Evaluation (Hermeneutics of Memory)*:

- Evaluate the context in which biblical texts were written, revealing that women also played significant roles and made contributions to biblical tradition.

(4) *Creative Imagination (Hermeneutics of Creative Imagination)*:

- Understand that the texts are influenced by an androcentric history and its dualisms. This step involves creating new interpretations of Scripture that foster a liberating relationship with women, acknowledging their struggles and restoring their rightful place in history.

Up to this point, we have explored the foundational elements and key paradigms of Feminist Theology. Now, it's time to focus on Latin America. The Liberation Theology of this region teaches us that there are diverse ways of being and expressing Christian faith. The unique perspectives from this part of the world offer a different lens through which to approach the divine. To further explore this evolution, we will examine the following experiences proposed by Velez (2001):

Evolution of Feminist Theology

The 1970s

Economic, Political, Ecclesial, and Theological Context:
- This era saw a surge in left-wing parties and popular movements.
- The CELAM's Medellín document laid the foundation for Liberation Theology, emphasizing the poor and the rise of grassroots ecclesial communities.
- Christians engaged actively in state issues, merging politics with theology, focusing on themes like exodus, liberation, and the historical Jesus.

Construction of Feminist Consciousness in Theology:
- Women began identifying as subjects of theological and liberative importance due to ongoing oppression based on social status and gender.
- There was mutual distrust between religion and theologians, complicating the development of a collaborative relationship.

Hermeneutics from a Woman's Perspective:
- God is seen as an ally of the oppressed, and the recovery of elements from classical texts is crucial for understanding liberation, highlighting Christology, the exodus, and justice.
- Central figures such as Deborah, Mary, and Hagar are emphasized, advocating for solidarity with the doubly oppressed and the need for new gender relations.

Reflection on Language:
- Terms like "feminist" and "inclusive language" were highly stigmatized and lacked validation.

The 1980s

Economic, Political, Ecclesial, and Theological Context:

- The period saw the end of dictatorships and the rise of restricted democracies, including the success of the Sandinista Front in Nicaragua.
- Foreign debt increased poverty, and liberation theology faced persecution while discussing themes like the Kingdom of God and the spirituality of liberation.
- An open dialogue about women's theological roles began, involving both men and women in the discussion.

Construction of Feminist Consciousness in Theology:

- More women entered the theological field, although their roles were not yet prominent. The generic focus on the poor was questioned, with women advocating for theology from a female perspective.
- Feminine perspectives began to be integrated into divine discourse, fostering dialogues with feminist traditions in Latin America and globally.

Hermeneutics from a Woman's Perspective:

- Efforts to interpret the entire biblical text from a woman's perspective included themes like God's feminine images and the reevaluation of women's virtues.
- There was a push to move beyond selective text interpretation, addressing patriarchal biases and considering non-normative texts when necessary.

Reflection on Language:

- Inclusive language started to be more explicit (using "he and she"), and the term "feminist" began to gain acceptance, although it faced resistance.

The 1990s

Economic, Political, Ecclesial, and Theological Context:

- The collapse of Eastern bloc countries and the Gulf War prompted ideological shifts.
- Neoliberalism emerged, marginalizing various groups, especially women.
- Grassroots ecclesial movements stagnated, and the rise of Pentecostalism reduced church polarization.
- Indigenous Theology grew, offering new biblical interpretations and perspectives. Feminist theology adopted a more radical, inclusive stance.

Construction of Feminist Consciousness in Theology:

- The effort to reclaim the feminine in theology was deemed insufficient. Ivonne Gebara called for a complete theological overhaul, incorporating gender theories to deepen feminist theological discourse.
- Black and indigenous women demanded that anthropological and symbolic theories be applied to their contexts.

Hermeneutics from a Woman's Perspective:

- Everyday life and the body became new interpretive categories, rejecting martyrdom and sacrifice themes.
- New epistemological frameworks were applied to Pauline texts and biblical themes like joy and corporeality.
- A radical challenge emerged to rethink Christian theology, causing discomfort due to its departure from orthodoxy.

Reflection on Language:

- Feminist and inclusive language remained stigmatized, but efforts continued to de-stigmatize and validate these terms.
- There was a shift toward describing God in non-gendered terms (e.g., grace, mercy, energy) and integrating gender theories.
- The term "feminist" gained acceptance, focusing on contextualizing contributions from global feminists for Latin America.

Feminist Theology's Objective

Feminist theology aims to combat exclusion while recognizing and preserving diversity. It seeks to end intolerance and foster mutual acceptance, acknowledging the equal dignity and diversity of both men and women as active participants in society and the Church (Huguet, 1988, pp. 105–123).

Feminist Theology (FT)

Reframing Women's Perspectives Feminist Theology (FT) aims to shift the perception of women from being a problematic issue to being a lens through which social, political, and theological realities can be reinterpreted. Theologians engage with texts through a feminist lens, reexamining established theological principles and offering a fresh perspective for analysis and reflection.

Initially, FT focuses on raising awareness of liberation, adopting a prophetic and transformative approach to reality. It operates independently of ecclesiastical institutions and engages directly with Revelation and its content.

A key tension exists between ideological feminism, which is centered on social and political struggle for women's rights, and feminist theology, which seeks a deeper understanding of God and humanity through Revelation.

A Critical Theology of Liberation Feminist Theology draws from the liberating principles of Liberation Theology, recognizing that women's experiences bring a new way of understanding theology and life. However, it diverges from traditional Liberation Theology, which is often seen as male-dominated and neglects the liberation of women.

Jakobs (1996) highlights that feminist theology must always address specific people and real-world political, historical, and social situations. If this connection is not visible, theology risks becoming mere ideology.

The exclusion of women from the Catholic priesthood underscores ongoing inequality. Despite the liberating intentions of Jesus' ministry, classical dogmatic theology has perpetuated oppression and discrimination. Castillo (2010) argues that any Christology that justifies suffering in Jesus' name is a distortion and misrepresentation of Jesus' true message. A divisive and confrontational Christology is inconsistent with Jesus' teachings.

Feminist theology critiques patriarchal norms, which are closely tied to male-dominated perspectives, and challenges the association of power with men. Theologians like Schüssler Fiorenza argue that patriarchal theology fails to recognize women's full dignity and humanity (1985). FT seeks to expose how androcentric language and theological frameworks support patriarchal structures within the Church.

Challenging Androcentric Interpretations Feminist Theology advocates for a Biblical interpretation free from sexist bias. It introduces a new hermeneutic approach, believing that a fresh examination of biblical texts can uncover liberating messages overlooked by traditional patriarchal theology (Porcile, 1988).

By unraveling patriarchal cultural roots, feminist theology allows for new interpretations. Works like Elisabeth Cady Stanton's *The Woman's Bible* highlight the need to reassess women's roles in religious texts. E.S. Fiorenza emphasizes the importance of rediscovering and reinterpreting traditions about women and exposing sexist translations and interpretations. Feminist theology seeks to recover female language, metaphors, and images of God (Bernabé, 2010).

Contributions and Challenges Feminist theology has been an ongoing process of recognizing and addressing the historical subjugation of women by theological concepts. It advocates for liberation on three levels: ideas and concepts, imagery, and language. This approach directly challenges classical theological methods by acknowledging an androcentric bias in traditional theology and emphasizing the importance of women's contributions throughout history.

FT emphasizes the need to incorporate women's experiences to develop more comprehensive theological insights. It has effectively used these experiences to create systematic theological knowledge. Recognizing the historical oppression of women within the Church, FT builds its narrative from this foundation. This connection aligns feminist theology with both liberation theology and the feminist liberation movement.

Feminist Theology (FT) follows the same structure as liberation theologies, which see themselves as a 'second act.' In this context, the 'first act' is the lived experience of faith, while theology is the reflective process that comes afterward, the 'second act.'

> In liberation theology, this second act rigorously builds upon a foundational experience of faith that is deeply rooted in a committed and demanding context—what is known as contextualized theology. It aims to transform unjust relationships characterized by dependency and domination. Similarly, FT functions as a second act, reflecting upon and assuming a prior commitment to and active involvement in women's liberation movements. (Gibellini, 1986, p. 55)

From Feminist Theology to the Latin American Ecofeminist Version

Overview and Evolution

We have explored the origins and development of feminist theology. However, it's important to highlight its current trajectory and evolution. Today, feminist theology critically examines the patriarchal and kyriocentric system that encompasses traditional concepts like Father, Religion, and Church. Theologians are now gaining recognition for proposing a new way of understanding and generating knowledge outside conventional contexts, focusing on a different relationship with the transcendent.

It's crucial to clarify that feminist theology does not simply make women the central theme. Instead, it positions women as active participants reflecting on their faith. This approach is inclusive, aiming to create a new social, political, and religious order that benefits both men and women. This systematic reflection has transformed the role of women from a marginal subject into a central focus in theological discourse, highlighting their thoughts, feelings, and relationship with the divine.

> It is important to note that there isn't just one type of feminist theology but rather a spectrum of feminist theologies. Latin American feminist liberation theology has developed over a long process and differs from other forms of feminist theology such as: American and European feminist theology, liberation theology by male theologians, northern feminist liberation theology, womanist theology by Black women in the U.S., womanist theology by Latin or Hispanic women in the U.S., Afro-American feminist theology by Indigenous and Black women in Latin America, and Latin American ecofeminist theology. (Rojas Salazar, 2015, pp. 30–36)

Key Contributions and Perspectives

One of the significant contributors to this theological reflection is Ivone Gebara, a Brazilian theologian who has integrated ecology and feminism into a Latin American context under the umbrella of Liberation Theology. Her work, although controversial and criticized by the Roman Catholic hierarchy, has led to what is known as Ecofeminist Liberation Theology. Key elements of this perspective, based on the work of Comesaña Santalices (2010), include:

(1) *Relationality*

- This involves developing a new way of relating to everything around us, recognizing ourselves as part of a greater whole that extends beyond our limited human perspective. It proposes an epistemology that sees humanity as part of a larger being, which constitutes the sacred body of the Earth and the cosmos. This approach advocates for a new ethic that respects indigenous peoples, their land, and their customs, while also challenging the exploitative aspects of the market economy.

(2) *Knowledge as a Process*

- This perspective rejects the patriarchal, linear view of knowledge construction. Instead, it embraces a circular understanding of events, where each occurrence builds upon the previous one in an ongoing, complex process of change. Gebara argues for an appreciation of the complexities that define us, emphasizing that knowledge is a dynamic, evolving process.

(3) *Unified Spirit-Matter*

- This concept represents a radical shift from the traditional anthropological, cosmological, and epistemological views that underpin classical dogmatic theology, which is predominantly heteropatriarchal. It posits that we are composed of both spirit and matter, intertwined without separation. We must embrace the transformation of our individual bodies into the mystery of our sacred body. Life's fleeting presence in the universe, which is both vital and mortal, demands intense love, respect for all beings, the pursuit of justice, and the right to happiness for everyone.

(4) *Gender and Ecology*

- Introducing these elements allows for a comprehensive analysis of human reality that moves beyond a narrow, masculine perspective, which often views humans as the pinnacle of creation with the authority to dominate it. An inclusive approach recognizes the diverse experiences of both men and women, providing a more holistic understanding of reality.

(5) *Holistic Perspective*

- This theological view values a diverse range of perspectives that are often overlooked by traditional, monotheistic interpretations. It champions the subjective, open, and diverse over the singular and objective. This includes valuing emotional aspects of knowledge, which brings a new dimension that contrasts sharply with traditional, reason-based approaches.

(6) *Inclusivity*

- Experiencing God or the divine is inherently inclusive of others. Religious experience is diverse and multifaceted, though there is a common underlying search for meaning, for that "mysterious" essence that dwells within and transcends us. Therefore, an inclusive epistemology welcomes the multitude of religious experiences as different expressions of a shared quest for unity and understanding.

By integrating these elements, ecofeminist theology fosters a deeper, more inclusive understanding of human and divine interconnectedness, challenging traditional theological norms and advocating for a more just and inclusive world.

Conclusion

In this work, my goal was to offer a historical perspective on the origins and development of theological thought, focusing specifically on the contributions of feminist theology. Rather than merely concluding this work, it is crucial to highlight the theological debt we owe to this paradigm. We must acknowledge and recognize the urgent and paramount necessity for the Church to open up, granting it space, respect, and value and honoring the epistemic approach that feminist theology offers. This perspective brings an undeniable shift in how we perceive women as bearers of God's revelation.

We must accept that feminist theology calls for justice in response to every instance where patriarchal attitudes within the Church have marginalized and undervalued women and their contributions. Moreover, as I discussed in the first part of this work, we must strive to create a world where women can feel whole, safe, empowered, dignified, and recognized as equals. The insecurity and unjust violence revealed by the statistics presented at the beginning of this work are a harsh reality that persists in our society, posing a challenge to theology, whether feminist or not, to actively foster a more just, fraternal, supportive, and sisterly environment—not just in rhetoric but also in concrete action. It is imperative to build bridges that enable faith to be lived in a manner that reduces structural and patriarchal violence against women.

Dedication I am writing from the perspective of a man committed to Feminist Theology who pays homage to a theological viewpoint that allows me to confront the stark reality of living in a country like Mexico, where women are still murdered simply because they are women. This viewpoint compels me to rethink my own masculinity and embrace a new understanding of God. I am reminded of the late Dr. Barbara Andrade, who, when I once asked her in class, "Who is God?" would often reply, "What if She is Black?" Thank you, dear Barbara, for planting the seed of a Father/Mother God and for opening my mind and heart to a new perspective.

References

Agencia Digital de Innovación Pública (ADIP). (2019). *Víctimas en carpeta de investigación en la Procuraduría General de Justicia. [Victims in investigation folder at the Attorney General's Office].* Retrieved from Portal de datos abiertos de la CDMX: https://datos.cdmx.gob.mx/explore/dataset/denuncias-victimas-pgj/table/?refine.ao=2019&refine.sexo=Femenino&refine.categoria=VIOLACION

Alison, J. (2000). *Una fé más allá del resentimiento [faith beyond resenment: Fragments catholic and gay]* (p. 5). Herder.

Bernabé, C. (2010). *Diez mujeres escriben teología. [Ten women write Theology]* (p. 31). Estella.

Castillo, J. M. (2010). *La humanización de Dios. Ensayo de Cristología. [The humanization of God. Cristology Essay].* Trotta. 207

Comesaña Santalices, G. (2010). *Ivone Gebara: una religiosa y teóloga ecofeminista. [Ivone Gebara: a religiuos and feminist theologician]* CLEPSYDRA. p. 41–68.

El Instituto Nacional de Estadística y Geografía (INEGI). (2018). *National Survey of Victimization and perception on public security.* Retrieved from INEGI: https://www.inegi.org.mx/contenidos/saladeprensa/boletines/2018/EstSegPub/envipe2018_09.pdf

Galván, M. (2019). *14 datos de la violencia de género que explican el enojo de las mujeres en Expansión. Política. [14 data on gender violence that explain the anger of women in Expansión. Politics].* Retrieved from https://politica.expansion.mx/mexico/2019/08/19/datos-sobre-violencia-contra-mujeres-mexico

Gibellini, R. (1986). Feminismo y Teología. Iglesia Viva. [Feminism and Theology. Live Church]. *Concilium, 121*, 55.

Huguet, M. A. (1988). Hacia una comprensión de la teología feminista. Cristo y el Dios de los cristianso. Hacia una comprensión actual de la Teología. [Towards an understanding of feminist theology. Christ and the God of Christians. Towards a current understanding of theology]. In E. J. e. Morales (Ed.), *XVIII Simposion Internacional de Teología de la Universidad de Navarra* (pp. 105–123). Servicio de Publicaciones de la Universidad de Navarra.

Jakobs, M. (1996). La Teología feminista en Europa, [The feminist theology in Europe]. *Concilium, 263*, 56.

Jerusalem, B.o. (1999) *Acts of the Apostles 9.* Doubleday.

Magdala M. M., & Ristine, J. (2018). *Mujeres más.* Retrieved from mujeresmas.mx: http://mujeresmas.mx/2018/07/18/maria-magdalena-no-fue-prostituta-jennifer-ristine/

Porcile, M. (1988). Mujer, espacio de salvación [Women, space of Salvation]. *Concilium, 69.*

Rojas Salazar, M. (2015). Teología feminista de la liberación [Feminist Theology of liberation]. *Revista de la Universidad Iberoamericana, VII*(39), 30–36. Obtenido de Revista IBERO: Rojas Salazar, Marilú (2015) Revista de la Universidad Iberoamericana Año VII Número 39 Agosto–septiembre 2015 www.ibero.mx/revistaibero/

Schüssler Fiorenza, E. (1985). *Romper el silencio. [Breaking the silence]* (p. 303). Concilium.

Schüssler Fiorenza, E. (1996). *Pero ella dijo. [But she said].* Trotta.

Velez, C. C. (2001). Teología de la mujer, feminismo y género. [Theology of women, feminism and gender]. *Revista Theológica Xaveriana, 140*, 545–564.

Femicide in Brazil

Jackeline Aparecida Ferreira Romio

Introduction

This chapter[1] is derived from the work carried out previously in a doctoral thesis on the subject of femicides in Brazil and the attempt to classify and measure their occurrence through secondary sources of information produced by the health sector and with the objective of assisting in the monitoring and diagnosis of the growing gender violence against women. The text analyzes and explains how the concept of femicides was modernized and amplified in the conceptual field and adapted to Latin American national realities as they spread as a law. In the end, it presents the author's understanding and a proposal for a new synthetic typology of the various paths that led to the current definition of femicide.

This article is derived from the Thesis Romio, JAF. "Feminicídios no Brasil, uma proposta de análise com dados do setor de saúde", UNICAMP. Campinas, SP, 2017.

[1] This chapter is a version in English of the paper of the author named "Feminicidio, o direito da mulher nomear suas eperiencias". Revista Plural. V. 26 N. 1 (2019): GÊNERO EM PERSPECTIVA INTERSECCIONAL/Dossiê: "Gênero em perspectiva interseccional."

J. A. F. Romio (✉)
State University of Campinas—UNICAMP, São Paulo, Brazil
e-mail: jackeline.romio@gmail.com

S. Castaños-Cervantes et al. (eds.), *Working with Vulnerable Populations*,
https://doi.org/10.1007/978-3-031-67710-6_18

Concept of Femicide

The concept of femicide emerged from the mid-1970s in the feminist movement, as a new way of naming the deaths of women by homicide because of their social status as women and in opposition to the apparent neutrality of the term homicide, which designated deaths by murder without the observation of the sex and gender differences in these deaths. The concept of femicide begins to dispute the epistemology of human rights, the word is a neologism.

The first time the term femicide was used occurred during the sessions of the First International Tribunal on Crimes against Women in Brussels, Belgium, in 1976. *In this court on the deaths of women in the United States and Lebanon, feminist activist Diana Russell testified and argued that such occurrences were the consequence of misogynistic actions and, as such, should be presented and judged as femicides.* The concept set forth in that court would encompass a variety of violence against women that result in death, from the practice of burning women considered witches in the past to infanticide of girls or cases of murders justified for reasons of honor. The activist aimed to demonstrate that this type of crime has been committed over time and for different reasons (Russell, 2011).

Later, in 1992, Diana Russell and Jill Radford launched the book *Femicide: The Politics of Woman Killing,* composed of several articles written by researchers and women's human rights activists on the subject of femicides, between 1980 and 1990. The authors analyzed the occurrence of the phenomenon in the United States, the United Kingdom, and India, adding discussions such as racism, systematic sexual violence, and lesbophobia as important dimensions to be considered (Russell & Radford, 1992).

In the introduction to the book, Jill Radford, co-editor of the work, defines femicides as follows:

> Femicide is the misogynistic murder of women by men, it is a form of sexual violence. As defined by Liz Kelly, sexual violence can be considered as "any type of physical, visual, verbal, or sexual act experienced by women or girls that has generated any effect that hurts, degrades, or takes away the ability to control intimate contacts." (Kelly, 1988: 41)

This definition is found in the book *Surviving Sexual Violence* (1988) in which she established the concept of the "*continuum* of violence," a framework for the development of the concept of femicide, which shows an outbreak of violence that can result in the death of women. Internal to this definition is the recognition of the dissonance between the perceptions and experiences of the social world and of sexual violence between women and men. The vision gives priority to women's experiences and understandings over the intentions of men and is consistent with one of the foundations of feminism: the right of women to name their experiences (Radford, 1992: 3).

For Radford (1992), this way of treating sexual violence developed by sociologist Liz Kelly expands the possibility of understanding, since it focuses on the desire for power, domination, and control. This conceptualization sees sexual aggression committed by men in relation to all the oppressions of women in a patriarchal society.[2] This also makes it possible to make connections between the various forms of sexual violence, that is, a "*continuum* of sexual violence," where rape, sexual harassment, pornography, and physical abuse of women and children are all different expressions of sexual violence committed by men and not discrete or disconnected from each other (Radford, 1992: 3).

The author believes that this resignification may be more sensitive to women's perceptions of violence compared to a legal vision of it, which tends to be biased by racist, heterosexist, and moralistic considerations embedded in the justice and public security apparatus, that is, the observation of the *continuum* of sexual violence against women makes it possible to identify and address the range of forced and coercive heterosexual experiences that women are subjected to, facilitating the analysis of sexual violence masculinity as a central form of maintaining patriarchy. The author locates femicide within this *continuum*, unmasking the tendency to portray and interpret aggressors as beasts or animals (a type of man who escapes the standards of "normality"), placing it in terms of sexual policies for the appropriation of women (Radford, 1992: 4).

Other factors highlighted by Radford concern the silence and trivialization involved in the overall treatment of these deaths by the justice system and the tabloid media. When a woman is murdered, there are no survivors to tell her story, there are no testimonies, and we are left with official documents notifying the deaths by the authorities and the accounts of relatives of the victim, the aggressor, and the witnesses. In cases of aggression against women, there is a tendency to make her the person responsible for the aggression she suffered (Radford, 1992: 6).

Addressing the structural issues of sexual violence perpetrated by men, the researcher clarifies that this type of violence has been defined as a characteristic of patriarchal society, the central way in which men hold power over women and children, expressing themselves as other forms of oppression, such as racism, in economic and legal discrimination, as every form of structural oppression is rooted in violence. Femicide serves to control women as a sex class and is fundamental to maintaining the *status quo* of patriarchy. Radford's definition is closely linked to the conceptions of violence in radical feminist theory, which seeks especially to highlight the patriarchal structures of women's oppression (Radford, 1992: 6).

In another text from the collection *Femicide (1992), Jane Caputi and Diana Russel define femicide* as follows:

> Like rape, many murders of women by husbands, lovers, parents, acquaintances, and strangers are not the product of some inexplicable deviation, they are femicides, the most extreme form of sexist terrorism, motivated by hate, contempt, pleasure, or a sense of ownership over women. Femicide includes deaths by mutilation, rape, beatings that end in death, immolation as in the case of women considered witches in Europe or widows in Asia, crimes of honor [...] naming them femicide removes the uncreated veil of terms such as homicide and murder. (Caputi & Russel, 1992: 15—own translation)

---

[2] Male domination + female subordination = patriarchal society.

For the authors,

> … femicide speaks of the extreme end of the anti-woman terror *continuum* that includes a variety of forms of physical and verbal violence and abuse, such as rape, torture, sexual slavery (particularly in prostitution), incest and extrafamiliar sexual abuse of children, physical and emotional violence, sexual harassment (by telephone, on the street, at work, and at school), genital mutilation (clitoridetomy, excision, infibulation), unnecessary gynecological operations (free forced hysterectomies), heterosexuality forced sterilization, forced motherhood (through the criminalization of contraception and abortion), psychosurgery, denial of food to women in some cultures, cosmetic surgery and other mutilation in the name of beauty. Whenever these forms of terrorism result in death, they become femicides. (Caputi & Russel, 1992: 15)

In another text in the collection, about the reinterpretations of the murders of women in European history, Marriane Hester deals with the persecution of witches in continental Europe, Scotland, and England, in the sixteenth and seventeenth centuries, a period in which thousands of women were sentenced to imprisonment and death on charges of witchcraft, which she called "historically covert femicide" (Hester, 1992: 30).

The author was attentive to the demographic context of the sixteenth and seventeenth centuries, when the population was changing and women were more numerous than men. For the lower classes, marriages took place increasingly later. Among small landowners and workers, the average age at first marriage was very high in the seventeenth century, rising from 27 years to 28 years for men and from 25 to 27 years for women. The circumstances of economic hardship meant that a marriage could not be financially maintained before that. The effect of this delay on marriage was the growth in the number of unmarried people, especially women, and of women living outside of male control. Within this context, women alone were actively competitive with men to survive in a situation of scarcity of resources, the particular case of peasant women, who were the most affected by the persecution of witches, especially the elderly (Hester, 1992: 30).

The proposals of the articles compiled in the book *Femicide: The Politics of Killing Women* have become conceptual frameworks for any research that seeks to understand the murder of women from a feminist point of view and that considers the interaction of oppressions, especially those of gender, race, class, and sexuality. The purpose of the compilation was to name femicide and identify it as an urgent topic both for feminists and for people fighting to end violence against women. For them, femicide is located in the context of sexual policies that guide patriarchal oppression.

In a more current discourse, Russell rediscusses his initial contributions to the concept of femicide and highlights the importance of choices regarding the spelling of the term. For her, the use of the prefix "Fem" refers to the English term "Female" and not "women," because in English the term "women" restricts the woman's age to the adult/reproductive period of the life cycle, which was not the intention of the author who wanted to include women of various age groups, whether girls, adolescents, adults, or the elderly, in the concept of femicide. This score could also be based on Brazilian Portuguese, where the word "woman" restricts a woman's age to the adult phase of the life cycle. Over the last 30 years, the term *femicide* began to be spelled in two ways in Castilian and Portuguese-speaking countries, sometimes as femicide, sometimes as femicide. For some authors, who later developed works on the subject, the differences do not only lie in the graphic form of the word but also in the concepts inherent to each chosen spelling. As an example, for some authors, the choice to spell femicide makes sense because it eliminates possible interpretations that equate femicide to homicide, which would result in a reductionism of the concept's potential (Russell, 2011). This last interpretation is also the option for this thesis, in which the concept is spelled as femicides, reducing to the maximum the noise that this new perspective may suffer.

Russell (2011) adds that femicides are the deaths of women due to unsuccessful abortions in countries with governments governed by patriarchal and religious premises that prohibit them in their legislation, as well as deaths resulting from the AIDS epidemics and the infection resulting from rape and sexist behavior, such as massacres with the majority of female victims.

In these texts, two forms of femicide are evident, one direct, specifically the murders of women by men, and the other indirect, which are the other forms of patriarchal violence that ends in death, especially institutional forms, such as the prohibition of abortion and other policies to control sexuality and the female body that ends in death, as well as the negligence of States to curb, punish, and eradicate direct forms, because State negligence promotes violence and the sense of security and justice is dislocated from the public sphere of the rights to become an individual responsibility.

The Dissemination and Translation of the Concept of Femicide in Latin America

At the beginning of the 1990s, the number of reports of the murder of young women maquiladora workers began to grow[3] in the border region between Mexico and the United States, Ciudad Juárez, Chihuahua. Sexual violence, mutilation, disfigurement, and abandonment of bodies on public roads and places, in the context of the deaths, drew the attention of the media and public opinion, causing outrage among the population. At that moment, a series of mobilizations began to defend women's human rights and to bring justice to the victims and their families. In this context, the concept of femicide has entered Latin America as a concept that defines this specific death of women.

The understanding given to the murders of Mexican women within the concept of femicide focuses on issues of social class and race/ethnicity and shifts the focus more on the intimate aggressor to the negligence on the part of the Mexican State in

[3] Companies that assemble and finish products for export, mostly from the USA and Japan, produce mainly electronics, car parts, and textiles. These types of companies are characteristic of the Mexican border region and have had expansion and tax incentives for their development since the 1960s. They are also the form of industrialization of this region of Mexico, a trademark of which are the low salaries and the high labor exploitation.

dealing with the murders, including the absence of investigation or assembly of rapid institutional responses focused on presenting culprits. Another debate that the Mexican case promoted was to reflect on structural issues related to the advancement of the neoliberal mode of production and its relationship with deaths, such as the installation of multinationals in the border region of Mexico and the subsequent internal migration of women in search of work in the region (Lagarde, 2006; Falquet, 2014).

The working conditions of women in the maquiladora factories and the absence of national policies aimed at the social development of this region make up the socioeconomic and political context of these deaths, in addition to the political aspects and military control throughout the country's history. Falquet (2014) points out that such contexts are comparable to similar stories of dictatorship and post-war history on the American continent (Falquet, 2014).

Dan La Botz (1999) dates back to the death of 13-year-old teenager Irma Angelica Rosales, who was raped and murdered on the way between her work and her home in Ciudad Juárez, on the border with the city of El Paso, Texas. For him, deaths like hers are symbols of corporate power, child labor, and the exploitation of women at the border. For him, the multinational maquiladora corporations (USA) were deployed on the USA–Mexico border as a result of exploiting the labor of young women like Irma. Young women were the majority of workers in these industries[4] at the time, and a dichotomous situation coexisted between the infrastructure offered by the government to the maquiladora companies and the social counterpart offered to the surrounding communities (La Botz, 1999).[5]

While multinational corporations such as General Motors, Ford, General Electric, and Johnson & Johnson obtained from their partnerships with the Mexican and American governments support for the construction of modern industrial parks with enormous parking possibilities for trucks, high-voltage electricity networks, and, in some cases, landscaped outdoor areas, the workers lived in subhuman conditions.

The US and Mexican governments, in partnership with private companies, built superhighways, railroads, and airports to serve the maquiladora zone. On the other hand, workers live in shacks and in the wreckage of industrial production, on unpaved streets, in places without running water, sewers, or electricity, with overcrowded schools and many young women working without attending school, in addition to the novelty of crack. Drug traffickers, police officers, and even the Mexican Army cooperated in the movement of drugs across the border. Police violence, shootings by rival factions, the widespread presence of private security for the rich, and factories threatened the safety of ordinary citizens (La Botz, 1999—free translation).

From the 1990s onwards, the concept of femicides began to be applied in Mexico and then disseminated to other Latin American countries. Among the voices is that

[4]Although young women can only be employed at the age of 16, it was common at that time for minors aged 12, 13, and 14 to be employed through false documentation.

[5]http://corpwatch.org/article.php?id=798

of the Mexican anthropologist and congressman Marcela Lagarde, who, influenced by the studies of Russell and Radford (1992), translated the term feminicide (*feminicídio*) from English into the Castilian form *femicide to understand and intervene politically in the deaths of* those young women.

Marcela Lagarde was the main Mexican feminist scholar to comment on femicides. She updated the concept of femicide to refer to the set of violations of women's human rights that exist in the deaths and disappearances of women in Mexico, in addition to understanding them as crimes against humanity (Lagarde, 2008: 216).

> Feminicide is genocide against women and occurs when historical conditions generate social practices that allow violent attacks against the integrity, health, freedom, and lives of girls and women. (Lagarde, 2008: 216)

According to Lagarde, the concept of feminicide addresses crimes against children and women to patriarchy, considering that they express the extreme end of gender domination against women. It identifies various types of agents of this violence, who may be people from various types of relationships with the victims, and highlights aspects of motivation linked to hate, such as:

> partners, ex-partners, boyfriends, spouses, companions, family members, visitors, colleagues and co-workers, or by the military, unknown and anonymous. The existence of criminal mafia groups linked to crime and their languages is also reported. A hallmark of these crimes is the high level of cruelty and in fact they are hate crimes against women. (Lagarde, 2008: 216)

For the author, "feminicide demonstrates the structural inequality between women and men and how the domination of men over women finds in gender violence a mechanism for reproducing the oppression of women." When the State and its authorities designated to prevent and eradicate these crimes act in a negligent, inefficient, and prejudiced manner and gender blindness or sexist and misogynistic prejudices about women coexist in society, the researcher considers that the condition for the existence of feminicides is created and that this becomes a State crime (Lagarde, 2008: 217).

Marcela Lagarde was a deputy from 2003 to 2007, in Mexico, for the *Partido de La Revolucìon Democratica (PRD)*, a period in which she acted to classify the crime of feminicide. In the period before her term of office, there was a special commission to investigate the homicides of girls and women in Ciudad Juárez. The commission used some information about existing homicides, even if in an incipient form. During this period, several complaints were filed about crimes against women from other parts of the country (Lagarde, 2008: 218).

To address the complexity of the cases in Mexican territory, under Lagarde's leadership, a special commission was created to monitor feminicides throughout Mexico. There were many conceptual and political advances during this process, first by dealing with cases throughout the country and not just in Ciudad Juárez and by naming the crimes with the terminology of feminicides and no longer as homicides, opting for the treatment of cases from a gender perspective. Little by little, the parliamentary committee began to work on the issue of accepting complaints and demanding justice (Lagarde, 2008: 218–219).

> The Diagnostic Investigation on Feminicidal Violence in the Mexican Republic was the first qualitative and quantitative scientific research on gender violence against women carried out in Mexico from a feminist perspective on gender and women's human rights. The main objective was to specifically document the situation of feminicide in the country, by locating feminicide as part of domestic violence and other forms of violence investigated. (Lagarde, 2008: 10—own translation)

The commission used official information from 1999 to 2006, with data on intentional and wrongful homicides. The crimes of feminicide were understood within the framework of gender violence and of relations with all forms of violence against girls and women. According to the research findings, the profile of these women varies according to their ages and social class but focuses on young, poor, and marginalized women. The victims suffered various forms of torture and violence (Lagarde, 2008: 222).

The theoretical perspective that the group adopted eventually demonstrated several other violent deaths of girls and women. The investigation uncovered alarming numbers of domestic accidents, traffic accidents, and suicides. A high number of women who died from reproductive health issues, such as cervical and ovarian cancer, was revealed, and it was confirmed that maternal deaths ranked first in the mortality rates of women of reproductive age. Regional studies showed marked differences between the various regions and cities of Mexico, revealing complex and differentiated realities by region (Lagarde, 2008: 224–225).

For Lagarde, the results of the Diagnostic Investigation of feminicides proved the various theoretical theses about them, including the fact that violence against women is "serious, complex and multifactorial, the result of the synergetic articulation of a set of determinations based on domination and sex." Alert to the issue of racism, classism, lesbophobia, and other related forms of oppression (Lagarde, 2008: 232).

Feminicide is one of the extreme forms of gender violence and is made up of a set of misogynistic violent acts against women, which entail the violation of their human rights, threatening their safety and endangering their lives. It culminates in the murder of some girls and women. There are countless survivors. Feminicide is consummated because authorities, who are silent, negligent, or in collusion with aggressors, exercise institutional violence against women by obstructing their access to justice and thereby contribute to impunity. Feminicide entails a partial rupture of the rule of law, since the State is unable to guarantee women's lives, to respect their human rights, to act legally and to ensure respect, to seek and administer justice, and to prevent and eradicate the violence that causes it. Feminicide is a state crime (Lagarde, 2008: 234).

Another study on femicides is the case of Costa Rica in Central America. Researchers Montserrat Sagot and Ana Carcedo analyzed the reality of the murders of women for the reality of Costa Rica. Like Lagarde, Sagot and Carcedo used Russell's original concept but chose to translate femicide with the spelling as in English.

Sagot and Carcedo say that violence against women has caused more deaths than malaria, AIDS, or war. The ideas of peace and security are strongly associated with the institution of the family in the Western world, but the authors argue that this is a conservative vision that does not reveal the experience of girls and women who have the most violent social group in their family and the home (casa), the most insecure place. According to her reflections, there is no exact estimate of the magnitude of violence based on gender inequality and its impacts due to high underreporting. However, many researches have made its existence increasingly evident (Sagot & Carcedo, 2006: 405).

For Sagot and Carcedo (2006), violence based on gender inequity is a significant cause of female illness and mortality. The researchers collected statistical information on the murder of women in Costa Rica for reasons associated with gender inequity, from 1990 to 1999. They analyzed the relationship between the victim and the aggressor, the place of the occurrence, the manner and conditions in which the women were killed, previous help requested by the women, and the answers found. The purpose of the study was to construct prevention and protection proposals for women at risk of death from violence based on gender inequity (Sagot & Carcedo, 2006: 409).

The research adopted as a theoretical framework knowledge about gender socialization, violence,[6] and femicide.[7] For Sagot and Carcedo, the concept of femicide "helps to dismantle the arguments that violence based on gender inequity is a personal or private matter and shows its profoundly social and political character, the result of power relations between men and women in society" (Sagot & Carcedo, 2006: 413).

The researchers understood femicide as:

> Femicide is understood to mean the murder of women for reasons associated with their gender. Femicide is the most extreme form of violence based on gender inequity, understood as violence exercised by men against women in their desire to gain power, domination, or control. It includes murders produced by intra-family and sexual violence. (Sagot & Carcedo, 2006: 414)

Starting from this initial definition, they develop the typology: intimate, non-intimate, and connected femicide. *Intimate femicide*[8] refers to murders committed by men with whom the victims had an intimate, family, cohabitation, or affinity relationship. *Non-intimate femicide* refers to murders committed by men with whom the victim had no intimate, family, or cohabitation relations, or affinity with them. It usually involves sexual assault. *Femicide by connection* refers to the murder of women who were murdered "in the line of fire" of a man trying to kill another

[6]All societies establish precise mechanisms for human beings to learn the behaviors and attitudes considered appropriate for each gender expectation, a process called gender socialization. A process that is not neutral and its main objective is to force people to adapt to the norms of a society structured based on gender inequality and oppression. Social control. Conceptual reference Andersen, 1988. (Sagot & Carcedo, 2006: 410).

[7]"Violence against women is also a structural component of the system of gender oppression" (Sagot & Carcedo, 2006: 2011).

[8]It is important to note that the type of intimate femicide already appears as a category in Diana Russell's (1992) assessments.

woman. Here are women in a family context, children, or other women who tried to intervene or who were simply caught up in the action of the femicide (Sagot & Carcedo, 2006: 414).

Therefore, according to the authors, the main defining characteristics of femicide are the type of connection between the victim and the aggressor and the circumstances of its occurrence. As a methodology, they drew up a list containing all the women who were killed intentionally from 1990 to 1999 and by reading each of the deaths, they reinterpreted the data that was not included in the official records. They used various sources to fill in the absence of specific information. They studied the records of the "Book of Diagnostic Cases" of the forensic pathology section of the Judicial Investigation Agency (OIJ); the news from Jornais Extra,[9] La Nación, La República, and La Prensa; the records of the Statistical Yearbook of the Judicial Investigation Organization (OIJ); the OIJ case book; the OIJ Homicide Files; the Vital Statistics of the Judicial Power[10]; and the yearbooks of the OIJ.

Second (Sagot and Carcedo, 2006), it is fundamental to study the relationship between homicides of women and homicides in general, the relationship between the homicides of women and the homicides of men, the relationship between homicides of women in general and femicides, characteristics of the murdered women and the aggressors, relationships and situations of greater risk, nationality, other people injured in the assault, weapons used, sexual assault associated with femicide, history of the murderers, suicides, frequency of femicides by province, relationship with the aggressor, place of death, and sentences condemnatory, for a complete tipification of the phenomenon (Sagot and Carcedo, 2006).

Later, in a study on femicides in Central America as a whole, Ana Carcedo developed the concept of femicide scenarios, defining them according to the territories that occur: family scenario, marital relations scenario, sexual assault scenario, commercial sex scenario, historical scenarios and new scenarios of femicide, scenario of trafficking in women for all types of exploitation, the scene of national and international mafias and criminal networks, the scene of gangs, women as a territory of revenge, the scene of misogyny, and intertwined scenarios (Carcedo, 2010).

Since the end of the 1990s, there has been a growing movement of Latin American and Caribbean feminist activists and intellectuals to establish local parameters for the analysis of specific deaths of women under the concept of femicide, especially feminist groups from Honduras, Guatemala, and Peru. There is an effort to relate the phenomenon to the absence of States in the prevention, punishment, and eradication of deaths and also the quest to highlight the relationship between these deaths and national political contexts, borders, insurgent wars (Colombia), military dictatorships, the disappearance of women in coup political contexts (Honduras), conflicts over land and the persecution of leaders of indigenous movements (Brazil), the

[9] Information about the death and possible suspects and relationship with the victims. In addition to information about instances of previous assaults, how this woman died or where her body was found, whether there were witnesses or other people injured, and what the killer did after the murder.

[10] Where data were sought about the murders and the relations between victim and murderer.

advance of neoliberalism, genocide, religious fundamentalisms, the sexual policies of female body control, and reproductive health of women. The argumentative effort thus far has been to place Brazil within the transnational framework of the phenomenon of femicides.

Adoption of the Concept in Brazil: Academic and Political Context

The first Brazilian publication on *femicides was the book Femicide: handcuffs of the (In) visible* by researcher Sueli Almeida, 1998. The book develops arguments about the category "intimate femicide." The term femicide was used to explain the sexist nature of marital crimes, "unmasking the apparent neutrality of the terms homicide and murder," in addition to revealing the phenomenon that is part of the sexual policy of appropriation of women. The references used are the studies proposed in the collection by Russell and Radford (1992) (Almeida, 1998).

Almeida first outlined the discussion in her PhD thesis in Social Sciences defended at the PUC in São Paulo, under the guidance of Marxist feminist sociologist Heleieth Iara Bongiovanni Saffioti, in 1996. For the author, "homicides or attempts are neither random nor isolated phenomena, they result from the intensive and extensive nature of gender violence, and in particular from its domestic version." For her, femicide was a term that highlighted the sexist nature of homicides in the heterosexual marital context (Almeida, 1998: 43).

The researcher points to the lack of records for the preparation of the history of femicides, because it was only in recent decades that data on homicides disaggregated by sex (since 1979 in the Mortality Information System) and the absence of information about the aggressors began to be compiled. Almeida concludes that the production of data on homicides by sex and type of relationship between victim and aggressor is a first for the development of femicide studies and, therefore, "By refusing to know the extent of the phenomena of domestic violence and femicide, the State collaborates to hide the history of extreme oppression of large segments of women" (Almeida, 1998: 43).

Another topic that inhabited the researcher's concerns was the murders of men by their (former) wives and (former) partners, which she named the "other face of femicide." His studies addressed the different forms of participation of the perpetrators of consummated and attempted marital homicides. The researcher analyzed 18 stories of which 7 women were victims of homicides in the context of marital relations; 4 were victims of attempted homicides, in which one was shot on the front line of the confrontation between her sister and her spouse; and 7 were homicides of men in marital relations; the information was captured in the courts of Rio de Janeiro. It found that in situations where men were victims of marital homicide, women were seeking to defend themselves from assaults or were suffering from a long process of aggression (Almeida, 1996: 44–45; 1998).

During the decade that followed, there was much struggle promoted by women's, feminist, and black women's social movements seeking to make the transition from the discussion about marital crimes to femicides with a focus on access to justice. An emblematic example is the publication of the book *From Silence to the Scream Against Impunity: The Marcia Leopoldi Case*, written by the victim's sister, Deise Leopoldi and the São Paulo Women's Union, from 2007 [12]. *The book complains about the femicide case of Márcia Leopoldi by her ex-boyfriend Lago, in 1984, and the saga of the family in conjunction with the women's movement for justice in the face of the negligence of the Brazilian justice system to investigate and prosecute crimes like this and the advocacy processes through international human rights organizations.*

A narrative about the complaint process to the OAS IACHR is transcribed below, because it is of paramount importance to understand this process, which has been the way in which social movements face the State's negligence in the face of the deaths of women:

> [in 1996], the São Paulo Women's Union, together with Cladem, Cejil and Human Rights Watch, drafted a petition reporting the Márcia Leopoldi case to the Inter-American Commission. It was submitted based on art. 12 of the Inter-American Convention to Prevent, Punish, and Eradicate Violence against Women (Convention of Belém do Pará). This article expresses the right of any person or non-governmental entity legally recognized in Member States of the Organization to submit to the Commission complaints or complaints of violation of policies designed to prevent, punish, and eradicate violence. (Leopoldi, 2007: 115)

The book mentions the concept of femicide in the terms of Russell and Radford, 1992. The text mentions the difficulties of finding the number of homicides that would be femicides in Brazil and that studies on them are scarce given the amount of media coverage about cases of murders of women:

> The subject is treated sensationally, as a 'show'. In view of the fact that situations of violence against women have been televised for hours and days, whose scenes the population follows as if they were a soap opera, imbued with fiction and sexist commentary. (Leopoldi, 2007: 177)

The femicide case suffered by Leopoldi is very similar to that of Maria da Penha, even in the process of seeking to activate international women's law mechanisms. In May 1983, Maria da Penha was asleep when her then-husband, Viveros, shot himself in the back. He pretended that the case was a robbery, and she became paraplegic. After four months in the hospital, upon returning home to Recife, he again suffered an assassination attempt, and the farce was discovered. In 1998, fifteen years after the crime, Maria da Penha's aggressor was tried and convicted twice, and both times he was released from the forum due to appeals. Because of this negligence of the Brazilian State in dealing with this and other various crimes against women, social organizations filed a complaint with the Inter-American Commission on Human Rights of the Organization of American States via the Center for Justice and International Law (CEJIL) and the Latin American and Caribbean Committee for the Defense of Women's Rights (Cladem).

In 2001, Brazil was condemned for the omission, tolerance, and impunity with which it treated cases of domestic violence and was instructed to initiate changes in legislation to curb violence against women and to pay reparations to Maria da Penha. Law No. 11,340 ended up being nicknamed Maria da Penha, because its drafting was both in dialogue with international agreements on women's rights and in response to measures that should be implemented after conviction by the Inter-American Court of Human Rights. In the case of the Maria da Penha Law, there is mention of deaths due to domestic violence, but there is no specific item using the term femicide, or feminicide.

In October 2008, the concept gained visibility and is now spelled as feminicide, in the text of two feminist activists, Maria Dolores de Brito Mota and Maria da Penha Maia, when they discussed the kidnapping and death of the adolescent Eloá Cristina Pimentel, 15 years old, by her ex-boyfriend, motivated by the "refusal to accept the end of the relationship." The case occurred in the ABC region, in greater São Paulo and was emblematic for Brazilian public opinion. During the 4 days that the young woman was kept in private prison, the press covered everything outside the housing complex on the outskirts of Santo André, where the young woman lived, where she was held captive and murdered.

The case occurred on October 13, 2008. The young Eloá was persuaded by her ex-boyfriend to let him enter her residence to talk after refusing to resume the relationship. At the time, the young woman was with her best friend, Naiara, and two other male schoolmates, Iago and Victor. The moment he came in, armed, he announced his intentions. After negotiation with the police, the young males were released, followed by her friend Naiara, with the exception of Eloá, who remained in prison and was assaulted and tortured. After a new police negotiation, the officers requested that Naiara try to negotiate the release of her friend with the aggressor, at which point she was recaptured. There was a lot of fraternal dialogue between the police officers and the aggressor. The officers committed successive failures and declared to the press their desire to preserve the life and moral integrity of the kidnapper, who, in their opinion, was just a young man in love (Vianna, 2010).

"(Lindemberg) hit the victim, accused, exposed, coerced and finally martyred her body with a gunshot to the groin, a place of representation of sexual identity, and to the head, a place of representation of individual identity"; the aggressor also victimized the young woman's friend with a gunshot in the mouth, during the time that he also held her hostage (Mota & Fernandes, 2008).

The authors understand that the murder of Eloa was a femicide that for them "is a hate crime, always carried out with cruelty, as the 'extreme of a *continuum* of anti-feminine terror, including various forms of violence until reaching the level of public death […] So femicide is a crime of power, it's a political crime. Legally, it is a heinous, triple-qualified crime: a futile motive, without conditions to defend the victim, premeditated" (Mota & Fernandes, 2008). In this way, the concept reappears but now spelled femicides, based on the study by anthropologist Rita Laura Segato, *Que é um femicide*, 2006, as a conceptual basis.

In the texts by Rita Segato (2006), it is possible to ascertain that the main discussion also concerns the question of whether the concept of femicide should include all murders of women or whether it should be a more restricted category. In his view, developing a specific typology for femicide cases would make it possible to create more accurate data and facilitate the identification of the culprits. Thus, precise legal categories regarding the authors would also be necessary to obtain more specialized information about femicides. For her, by defining these specificities, it would be possible to draw a parallel between the categories of femicide and genocide. In a 2011 text, Segato defends femicide as a "group of violence aimed specifically at the elimination of women because of their status as women," making it necessary to raise the category of femicide to a level equivalent to that of "genocide" (Segato, 2006, 2011: 6).

In the field of public policies, since 2010, there has been an amplification of efforts in the context of feminist policies and struggles for women's rights to include femicides as a legal category in several countries, including Brazil. A first sign of the transnationalization of the concept in Latin American and Caribbean countries can be seen in the documents prepared by *the XI Regional Conference on Women in Latin America and the Caribbean*, held in Brasilia in 2010, with the participation of women from state politics and activists dedicated to the promotion and defense of women's rights in favor of gender equality with an emphasis on autonomy and economic empowerment. In the document, the terms femicide and feminicide appear in the topic intended for recommendations to expand women's participation in decision-making processes and spheres of power. In it, femicidal violence against women appears as an obstacle to achieving this participation, in the following terms:

> f) Incorporate into public security policies specific measures to prevent, investigate, punish, penalize and eradicate femicide and femicide, understood as the most extreme form of gender-based violence against women. (Cepal De Las Mujeres, 2010: 8)

Wânia Pasinato discusses the political implications of choosing the femicide category (the author believed that there were two ways of graphing the category and that the choice of femicide or feminicide had no impact on conceptual differences for the Latin American and Brazilian reality, in the 2011 article "Femicides and the deaths of women in Brazil"). The researcher brought with her article a bibliographic review on the subject, referring to the reflections of Russell and Radford (1992), pointing to the lack of or lack of access to available information that would enable the analysis of cases in Latin America. According to Pasinato, to overcome this obstacle, most studies have been using information disseminated in print and multiple official and social sources, such as criminal cases and international reports. The article seeks to define, delimit, and consider what advances the category "femicides" may or may not bring (Pasinato, 2011).

Pasinato (2011) compares the category femicide and its tendency to encompass all deaths of women to the "amalgam method" by Elisabeth Badinter (2005), which according to her is applied whenever an attempt is made to give numerical expression to crimes against women by unifying them. The homogenization of all murders of women in a single category is the author's greatest criticism, who argues about the fragility of their political impact, if specific characteristics of the victims are not considered, such as age, race/color, and socio-occupational group to which they belong, for example, and the context in which the crime occurs (Pasinato, 2011).

From 2010 onward, academic studies and initiatives by social movements on feminicides multiplied. Another example was the text by IPEA researchers Leila Posenato Garcia, Lúcia Rolim Santana de Freitas, Gabriela Drummond Marques da Silva, and Doroteia Aparecida Höfelmann, who explore the data on deaths due to aggression provided by the Mortality Information System (SIM/DATASUS), from 2001 to 2011 (Garcia et al., 2013).

For them, femicides/feminicides are the deaths of women resulting from gender conflicts, because they are women. They describe that these deaths are generally perpetrated by men in relation to women and result from situations in which women have less power compared to men (Garcia et al., 2013).

In 2013, at the legislative and legal levels, the Joint Parliamentary Committee for the Investigation of Violence Against Women, CPMIVCM, was appointed with the objective of "investigating the situation of violence against women in Brazil and investigating allegations of omission by the government regarding the application of instruments established by law to protect women in situations of violence." Among the proposals of the final CPMI report, a bill was invested in a bill to classify and include feminicide in the Brazilian Penal Code. The CPMIVCM had already occurred on two other occasions in 1992 and 2003 (CPMIVCM—Senado Federal, 2013).

The bill proposed that feminicide be aggravated by homicide in the Penal Code, with a prison sentence of 12 to 30 years, typifying it as murders of women with circumstances of domestic or family violence, sexual violence, mutilation, or disfigurement of the victim (CPMIVCM—Senado Federal, 2013: 998 & 1002).

For the commission,

> The importance of typifying feminicide *(feminicídio)* is to recognize, in accordance with the law, that women are being killed for the reason that they are women, exposing the fracture of gender inequality that persists in our society, and is social, by combating impunity, preventing feminicides from benefiting from anachronistic and morally unacceptable legal interpretations, such as having committed a "crime of passion". It also sends a positive message to society that the right to life is universal and that there will be no impunity. It also protects the dignity of the victim, by preventing strategies to disqualify, through the media, the condition of brutally murdered women, ascribing to them the responsibility for the crime of which they were victims. (CPMIVCM—Federal Senate, 2013: 1004)

As a result of the debates and actions, on March 9, 2015, the law against feminicides was approved in Brazil, within the Criminal Code, as an aggravating factor for homicide cases, Article 121 of the Criminal Code. Thus, feminicide was defined as homicides committed against women because of their female status, defined as: domestic and family violence and disregard or discrimination against the status of women. The penalty may be increased from 1/3 to half if the crime is committed against a woman during pregnancy or within 3 months after giving birth or against a person under 14 (fourteen) years of age, over 60 (sixty) years of age, or with disabilities, in the presence of a descendant or ascendant of the victim (UN, 2016; Brazil, 2015).

Brazil was the 16th Latin American country with laws that punish feminicides. The discussion about feminicides has already gained visibility in the judicial and political spheres in several countries in Latin America and the Caribbean. In some countries, such as Mexico, the State has, in addition to the law, mechanisms for monitoring and diagnosing feminicides (ENDIREH). Uruguay now approved it in 2017, becoming the 17th country to have punitive legislation for femicide/feminicides.

In view of the above framework, it is considered that there is an effort to define which parameters are central to the concept of feminicides within feminist criticism. In the legal sphere, we note a transnationalization of the criminal concept of feminicide as a crime in LAC and a history of works that seek to define ways of measuring them as a social phenomenon. It is possible to find different spellings of the term (femicide and feminicide). It is agreed that in Castilian- and Portuguese-speaking countries, the form feminicides eliminates the direct association with the female version of homicide, which would be a reductionism and would remove the power of the category, which is precisely to question the apparent neutrality of legal terms, such as homicide.

Feminicides are considered to be deaths specific to women. It is emphasized that the perpetrators of the deaths are male in the direct case and of the State, through its institutions and organized groups, in the indirect case. Objectively, we can see from the above in the analyzed bibliography that the case of indirect authorship has to do with deaths linked to sexual policies of control of the female body and reproduction (procreation), systematic sexual violence in the case of wars and conflicts, and omission in the face of direct cases. The case of direct authorship is composed of deaths caused by violence, such as suicide, homicide, and undefined external causes. They do not correspond to the total of these deaths but represent a large part of them.

The author of this article presents as a proposal for analysis a new typology aimed at an interpretation of the most basic forms of feminicide (Romio, 2017). Thus, a feminicide is considered when it meets one or more of the following conditions:

Reproductive feminicide—linked to policies to control women's bodies and sexuality, whose minimum expression is deaths due to abortion.

Domestic feminicide—lethal violence due to physical aggression against women in the home, marital, or family context.

Sexual feminicide—lethal violence due to physical assault against women through sexual means.

References

Almeida, S. S. (1996). *Gender violence: Public vs. private* (p. 355). Thesis (Doctorate)—Pontifical Catholic University of São Paulo.

Almeida, S. (1998). *Femicide: Handcuffs (in) visible to the private public*. Revinter.

Caputi, J., & Russell, D. (1992). Femicide: Sexism against women. In Radford & Russell (Eds.), *Femicide: The politics of woman killing*.
Carcedo, A. (2010). Concepts, contexts, and scenarios of femicide in Central America. In A. Carcedo (Ed.), *We don't forget or accept: Femicide in Central America 2000–2006* (1st ed.). CEFEMINA.
da Fernandes, M., P. M., & de Mota, M. D., B. (2008). *Live femicide: What Eloá calls us*. Adital Website, 20/10/2008.
Falquet, Jules (2014) From the murders in Ciudad Juárez to the phenomenon of femicides: New forms of violence against women?
Garcia, L. P., de Freitas, L. R. S., da Silva, G. D. M., & Höfelmann, D. A. (2013). *Violence against women: Femicides in Brazil*. Text for discussion—TD. Ipea.
Hester, M. (1992). The witch-craze in sixteenth-century England as social control of women. In Radford & Russell (Eds.), *Femicide: The politics of woman killing*.
Kelly, L. (1988). *Surviving sexual violence*. Polity Press.
La Botz, D. (1999). *Mexico: Girl's murder sad symbol of corporate power, child labor, female exploitation on the border*. Mexican Labor News and Analysis March 2nd, 1999.
Lagarde, M. (2006). Presentation. In *Feminicidal violence in 10 entities of the Mexican republican*. Congress of the Union, Chamber of Deputies.
Lagarde, M. (2008). "Antropología, feminismo y política: Violencia feminicida y derechos humanos de las mujeres". In BULLEN, Margaret y DÍEZ, Carmen (coords.) RETOS TEÓRICOS Y NUEVAS PRÁCTICAs. Serie, XI Congreso de Antropología de la FAAEE, Donostia, Ankulegi Antropologia Elkartea.
Leopoldi, D. (2007). *From silence to the cry against impunity: The Márcia Leopoldi case*. São Paulo Women's Union.
Pasinato, W. (2011). *'Femicides' and the deaths of women in Brazil* (pp. 219–246). Cadernos Pagu (37), July–December. 2011.
Radford, J., & Russell, D. E. H. (1992). *Femicide: The politics of woman killing*. Open University Press.
Romio, J. A. F. (2017). *Femicides in Brazil, a proposal for analysis with data from the health sector*. [doctoral thesis]—Campinas.
Russell, D. (2011). *Talk about the origins of femicides*, December 2011. http://www.dianarussell.com/origin_of_femicide.html
Sagot, M., & Carcedo, A. (2006). When violence against women kills: Femicide in Costa Rica, 1990–1999. In Corrêa et al. (Eds.), *Family life: A comparative perspective on "crimes of honor"*.
Segato, R. L. (2006). Que és un feminicídio. Notas para un debate emergente. Brasília: UnB.
Segato, R. L. (2011). Femi-geno-cidio como crimen en el fuero internacional de los derechos humanos: el derecho a nombrar el sufrimiento en el derecho. In: FREGOSO, Rosa-Linda; BEJARANO, Cynthia (Eds.). Feminicidio en América Latina. Mexico, DF: Centro de Investigaciones de Ciencias Sociales y Humanidades; Universidad Nacional Autónoma de México.
UN. UN Women Brazil. (2016). *National guidelines for investigating, prosecuting, and judging violent deaths of women—Femicides from a gender perspective*. UN Women.
Vianna, C. S. M. (2010). *The Eloá case: Analysis of the approach to femicide in the media*. Paper Presented at Fazendo Gênero 9, UFSC, September 2010.
Women's Cepal. (2010). *Brasilia Consensus*. XI Regional Conference on Women in Latin America and the Caribbean.

The Training of Psychologists in Childcare and Protection

Hilda Paredes-Dávila

Introduction

In Mexico, as in other parts of the world, childhood is considered a foundational period in the life of an individual. The Universal Declaration of Human Rights of the United Nations states that children under 18 years of age have the right to special care and assistance due to their lack of physical and mental maturity (UNICEF, 2018). In the year 2000, the fourth article of the Political Constitution of the United Mexican States was modified so that all children and adolescents have their food, health, education, and recreational needs met for their comprehensive protection. Together with this, the Law for the Protection of the Rights of Children and Adolescents was created, which was subsequently replaced on December 4, 2014, by the General Law of the Rights of Children and Adolescents (GLRCA).

The GLRCA is mainly focused on guaranteeing substantive equity, which ensures that all children and adolescents have the same treatment, rights, and opportunities. Likewise, it establishes that all children and adolescents will have access to quality education, health and protection, and new technologies and the right to participate in everything that concerns them. In this sense, children and adolescents have the right to express their opinions and to have them heard and taken into account in all acts and decisions that affect their lives. However, unlike other countries, in Mexico, there are various cultural and social factors that frame the education and upbringing of children and adolescents that do not favor child well-being, such as poverty, lack of access to social security, food, health services, basic services in the home, and a lack of quality education. Additionally, there are high rates of childhood mortality, teenage pregnancies, violence, migration, work, and child

H. Paredes-Dávila (✉)
Faculty of Psychology, National Autonomous University of Mexico, Mexico City, Mexico
e-mail: hildapd@unam.mx

S. Castaños-Cervantes et al. (eds.), *Working with Vulnerable Populations*,
https://doi.org/10.1007/978-3-031-67710-6_19

marriage, among other threats to healthy development (CONEVAL, 2014 cited by UNICEF 2016; National Human Rights Commission-CNDH, 2016; National Institute of Health Public, cited by UNICEF, 2016).

Child welfare is a responsibility that families, the community, and educational and government institutions must assume. For this, it is necessary to favor collaboration networks that allow us to learn about others and ourselves and to learn from and with each other (Baistow, 2000) to broaden horizons and expand frames of reference, stimulate creativity, and inspire new strategies and good practices for childcare and protection.

The Role of Universities in Promoting Child Welfare

Since their inception, universities have provided education and professional training in various professions according to the economy and the needs of society, so universities play a fundamental role in the social, cultural, scientific, and technological development of a country. However, with regard to child and well-being, there are few universities in Mexico that train professionals in this area Rather, there are isolated efforts by some teachers to train their students in the theoretical and methodological content regarding care and child protection, primarily in disciplines such as medicine, nursing, law, pedagogy, social work and psychology.

It should be noted that the work that different professionals provide in terms of child protection depends on the relationship they have with families and/or the community (Gilbert, 2012; Gilbert et al., 2011). In child safety-oriented systems, the relationships that are established tend to be more asymmetric; the professional has power and knowledge, and the family and/or the community acquires a subordinate role. Under this orientation, abuse is conceived as a threat to child welfare caused by inadequate parents, incapable of protecting and meeting the basic needs of their sons and daughters. In these systems, the principle that guides protective action is to safeguard children and adolescents from the possible harm caused by an abusive family, often revealing disciplinary attitudes toward fathers and mothers. This asymmetry of roles gives rise to relationships between professionals, families, and/or community which can become tense and conflictive at times.

On the other hand, in systems oriented toward family support, a spirit of collaboration is observed more frequently, promoting to a greater extent the participation of children and adolescents and their families and community in decision-making. In this orientation, abuse is conceived as the result of family or community stress caused by social, psychological, and/or economic difficulties (problems of poverty, substance abuse, gender violence, untreated mental health problems, among others). Therefore, the response from the protection system is to try to reduce the risk factors that may be affecting families, establishing voluntary agreements with families to enable protective intervention and keeping, as far as possible, children within their own family and/or community through foster care.[1]

In the continuum that goes from an orientation focused on child safety to an orientation focused on family support, competent, autonomous, and reflective professionals are required, capable of developing innovative models that have an integral impact on the problems faced by children and adolescents, their families, and community to help them co-manage childcare and well-being. Next, the training of psychologists in the Faculty of Psychology of the UNAM is described, the actions that have been carried out to promote childcare and well-being among students and other professionals, as well as the challenges to face for the creation of conditions that contribute to the processes of care and protection in the twenty-first century from psychology.

The Training of Future Psychologists

Currently, the Faculty of Psychology of the National Autonomous University of Mexico (UNAM) is the educational institution that trains the largest number of psychology undergraduate and graduate students in the country. The said training is centered on a study plan and program in which supervised internships are emphasized. These internships, which involve continuous supervision, occur in places and situations where the professional business of the psychologist is carried out in order to promote the development of various professional skills by linking the theoretical advances of the discipline and related areas with the ability to select, adapt, and create techniques and procedures relevant to the real needs of society. There is also an emphasis on reflective, responsible attitudes and an ethical commitment in their professional work (Faculty of Psychology, UNAM, 2008a, b). Unfortunately, there is no line of professional training in childcare and welfare systems to meet the practical requirements in the professional training of undergraduate and postgraduate students, as well as to meet the problems regarding childcare and protection. However, steps are being taken to address this issue, including international collaboration and the creation of several books designed to address the paucity of research and provide resources for training future generations of professionals.

[1] For the purposes of this work, "community" is understood as the group of people who interrelate with each other and who have common goals; therefore, the community goes beyond the framing of a physical space. What is relevant about the community is that shared meanings are built in it through interaction with others and through childcare and well-being practices that are carried out in the social and cultural environment (Seda & Torres, 2013).

Moving Forward

"Bridges to Grow"

From 2007 to 2011, the "Bridges to Grow" project was carried out by Dr. Ileana Seda Santana, which was financed by the Van Leer Foundation in The Hague, Holland. As a result of this project, the book *Multiple Perspectives on Child Care and Well-Being* (Seda & Pastor, 2013) was published, which describes specific developmental problems in children and adolescents. The book compiles articles written by various authors who address childcare and well-being from various perspectives, emphasizing that there is no single way to promote childcare and well-being practices. It should be noted that the book addresses the challenges that the various agents involved face, as well as the need to reflect on the various daily situations in which children and adolescents develop and on the skills that professionals in psychology and medicine possess education to create environments that promote the comprehensive development of children and adolescents. "This work documents theoretical aspects, research and practices within countless spaces such as families, communities, classrooms, children's centers and higher education institutions that train professionals in psychology and teacher education. Additionally, the authors emphasize the role of educational agencies and their responsibilities regarding the rights of children and their families, as well as the skills required for the care and well-being of children and adolescents" (Seda & Pastor, 2013, p. 11).

Collaboration with the University of Groningen, the Netherlands, and the Universidad de la Frontera in Temuco, Chile

Since the signing of the agreement between the University of Groningen and UNAM in 2017, with the aim of intensifying cooperation in research and teaching between both institutions, the International Colloquium is held in August 2018: "The future of child protection," organized by the members of the Hestia research project and carried out at the Faculty of Psychology of the UNAM. Over the course of five years, various exchanges have been carried out by the collaborators of the three universities, in academic events such as the international congress of EUSARF (European Scientific Association on Residential and Family Care for Children and Adolescents) held in Oporto, Portugal, and the "Child Protection Systems Seminar: Current Challenges in Chile," organized by the Universidad de La Frontera in Temuco, Chile. Likewise, the collaborators have had constant informal conversations and extensive online contact, given the new scenario generated by the SARS-COVID-19 pandemic, which resulted in the preparation of the book: *The future of Child Protection Systems in Latin America and Europe: Lessons and Impacts* (López et al., in press).

The fundamental objective of the book is the comparative analysis of policies, practices, and research regarding child protection systems in various countries in

Latin America and Europe. It is expected that the different experiences collected in the text contribute to the scarce existing literature on the subject in Ibero-America, despite its enormous relevance for the different participants, researchers, professional community, and decision-makers.

The book is organized into two sections. The first section takes an international look at the historical development of child protection systems in various countries in America (Argentina, Chile, Colombia, Guatemala, and Mexico) and Europe (Germany, England, and the Netherlands), in order to understand the current situation, pointing out challenges and perspectives in the creation of conditions that contribute to care and protection processes in the twenty-first century. In the second section of the book, different experiences of intervention for the practice of child protection in various international contexts are presented. They are articulated around certain patterns of analysis where the practice of childcare and protection acquires a central role in its reflection and transformation.

Collaboration Agreement with the National System for Comprehensive Family Development (National DIF)

During the first quarter of 2022, a collaboration agreement will be signed between the Faculty of Psychology of the UNAM and the National System for the Integral Development of the Family (DIF Nacional) in order to build new learning networks between students, research teachers, and administrative staff of both institutions regarding the area of protection of the rights of Children and Adolescents, through prevention, intervention, and evaluation of quality strategies that favor the comprehensive development of children and adolescents and facilitate a better process transition of DIF graduates to society through accompaniment and training for families, caregivers, directors, and the community. The participation of undergraduate and graduate students in the three experiences mentioned above has led to the acquisition and/or development of the following skills related to childcare and protection in their training process as psychologists, namely:

I. Psychoeducational Evaluation: To select, adapt, apply, and qualify various instruments and/or assessment techniques that allow detecting intervention needs, monitoring their progress, and evaluating their impact on children, families, caregivers, managers, and the community.
II. Psychoeducational Intervention: To select, adapt, and/or design intervention programs and support materials that favor the well-being of children and adolescents, considering the context shared by all the people involved but also those that differentiate them in order to promote learning networks between the same, continuously monitoring and evaluating the effectiveness, efficiency, impact, and permanence of the implemented intervention programs and communicating in an eloquent and clear way, the results of the implementation of programs through oral and written reports presented to different audiences, in different times and for different purposes.

III. Educational Innovation: To continuously document, justify, and evaluate the intervention process, each of the strategies used, and the results obtained, through the collection of multiple and diverse evidence, with the purpose of identifying the essential elements (theoretical and methodological) of an effective and efficient intervention that allows the extraction of innovative intervention models or guidelines to promote child well-being and favor changes and improvements in childcare and protection.
IV. Professional Identity - Being and acting as a psychologist: To identify their own training needs with an open, critical, and reflective attitude about their professional performance that allows them, on the one hand, to look for the ideal updating and improvement options, considering the advances in the psychological discipline and, on the other hand, to work together with professionals from the discipline itself and from other disciplines to find solutions to the needs of childcare and well-being, using a wide variety of teamwork, communication, and communication skills in a flexible way and social interaction, as well as assuming the professional role of psychologist with responsibility and ethics.

The acquisition and/or development of the aforementioned skills has been achieved through: (a) the delivery of theoretical-methodological seminars that allow psychologists to articulate the knowledge of the discipline with the skills to select, adapt, or create techniques and procedures relevant to child welfare; therefore, conceptual knowledge is significant because it is related to the situations in which it is applied; (b) a supervised practice by the expert supervisor, who is in charge of observing, providing feedback, modeling, and evaluating the activities carried out by the students in the different practice scenarios; (c) promote continuous reflection through discussions, documentation of the activities carried out and the weekly preparation of a log or field diary; (d) the development of intervention-research projects according to the needs of child care and well-being, to provide a quality service and generate applied research proposals; and (e) the performance of collaborative work with their undergraduate and master's classmates, as well as other professionals with whom they share their own approaches to the problems encountered (Macotela & Paredes, 2003; Schön, 1992; Richardson, 1990; Coll et al., 2006).

Final Considerations

Training professionals in the field of child protection is quite a challenge. In addition, carrying out training based on practical work, as outlined in the curriculum and programs of the Faculty of Psychology at UNAM, is made difficult by the false conception that practice is subordinate to theory and that the former represents only an application of the latter; the lack of professional settings where students can practice the knowledge and skills that will be required in their professional practice; the lack of criteria that allow for the evaluation of the competent performance of students at various times during their training; the absence of the implementation of a model for supervising practical training; and a poor sensitivity to work in and with the circumstances that arise in child protection systems, among others.

Sometimes, there seems to be a distance between the training given in universities and the needs that graduates face in their professional and working life. Both camps seem distant and often cause mutual frustration. In universities, there is a tendency to design models and methods based on theories to be implemented in the long term, while in the workplace, professionals generally tend to provide short-term solutions to meet individual needs or improvements at the local level. Professionals in the workplace act from the need to change something in the present and immediately, relegating or ignoring much of the research carried out in universities. "These differences lead to assumptions about the other. Researchers are considered agents with authority over knowledge (Sholoch, 2012), while professionals in the workplace are often considered agents resistant to change" (Vincent, in López et al., in press).

However, to produce changes, so that progress is noticed, it is necessary that educational institutions, in this case, the UNAM Faculty of Psychology, promote training based on the development of various professional skills (knowledge, skills, and attitudes) derived from their participation in authentic and real scenarios, and with the support of tutoring and continuous supervision, and promote in students a progressive mastery and a link between theory and practice so that they can address the problems faced by the different people involved in child care and welfare.

Although there are examples of links between the University and the professional field in the field of child protection, such as those described in López, Paredes, and Vizcarra (in press), the challenge lies in the need to incorporate and collaborate together in the implementation of strategic actions that support the comprehensive development of children and adolescents, who will be the generation of adults in the future. Therefore, today's children cannot live in situations of fear and/or abuse if we want them to have the cognitive, physical, and emotional skills that allow them to develop in a community where mutual respect among all prevails.

References

Baistow, K. (2000). Cross-national research: What can we learn from inter-country comparisons? *Social Work in Europe, 7*(3), 8–13.

Coll, C., Mauri, T., & Onrubia, J. (2006). Análisis y resolución de casos-problema mediante el aprendizaje colaborativo. *Revista de Universidad y sociedad del conocimiento, 3*(2), 29–40.

Comisión Nacional de Derechos Humanos México. (2016). *Informe Anual de Actividades*. 2016. Recuperado de http://informe.cndh.org.mx/menu.aspx?id=10044

Facultad de Piscología, UNAM. (2008a). *Plan de estudios de la carrera de Psicología de la UNAM*. UNAM. Recuperado de: http://www.google.com.mx/search?sourceid=navclient&aq=&oq=facultad+de+ps&hl=es&ie=UTF8&rlz=1T4TSHL_esMX326MX326&q=facultad+de+psicologia+de+la+unam&gs_l=hp..5.0l5j4l13.0.0.0.4696...........0.yFEc_P0YibM

Facultad de Piscología, UNAM. (2008b). *Propuesta de Modificación al Plan y Programa de Estudio de la Licenciatura en Psicología Para el Sistema Escolarizado y Abierto*. UNAM.

Fondo de las Naciones Unidas para la Infancia UNICEF (2018). *América Latina y el Caribe a 30 años de la aprobación de la Convención sobre los derechos del niño*. Recuperado de: https://repositorio.cepal.org/bitstream/handle/11362/44271/1/S1800977_es.pdf

Fondo de las Naciones Unidas para la Infancia UNICEF, Consejo Nacional de Evaluación de la Política de Desarrollo Social (CONEVAL). (2014). *Pobreza y derechos sociales de niños, niñas y adolescentes en México*. Citado por UNICEF México (2016) Informe anual 2016. Recuperado de https://www.donaunicef.org.mx/informe-anual/?utm_source=mpr_ons&utm_campaign=informe-anual16-web&utm_medium=ons&utm_content=informe-anual16-web&utm_term=informe-anual16website#

Gilbert, N. (2012). A comparative study of child welfare systems: Abstract orientations and concrete results. *Children and Youth Services Review, 34*(3), 532–536. https://doi.org/10.1016/j.childyouth.2011.10.014

Gilbert, N., Parton, N., & Skivenes, M. (2011). *Child protection systems: International trends and orientations*. Oxford University Press. https://doi.org/10.1093/acprof:oso/9780199793358.003.0012

Instituto Nacional de Salud Pública & UNICEF México. (2016). *Encuesta de indicadores Múltiples por conglomerados 2015, Informe final*. Citado por UNICEF México (2016) Informe anual 2016. Recuperado de https://www.donaunicef.org.mx/informe-anual/?utm_source=mpr_ons&utm_campaign=informe-anual16-web&utm_medium=ons&utm_content=informe-anual16-web&utm_term=informe-anual16website#

López López, M., Paredes Dávila, H., & Vizcarra Larrañaga, M. B. (Eds.). *El futuro de los sistemas de protección infantil en América Latina y Europa: Lecciones e impactos*. Fomento Editorial UNAM.

Macotela, S., & Paredes, H. (2003). Formación de psicólogos escolares con base en un modelo de supervisión experta en campo. *Enseñanza e Investigación en Psicología., 8*(1), 5–23.

Richardson, V. (1990). Significant and worthwhile change in teaching practice. *Educational Researcher, 19*(7), 10–18.

Schön, D. A. (1992). *La formación de profesionales reflexivos*. Paidós.

Seda, I., & Pastor, R. (2013). *Perspectivas Múltiples en el cuidado y bienestar infantil: Investigación, teoría, práctica fundamentada*. UNAM.

Seda, I., & Torres, G. (2013). La comunidad, un espacio de aprendizajes en lo cotidiano. In *Perspectivas múltiples en el cuidado y bienestar infantil: Investigación, teoría y práctica fundamentada*. Facultad de Psicología, UNAM y Proyecto "Puentes para crecer".

Pedagogical Guidelines for Vulnerability in Postmodernity

José de Jesús Alcalá-Anguiano

Dialogs Between Postmodernity and Human Vulnerability

Araujo-Olivera (2002) affirms that education has been present in the historical development of all peoples, albeit not uniformly, due to the variation in their expressions according to the circumstances in which it develops and tries to respond to particular components of the cultural system. It is imperative to understand the cultural characteristics of each society to respond effectively to the demands posed by each era; this is why the issue of vulnerability in postmodernity is contextualized. Moreover, based on an anthropological approach of vulnerability, it is understood that human beings seek to bond with the environment they belong or seek to belong to; however, due to numerous imbalances and tensions, both on an individual and social level, this connection is not always achieved in a functional and harmonious way, creating a state of insecurity and defenselessness that affects multiple dimensions of people. Consequently, it is observed that vulnerability is a part of our human condition (Torralba Roselló, 2010) that does not have a single manifestation; therefore, we can address it from different fields or knowledge areas.

Torralba Roselló (2010, p. 25) states that "the human being, like any mundane entity, is vulnerable" due to the link of this condition to our finitude (Jaspers, 1989), and although we try to hide or ignore it, we can consciously embrace it. This appropriation applies both to the perception of one's own vulnerability and that of others, and although it is made of fundamental elements, it is nuanced by different conditions, including the social, historical, and cultural context in which it manifests, as

---

Translated by Samantha Legy Espinosa, Kenia Romero, Paula Castellanos, and Andrés Escobar.

J. de Jesús Alcalá-Anguiano (✉)
Universidad Popular Autónoma del Estado de Puebla, Puebla, Mexico
e-mail: josejesus.alcala@upaep.mx

S. Castaños-Cervantes et al. (eds.), *Working with Vulnerable Populations*,
https://doi.org/10.1007/978-3-031-67710-6_20

it provides certain circumstances that affect its morphology. In this regard, this text seeks to analyze the problem of vulnerability in a particular age, the current one. According to Pizarro (2001), vulnerability has developed as one of the outstanding features of the contemporary world, especially because of prevailing economic models, where consumption criteria rule out those who are not capable of solving the fast, spectacular, and extremely demanding dynamics of the present.

As previously mentioned, within a philosophical and sociological perspective, the contemporary era is known as *postmodernity* (Lyotard, 1991). To understand this term, it is wise to remember, as a preamble and inspired by the philosophical anthropology proposed by Cassirer (2016), that the human, as a symbolic being, seeks the meaning of its existence, assigns meanings, and provides explanations of the natural and social phenomena that surrounds it, constructing these narratives and stories that respond to multiple questions, whether fundamental or instrumental. These explanations are diverse and are constructed by different sources. It has been observed that, at least in the West, there are certain all-encompassing stories that have sought to explain and justify the essential issues of being and life (Bustos, 2009), offering absolute answers and thus founding the institutions that govern people's social and cultural life. These totalizing discourses are called *meta-narratives* (Lyotard, 1991), and although they offer a meaning to the existence and teleology of history, they have lost strength in the present day; they have been fragmented, constituting what today is precisely known as postmodernity and could be characterized as the end of unitary history (Vattimo, 1990, 1991, 2013).

In addition to the above, postmodernity implies a paradoxical meaning through the renunciation to the search for meaning, or at the least the desire for an absolute one, leaving aside global explanations and causing the proliferation of partial explanations of equally partial realities (Bustos, 2009). It is pertinent to illustrate that, tempting as it might be, it is not assertive to analyze postmodernity from a polarized perspective. That is to say, it is not a completely desirable or undesirable phenomenon, right or wrong, but it involves different nuances that break with the perception of a one-dimensional world. On the one hand, it can bring characteristics such as disenchantment and intellectual and moral relativism and, on the other, greater plurality and tolerance for what breaks with the established schemas, opening a door to multiculturalism. The meta-narratives are equally polyvalent, since they provide answers, security, and confidence, but only if the proposal fits with one's own values and life expectations; otherwise, being totalitarian means they are aggressive (Vattimo, 1991) by excluding the voices of those who do not align with the majority. This way, we can foresee that the rupture of the meta-stories moves toward the diversity of narratives, breaks ethnocentrism, and generates a multiplicity of discourses.

One of the first concerns that arise when addressing postmodernity is its plurality, because its story lies precisely in the non-story, or at least not from an absolute perspective. This condition implies the possibility of studying the postmodern phenomenon from different disciplines and in multiple dimensions. However, in this case, we will base our analysis on an ethical framework to offer pedagogical guidelines that facilitate attention to vulnerability in postmodernity. While the subject of vulnerability is inherently complex, we will now focus on explaining what concerns human action, because it is in this field that we observe trends that, paradoxically, can claim the place of people in vulnerable situations or, on the contrary, sink them into exclusionism.

The Consideration of the Other, a Paradoxical Point

Although not exclusively, but significantly, hyperconsumption has shaped one of the dominant ethical features in postmodernity: The exaltation of the individual above the community. This approach values individual qualities and the virtuosity of those who excel in social competition through their creativity, innovation, and entrepreneurship. However, strong tensions can also be discerned in this way of life, which leads the human being to cease "being a subject of ties that bind him to the society to which he belongs, to the rest of its members, and to the past, to become someone who (...) is self sufficient, although he can only do so apparently" (Bustos, 2009, p.127).

This emphasis on individual action uproots the human being from their community, and it is expected that the effect will be more pronounced on people whose vulnerability is greater, because they not only face a competitive and exclusive world but are also treated with a utilitarian criteria, from mere appearance and, in certain cases, even indifferently. This is because in a society where capital has become the driving force of human action, those who break with the logic of consumption are excluded or instrumentalized, using their faces and life stories as mere emotional catalysts, without a genuine interest. Below, two approaches that explore this social dynamic are presented, that of Lipovetsky and Bauman's, who, through the terms *hyperindividualism* and *adiaphora*, seek a reflection on the exaltation of the individual and the omission of the other.

The first of these authors, Lipovetsky (2013), who prefers to substitute the term postmodernity for *hypermodernity*, affirms that throughout history the human being has identified with different mythological figures, since he asserts that "each generation recognizes itself and finds its identity in a mythological figure which it reinterprets according to the problems of the moment: Oedipus as a universal emblem, Prometheus, Faust or Sisyphus as mirrors of the modern condition" (Lipovetsky, 2013, p. 43); and currently, authors such as Lasch and Sennet (on Lipovetsky, 2013) agree that Narcissus is the symbol that represents our times.

According to Lipovetsky (2013), hyperindividualism is the result of a state of emptiness that manifests the loss of meaning and the detachment of the present from the past and the future, thus sacrificing the continuity and teleological character of history. These conditions emphasize the hedonistic character of the contemporary individual, who, in his effort to enjoy the present fleetingness, succumbs to the seduction of spectacular media and seeks to define his persona through consumption. In this way, individual desires are experienced as the criterion that apparently guides human action, shaping new forms of relationship with oneself and with others but actually responding to the interest of hyperconsumption.

Hyperindivudualism presents desirable components for today's practical criteria, such as creativity, proactivity, and entrepreneurship, because of the possibility they offer to achieve personal goals and facilitating autonomy. However, the criticism to hyperindividualism does not rest on these features, since it is not about overshadowing personal virtues, or going against personal development, but rather its dissociating character from the individual to his community, because in this process unhealthy and excessive competition easily arises, leaving aside those who are in a more vulnerable position.

The tension between the desirable and undesirable character of hyperindividualism could emerge at this time when trying to verify what is exposed here with what we observe in our daily lives, especially what is mediated by a screen, since the information given in technology and communication shows us a panorama in which care to people in conditions of vulnerability is provided, and possibly in many cases these actions have authentic and desirable motives, means, purposes, and consequences. To achieve a better discernment in these situations, it is necessary to consider that hyperindividualism can be misleading when it comes to the relationship with the other, especially with the vulnerable. This happens because we are presented with more charitable, fraternal, and cooperative organizations behind the screen, in a spectacular context, exploiting the individual's needs with a utilitarian purpose.

In addition to Lipovetsky's contributions, Bauman makes a sociological critique of postmodernity, although it is common in his work to be named by the term *liquid modernity* (Bauman, 2015), due to the fast and fluctuating nature of the present, in contrast to the solidity of modernity. This condition emphasizes what Lyotard (1991) explains as the fragmentation of meta-narratives, causing the decay of the normative systems of human action, or at least the most traditional ones, and generating a new perspective of ethics in the postmodernity (Bauman, 2013), in which there are no absolutely right or wrong actions, but there is a constant capitalization of human behavior, for example, service and charity.

Furthermore, adiaphora is linked to hyperindividualism as one of the predominant ethical trends in postmodernity, emphasizing the desire to overcome normative systems and the restructuring of the criteria that govern over individual and social human action. This is analyzed by Bauman and Donskis (2015) and is understood as indifferent and moral evaluation lacking human action, in a way that a disconnection between the use of freedom and the responsibility that comes with it occurs. In turn, the moral numbness generated by adiaphora exalts the needs of a few individuals, while belittling those of vulnerable groups, rewarding individual success and displacing genuine attention to those in need.

As can be seen, the adiaphora shares a superficial character with hyperindividualism and is largely shaped by the same components: hedonism, consumerism, and detachment from the community. Actions in favor of people in need or in conditions of vulnerability are subrogated to self-interest, exalting the individual and their personal motivations. Human action is mediated by mass communication devices, presenting us with supposedly charitable and selfless actions, whether by politicians or celebrities, unleashing emotional and spectacular components, apparently "good" but not authentic, causing a masked individualism. It should be noted that this ethical landscape, despite its complications, also shows milestones of hope, since it is not a society that is entirely indifferent to others or devoid of any symptom of morality but rather provides opportunities to rethink the world in which we live and the actions we take (Bauman, 2013).

So far, we have approached the postmodern phenomenon from a standpoint focused on ethical trends that enhance indifference, detachment, and the denial of the other. Nevertheless, it is necessary to explore other positions, because there are multiple contributions that rescue the desirable value of our contemporary setting, among them, Vattimo (1991), who perceives the totalizing structures, in this case, the metanarratives, as aggressive entities based on so-called *strong thinking*, characterized by its lack of flexibility. This is so because every all-encompassing story, in its effort to provide a vision of history as a unitary entity, eliminates the discourses of the minority and becomes exclusive.

Blanco Gálvez (2007) explains that Vattimo stands as an alternative to the pessimistic views regarding postmodernity, through an ethical perspective that renounces the strong thinking so characteristic of the metaphysical tradition. This stance is grounded in nihilistic hermeneutics, an ethics of interpretation rooted in the philosophy of Nietzsche and Heidegger, which advocates for *weak thought*, distinguished from its counterpart by its interpretive and tolerant structure. In this way, the emancipation of minorities is built, and the voice of the vulnerable is heard, renouncing to the aspiration for a single sense of history and a totalizing vision of human teleology.

Unlike authors such as Lipovetsky and Serroy (2009, 2014), Bauman (2013) or Spitzer (2018), who identify in media culture the potential to emphasize many of the features of postmodernity, especially in the logic of the spectacle proposed by Debord (2018), Vattimo (1990) opts for a more hopeful aspect of the media. This perspective considers the possibility of expanding the diversity of voices that arise in postmodernity, so that it is not solely the narrative constructed by the hegemonic position. Consequently, we understand that postmodernity, approached from the ethical and hermeneutical contributions of Vattimo (1990), opens the possibility of listening to the voices of people in conditions of vulnerability by favoring a more communicative and transparent society. This position is revisited in the *Ethics of Interpretation* (Vattimo, 1991), by developing a philosophical reflection carried out from weak thinking, to achieve the inclusion of less privileged communities.

The transparent pluralistic conception proposed by Vattimo (1990, 1991, 2013) considers the non-predominant stories, the least heard voices, moving away from the major legitimizing authorities and valuing a cultural heritage that is far from being homogenous and that must be interpreted responsibly, in order to renounce a totalizing vision of human teleology and opt for a participatory, tolerant, and transformative stance. This openness to generalized communication and the plurality of cultures favors the awareness that there are other worlds, other forms of life, in such a way that "living in this multiple world means experiencing freedom as a continuous oscillation between belonging and estrangement" (Vattimo, 1990, p. 86). It is pertinent to mention that Vattimo highlights the value of diversity, tolerance, and plurality; however, some of his contributions have been described as relativistic, because some of his detractors affirm that he places the value of charity above the value of truth, offering an experience of apparent development that masks the real attention that the problems of our time demand.

To conclude this section, emphasis is placed on the paradoxical character that postmodernity offers us regarding the consideration of the other, especially the vulnerable, by balancing between the exaltation of the individual and the opening to the plurality of ways of life. As Giroux (2006) explains, private issues are extolled at the same time that disinterest in values such as empathy, compassion, love, and solidarity grows, subrogating the human condition to the logic of consumption and, consequently, leaving away those who fail to satisfy themselves with these cultural criteria. Additionally, the role of education in all of this is essential, due to the reproductive or critical capacity that it can play and the influence that this entails in the life course of people in vulnerable conditions.

From Reproductionism to Criticism

Before proceeding, it is pertinent to remark that complexity has been a transversal element in the phenomena that have been addressed in this text, and it is that both vulnerability and postmodernity are multidimensionally composed, with various areas of impact and paradoxes that surround us in a wake of uncertainty. Therefore, we could address the problem of vulnerability in postmodernity through various disciplines, but on this occasion the pedagogical approach has been chosen, since, as Bauman (2014) refers, education is part of culture; however, it has the potential to transform it. It is important to highlight that education is not oblivious to postmodernity; it has even been a prolific entity in the production of new narratives (Carbonell Sebarroja, 2016) or, on the contrary, as the reproductionists claim, in the perpetuation of the dominant narratives.

This is why the role of education in attention to vulnerability in postmodernity is emphasized, given that its cultural potential allows to support the human being in the construction of a pertinent ethical scheme in the face of today's social demands. Consequently, within it lies a way to promote charity, justice, and tolerance, although it is also necessary to consider that this change is not exclusive to education but rather requires the sum of multiple efforts. In this regard, Bourdieu (2013, 2018) affirms that within the school inhabits the capacity to build social order; however, this does not mean that the said order is always based on a supportive axiological structure, because sometimes it replicates the existing differences and inequalities in society via "extremely complex mechanisms through which the school institution contributes to reproducing the distribution of cultural capital" (Bourdieu, 2007, p. 33), causing the separation of the heirs of said capital from those who lack it, privileging the former, harming the latter.

In agreement with Bourdieu, Giroux (2014) states that it is necessary to analyze the reproduction systems, due to the enormous responsibility that rests on schools by perpetuating the benefits of the dominant society and the conditions of vulnerability of those who, as a result, are oppressed within this social order. In accordance to the aforementioned and according to Araujo Olivera (2002), the ability to transmit culture is perceived in the school, and it often does so through the narrative of the hegemonic class, reinforcing socially produced inequalities, concealing injustices, and legitimizing an interpretation of learning difficulties as a product of a lack of effort or talent on the part of people from vulnerable groups. It should be noted that, as Bourdieu (2007, 2018) states, the social structure generated through the reproduction of hegemony also subjects those who apparently benefit from this social dynamic, so that, sooner or later, in the culture of abuse and oppression, no one wins.

Although schooling constitutes one of the primary indicators in measuring human development (Rodríguez, 2009), it requires assertive orientation, in accordance with the demands of the current era and guided by a continuous ethical discernment, because, as it has been demonstrated, the school, as an institution entrusted with the social function of teaching, has the potential to define what is legitimate to learn (Bechelloni on Araujo Olivera, 2002). Likewise, schools have a significant influence on the construction of axiological hierarchies, establishing social value and personal value, in addition to the recognition and sense of human dignity (Bourdieu, 2013, 2018). Repeatedly, it is associated with education as the means to access a certain culture that, in the words of Bourdieu (2013, p. 459), "is one of the fundamental components of what makes men consummate in his dominant definition."

In addition, from the criticism of reproductions, concordances with the ethical theses of Lipovetsky and Bauman are found when they affirm that "there seems to be a growing lack of interest on the part of the general population in non-commercial values, such as empathy, compassion, love, and solidarity" (Giroux, 2006, p.120). It is, therefore, not surprising that in postmodernity hyperindividualistic and adiaphoric people can be easily related to the oppressor who seeks the reproduction of the hegemonic system, because both categories exalt the demands of a few above the needs of the community, behaving with indifference toward those who need a fairer management of cultural and economic capital. This is because they have found in the educational institutions a mechanism that can easily be ordered to their own interest, and, as stated by Lipovetsky (2013), the school is one of the main social spaces in which indifference is present. Because of this, as we understand the great influence that education has in both the economic and cultural sector, it becomes easier to perceive the inequalities that are generated and affect those who are more vulnerable (Apple, 2008).

It is true that education in postmodernity, in addition to adopting a fleeting, changing, and consumerist character (Viveros Plancarte, 2005), may perpetrate hegemonic narratives and pronounce inequality and injustice. However, it is equally true that there is an enormous potential in the creation of new narratives that can be constructed through a reflexive and transformative practice. It is essential to clarify that being conscious of the reproductionist characteristics of the school and its potential for violence, both in the material and symbolic spheres, must not overshadow the attention placed on educational institutions. Otherwise, we would fall into a bias that would numb our perception of the hopeful efforts made in schools day by day, and we must not forget that, in the end, the school constitutes one of the primordial factors for the individual and collective development of people (Rodríguez, 2009).

As a result, there is a need for a guiding pedagogical movement that advocates for the transformative and critical nature of education (Carbonell Sebarroja, 2016), in order to bring together the demands of different strata of society for the benefit of a fairer and more equitable community. It is evident that education has a great social responsibility in postmodernity, and the prevailing narratives in culture largely depend on it. Nevertheless, one aspect that cannot be overlooked is that there are various pedagogical approaches that have sought to address the demands of the contemporary world, creating stories that genuinely focus on people in vulnerable conditions, grounded in anthropological perspectives that, albeit with certain specificities and nuances, recognize human dignity, the responsible exercise of freedom, and the creative potential within each person, orienting educational efforts toward a teleology that seeks the development of human potential, the creation of communities, and the happiness of individuals. All of this from an axiological structure based on respect, freedom, fraternity, and, on some occasions, inclusivity.

In response to the ethical conditions and needs posed in both modernity and postmodernity (Viveros Plancarte, 2005), there arises an educational current that serves as a narrative that, in turn, transforms narratives: Critical Pedagogy. This approach emerged toward the end of the twentieth century through the reflexive conjunction of philosophy, sociology, and pedagogy (Araujo Olivera, 2002), hoisting a strong critique against the reproductionist role assigned to the school and recognizing the dignity of minorities by managing structures that promote the vindication of marginalized and less-favored groups. Below, some of the main propositions of perhaps the most representative authors of critical pedagogy are exposed, not without warning the reader that this is a cursory approach.

Definitely, one of the key pedagogues who critically analyzed the responsibility of education in the formation of social order was Paulo Freire. His thinking diverges from totalitarian and unquestionable stances and is open to any ideas that favor a better comprehension of social reality, starting from an anthropological conception that unites the human being with their environment, not as a *subject in the world* but as a *subject with the world* (Freire, 2006), capable of transforming the reality from equality and considering the most vulnerable. However, as Freire (2011) exposes, this process cannot happen without two key elements: awareness and shared experience. Freire's (2007) critical proposal is inspired by Gramsci, who had already denounced the transmissionist and inhumane character of working-class education (Maldonado García, 2014); however, the Brazilian pedagogue highlights the participatory and conscious nature of personal and social development. This allows us to visualize that the path leading the oppressed toward liberation and hope is walked in the community, and it is obvious that this stance opposes hyperindividualism and the adiaphora that are so prevalent in postmodern society.

Furthermore, Freire underpins his pedagogy in an emancipatory social scheme that promotes the recognition of individuals in vulnerable circumstances and aims for the liberation of the less privileged from his own reality, by rejecting the pre-established formulas set by the dominant powers and proposing a situated learning capable of bringing better life opportunities. In the words of Freire himself (2006, p. 73–74): "When reaching this understanding of reality, through collective action and reflection, they discover themselves as its true creators and recreators," thus fostering not just apparent participation but a genuine commitment from the oppressed in their own process of liberation. It's important to clarify that this stance does not wield romanticization or victimization of the people in vulnerable conditions, but it does criticize the structure that makes it more difficult to fight for their rights (Freire, 2007).

Another aspect postulated by Freire (2007) that opposes hyperindividualism and adiaphora, while strengthening the recognition and the freedom of the oppressed, is the dialogue, due to the possibility it offers to encourage the encounter between human beings, especially those who look to transform the world (Palacios, 2014). Moreover, dialogue constitutes an essential element of education, but not from a banking or oppressive perspective rather from a practice of community and freedom, since its exercise allows the reflection and stimulates the awareness of the vulnerable, helping them move beyond their passive and lethargic stance and propelling them toward the practice of transforming reality.

From this perspective, the labor of the professors renounces the exercise of banking education, characterized by the reproduction of content, positioning the Magisterium as a dynamic entity, capable of enhancing conditions that allow the voices of the oppressed to be affirmed. Maldonado García (2014) explains that in Freire there is also a rethinking of the teaching vocation when recovering the integral intention of the critical and transformative intellectual. It consists of a pedagogy substantiated not only in the participatory action but also in the research work. This teaching concept is key in the pedagogical consolidation of methodological approaches such as action research.

While Freire is one of the icons of critical pedagogy, it's important to consider he is not alone and is accompanied by other thinkers who, from different stances, advocate for the same cause. Among these pedagogues, we find the aforementioned Giroux (2014), who stated the idea that schooling requires connecting with other processes of social emancipation and that the school is responsible to competitively prepare students to be critical of themselves and participants of a democratic society, breaking, in this manner, with patterns of indifference and oppression that excluded the underprivileged from political and economic systems.

Giroux explains that to achieve the exercise of a pedagogic discourse that provides opportunities for development and break with the traditional pedagogical proposals, it is necessary for schools to contemplate the dialectic relationship between the students and the historical and cultural context that surrounds them (Bórquez y Bustos, 2015), in this case, the postmodernity and the vision of the school as a contradictory place. This, in light that the school should not precisely embody the same cultural criteria as the rest of the social spaces, as it needs to be a place marked by critical dialogue, composed of both the struggle and adaptation.

In order to achieve a better understanding of the relevance of critical pedagogy under the ethical conditions of vulnerability in postmodernity, it should be noted that Giroux (2006) coincides with the social and political vision of Bauman (2001), especially in the analysis he made on the criteria that govern the democratic life. He states that the pressure of the market has exalted the privatized notion of citizenship, shifting the value of the public compromise and the possibility to collectively resolve urgent problems. To reach this commitment, the radical pedagogy (Giroux, 2014) proposes a technical, hermeneutic, and emancipatory rationale, sustained in the social critical theory.

The dialogue between these two authors facilitates the understanding of social dynamics and the construction of an educational model that contributes to the emancipation of the human being by favoring a better positioning of the community from an axiology that, based on respect and commitment to the other, contrasts with the previously mentioned hyper-individualistic and adiaphoric tendencies. Giroux also highlights Bauman's proactive stance, for whom "one of the central educational obligations in the current era is to provide forms of pedagogy that encourage a respect for public life and provide the conditions to convert private problems to public considerations" (Bauman en Giroux, 2006, p. 123). From this standpoint, the proactive character of struggle and conflict is highlighted as an essential part of educational analyses, because, in their absence, schools would be limited to mere instructional exercises.

We cannot conclude without mentioning Jürgen Habermas, who, through his philosophical and sociological contributions in the *Theory of Communicative Action* (Habermas, 1987), has strongly influenced critical pedagogies. In accordance with Maldonado García (2014), Habermas proposed the rational fusion between the objective world and the intersubjective world, through the construction of knowledge as a result of the actions that the subjects execute and the arguments they build around said actions, thus constituting the exercise of a communicative rationality. Likewise, the concept Habermas (1987) made about society stands out; it is understood as an organic structure composed of the life of the private sphere and the sphere of public opinion, as well as a system, whose political and economic dimensions build an energized network via relationships based on money and power (Carbonell Sebarroja, 2016).

This systemic composition reformulates the consideration of collectivity, in which people are capable to hold a dialogue that deals with the differences and promotes consensus, in order to generate agreements and promote actions that facilitate the transformation of social life through communicative action where language behaves as a mediating element and promoter of criticism, reflection, and understanding. Some of these constructs proposed by Habermas (1987) have been transferred to the educational field via the *Critical Theory of Education* (Karr & Kemmis, 1988), who fundamentally fosters critical awareness of people regarding the social and historic dispositions that have affected the subjective meanings and that have led to a distorted self-perception of vulnerable individuals. This is, therefore, a self-critique that, along with a critique of the system, allows the development of an ethic of self-realization and collaboration, always from a dialectical relationship between theory and practice as motor axes of social transformation.

As shown, albeit briefly, the practices proposed by critical pedagogies promote social transformation and the liberation of the oppressed through awareness, dialogue, participatory action, and different forms of rationality, reconfiguring self-perception and positioning of vulnerable individuals within the system, helped by the investigative and reforming action of teachers, who become transformative intellectuals. However, it is important not to overlook that one of the elements that has the most influence on these processes is the curriculum, as its composition will be almost decisive in shaping the direction of learning. Carbonell Sebarroja (2016) explains that to achieve this path of emancipation, a curriculum is required to, in accordance with the ideas of Vattimo (1991), respect social and cultural diversity, especially that of the marginalized and excluded strata, always in consideration of the environment and with a hopeful vision of reality.

On the Pertinence of a Dynamic Conclusion

> The new critical conception of education conceives students as cultural producers and not as simple passive consumers. Thus, educators and students must regain confidence in education as one more means to fight against the current situation of growing inequality and injustice. (Viveros Plancarte, 2005, p.67)

If something has characterized this writing, it is the plural and dynamic nature of the phenomena presented here, which is why it would be contradictory to establish a static conclusion, at least from a determining perspective. The problem of vulnerability is far from over and its anthropological inherence invites us to maintain constant reflection. Because of this, only a dynamic conclusion can be offered, subject to the changes to come. Hence, it is conceived that postmodernity, in its different discourses, offers a multiform and diverse panorama, incapable of being valued from a single ethical position. We find elements that, receding from a polarized vision, can favor or harm the relationship we have with the other, particularly with the most defenseless. This means that, in postmodernity, the direction that human action takes is of the utmost importance, as the attention given to people in conditions of vulnerability will oscillate between the different ethical nuances that comprise it, so that it is recognized through an attitude that embraces the least favored, promotes common responsibility, and respects for differences or that, on the contrary, it indifferently excludes those who are not capable of living up to the individual competition legitimized via the criteria imposed by the logic of consumption.

The problem of vulnerability in postmodernity is complex in composition, which is why it can be interpreted through different disciplines and at multiple levels of epistemological relationship, but on this occasion, an approach from pedagogy has been chosen, not because it holds the exclusive answer but because it identifies the potential to influence the processes of shaping individual and collective consciousness, as well as promoting social order and the fair distribution of the different types of capital. For this reason, it is necessary to estimate the vital responsibility of education in the attention to vulnerability, since just as it is capable of behaving as a means of reproducing the hegemonic system for the benefit of a privileged few, increasing inequality and injustice, it can promote awareness, inspire reflection, and promote transformation from a critical pedagogy that, rather than seeking the interest of a few, is committed to dialogue, collaboration, tolerance, and respect for the other.

To conclude, it is pertinent to mention that, although critical pedagogies assertively address the demands presented here, they do not exhaust the problem of vulnerability in postmodernity; thus, there is an appeal to review other contemporary educational currents whose theoretical and methodological principles favor an increasingly deep and complete approach to the subject, for example, the pedagogies of inclusion and cooperation, the slow pedagogies, or the pedagogies against cruelty. Additionally, it has been emphasized that education is not the only way to care for people in conditions of vulnerability, which is why interdisciplinary or transdisciplinary work is required and, above all, a personal commitment so profound that it has no other option but to manifest through testimony. We must not forget that the problems exposed here are not foreign to us; we are not talking about a distant reality but about a problem that escapes the pages of books and that takes shape in faces and concrete life stories.

References

Apple, M. (2008). *Ideología y currículo*. Akal.

Araujo Olivera, S. (2002). *Paulo Freire: Pedagogo crítico*. UPN.

Bauman, Z. (2001). *En busca de la política*. Fondo de Cultura Económica.

Bauman, Z. (2013). *Ética posmoderna*. Siglo XXI.

Bauman, Z. (2014). *Sobre la educación en un mundo líquido*. Paidós.

Bauman, Z. (2015). *Vida líquida*. Paidós.

Bauman, Z., & Donskis, L. (2015). *Ceguera moral*. Paidós.

Blanco Gálvez, J. (2007). *La ética de la interpretación de Gianni Vattimo en el contexto de la posmodernidad*. A Parte Rei.

Bórquez Bustos, R. (2015). *Pedagogía crítica*. Trillas.

Bourdieu, P. (2007). *Razones prácticas: Sobre la teoría de la acción*. Anagrama.

Bourdieu, P. (2013). *La distinción*. Taurus.

Bourdieu, P. (2018). *La reproducción: Elementos para una teoría del sistema educativo*. Siglo XXI.

Bustos, M. (2009). *La paradoja posmoderna: Génesis y características de la cultura actual*. Encuentro.

Carbonell Sebarroja, J. (2016). *Pedagogías del siglo XXI: Alternativas para la innovación educativa*. Octaedro.

Cassirer, E. (2016). *Antropología filosófica*. Fondo de Cultura Económica.

Debord, G. (2018). *La sociedad del espectáculo*. La marca editora.

Freire, P. (2006). *Pedagogía del oprimido*. Siglo XXI.

Freire, P. (2007). *Pedagogía de la esperanza*. Siglo XXI.
Freire, P. (2011). *La educación como práctica de la libertad*. Siglo XXI.
Giroux, H. (2006). *Estudios culturales, pedagogía crítica democracia radical*. Popular.
Giroux, H. (2014). *Teoría y resistencia en educación*. Siglo XXI.
Habermas, J. (1987). *Teoría de la acción comunicativa I. Racionalidad de la acción y racionalización social*. Taurus.
Jaspers, K. (1989). *Introducción a la filosofía*. Círculo de lectores.
Karr, W., & Kemmis, S. (1988). *Teoría crítica de la enseñanza*. Martínez Roca.
Lipovetsky, G. (2013). *La era del vacío*. Anagrama.
Lipovetsky, G., & Serroy, J. (2009). *La pantalla global: Cultura mediática y cine en la época hipermoderna*. Anagrama.
Lipovetsky, G., & Serroy, J. (2014). *La estetización del mundo: Vivir en la época del capitalismo artístico*. Anagrama.
Lyotard, J. (1991). *La condición postmoderna*. REI.
Maldonado García, M. (2014). *Pedagogías críticas: Europa, América Latina, Norteamérica*. NEISA.
Palacios, J. (2014). *La cuestión escolar: Críticas y alternativas* (4th ed.). Coyoacán.
Pizarro, R. (2001). *La vulnerabilidad social y sus desafíos: Una mirada desde América Latina*. CEPAL.
Rodríguez, M. (2009). *La educación básica como derecho social fundamental*. FLAPE.
Spitzer, B. (2018). *Demencia digital*. Ediciones B.
Torralba Roselló, F. (2010). Hacia una antropología de la vulnerabilidad. *Forma, 2*, 25–32.
Vattimo, G. (1990). *La sociedad transparente*. Paidós.
Vattimo, G. (1991). *Ética de la interpretación*. Paidós.
Vattimo, G. (2013). *Adiós a la verdad*. Gedisa.
Viveros Plancarte, G. (2005). *Enfoques pedagógicos para la enseñanza de hoy*. Pax.

Part IV
Conclusion

Working with Vulnerable Populations: Final Reflections and Implications

Susana Castaños-Cervantes, Angélica Ojeda García, and Cristina L. Reitz-Krueger

Living in emerging and developing countries is characterized by multiple social disadvantages, inequities, injustice, marginalization, and exclusion that increase the risk of becoming vulnerable. People who grow up in these countries struggle to cope with hardships in the face of recurring illness, natural disasters, and other hazards without adequate systems, structures, and internal resources. In this context, resilience is undermined and paves the way for vulnerability (Proag, 2014), leading to the existence of vulnerable groups such as indigenous groups, migrants, the mentally and/or physically impaired, individuals with low income and education, and those in rural and remote countries, which suffer from social deprivation and disadvantages and multiple inequities. Hence, a vulnerable group is one whose specific characteristics place it at a higher risk of needing humanitarian assistance than others or is more susceptible to damage or risks due to social disadvantages (Barros-Ferreira et al., 2021).

However, what does it mean to be vulnerable? According to the Oxford English Dictionary (2018), vulnerability is the quality or state of being exposed to the possibility of being attacked or harmed, physically or emotionally. Thus, vulnerability is a conditional characteristic of human beings because it is dependent on the internal resources (e.g., personality, attitudes, strengths, capabilities) of an individual and on the environment, which alludes to external resources (access to quality healthcare, education, job opportunities, public policies) (Clark & Preto, 2018).

S. Castaños-Cervantes (✉)
Escuela de Psicología, Facultad de Ciencias de la Salud, Universidad Panamericana, Ciudad de México, Mexico
e-mail: scastanos@up.edu.mx

A. Ojeda García
Universidad Iberoamericana, Ciudad de Mexico, Mexico

C. L. Reitz-Krueger
Department of Psychology, Warren Wilson College, Asheville, NC, USA

S. Castaños-Cervantes et al. (eds.), *Working with Vulnerable Populations*,
https://doi.org/10.1007/978-3-031-67710-6_21

In this context, vulnerability plays a prominent role in academic, governmental, and everyday accounts of the human condition. Policymakers and practitioners are now concerned with addressing vulnerability through various interventions.

Therefore, as the world becomes increasingly connected and localities become more diverse, researchers and practitioners working to ameliorate human suffering cannot rely on one-size-fits-all solutions, particularly for the most vulnerable members of society. This edited collection, broken into three sections—Physical, Psychological, and Social Vulnerability—explores vulnerability in many forms and among diverse populations.

Part I of the Book explored physical vulnerability across several domains, such as disabilities and employment (Chap. 1), effects of pathogens in hospitals (Chaps. 2 and 3), doctor-patient communication (Chap. 4), physical activity with vulnerable children (Chap. 5), and chronic illness and the internet (Chap. 6). This part of the book adds to the growing body of literature on physical vulnerabilities. It paves the way for designing research-based and culturally competent programs to help improve the quality of life of physically vulnerable groups, particularly in the context of low- and middle-income countries.

Part II delved into characteristics and situations that may render someone psychologically vulnerable (e.g., high-stress work environments, extreme poverty, exposure to organized crime) and also examined promising approaches to working with individuals who are at risk of being psychologically vulnerable such as medical students (Chap. 7) and who are already psychologically vulnerable like indigenous communities (Chap. 8), children with autism disorders (Chap. 9), mentally ill patients (Chap. 10), Palestinian refugees (Chap. 11), and Mexican homeless females (Chap. 12). We hope this growing body of knowledge can help inform policies and interventions for at-risk groups that can positively impact their well-being and mental health and that have the potential to increase psychological resources and better adaptation to stress and adverse circumstances, prevent psychopathology, and enhance resilience and traumatic healing.

In the final section (Part III), our authors examined vulnerabilities that are partly due to sociocultural conditions and identities. In many ways, this section unites the other two by considering how individual identities and life circumstances interact with culture and other environmental factors to exacerbate both physical and psychological risk potentially. In this vein, it is essential to note that what may create a vulnerability in one culture could be a neutral or even protective factor in other cultures. As such, one cannot examine any vulnerability without considering the broader context in which it exists. This also speaks to the importance of intercultural competence for human service providers and cross-cultural collaborations in the research domain. Being too immersed in one's own culture may inadvertently close our eyes to the vulnerabilities of others. Therefore, this section covers a broad spectrum of social vulnerabilities from children placed in residential care (Chap. 13), ancient Nahuatl-speaking people (Chap. 14), inmates (Chap. 15), victims of sexual assault (Chap. 16), women and religion (Chap. 17), and femicide (Chap. 18) to training of psychologists (Chap. 19) to pedagogical guidelines (Chap. 20) for appropriately addressing these vulnerabilities mentioned above. This section highlights how vulnerability is a complex construct needing various interventions and approaches to tackle social problems effectively. Therefore, we propose, aligned with the statements of Kuran et al. (2020), that intersectionality be used as a guiding principle in risk and crisis management to provide a better and more nuanced picture of vulnerabilities and vulnerable groups. As a result, national and local authorities and agencies will be able to develop culturally competent and specific actions to address the needs and specific characteristics of those deemed vulnerable and to clearly identify differences between the same vulnerable groups and among different vulnerable groups, avoiding homogenization and inappropriate representation.

Consequently, this book aims not to present exhaustive solutions to any of the problems discussed therein but to offer examples of the considerations that should be afforded when working with groups with unique vulnerabilities. Through the case studies, original research, and literature reviews presented in this collection, students and professionals interested in public health, social work, psychology, and other helping professions will gain insight into how work being conducted in various localities speaks to the challenges they may face on their own. By exploring the unique issues facing vulnerable populations around the globe, we can apply those same considerations in our own communities.

Once again, this edited collection explores diverse, understudied, vulnerable populations worldwide from different perspectives. With interdisciplinary contributors from four continents, working in diverse fields such as social psychology, pedagogy, community psychology, medicine, sociology, clinical psychology, anthropology, and social work, the collection brings together theoretical and applied research evidence on three vulnerable population categories: physical vulnerability, psychological vulnerability, and social vulnerability. The collection explores characteristics and profiles of diverse, vulnerable groups, intervention strategies, and recommendations for public policy actions, particularly in developing and emerging countries. It does not focus on a specific vulnerability parameter or a particular population group. It argues the need for interdisciplinary research and action and challenges popular discourse on vulnerable groups in Western societies and developed countries. It provides experiences and health and social needs of critical vulnerable groups. It presents an engaging social science perspective relevant to everyone, exploring how we and society care for the vulnerable. Each chapter defines and explores a vulnerable group, bringing theoretical, policy, and practical perspectives together. Furthermore, each chapter provides knowledge and understanding of critical vulnerable populations and intervention strategies that may help diminish vulnerable conditions and enhance quality of life.

Lastly, in this book, we sought to explore and elucidate the multifaceted nature of vulnerability, examining its manifestations across different contexts, particularly from non-Western environments, its underlying determinants, and its implications for policy, practice, and social change. We aim to deepen our understanding of physical, psychological, and social vulnerability through interdisciplinary and multicultural perspectives, foster critical dialogue, and inspire meaningful action toward building more equitable and resilient societies, including challenging current Western perspectives about vulnerable groups and intervention strategies.

We conclude here by highlighting three key features of vulnerability across non-Western societies. First, there is a need to apply an intersectionality lens to understand and tackle vulnerability since although characteristics like poverty, ethnicity, disability, age, and gender have received some attention concerning the notion and realities of vulnerability in policy and practice, less is known about how these may shape other dimensions of difference, such as household status, migration, religion, and sexuality. Second, we argue the importance of developing specific policies and practices that consider context and vulnerability and include the perspectives and experiences of stakeholders, practitioners, service managers, and staff of institutions providing services for vulnerable groups. Third, there needs to be more focus on vulnerability research in low- and middle-income countries, which reveals policy and practice shortcomings and biases that need to be addressed and critically approached, especially with how vulnerability is lived and experienced in contemporary society.

References

Barros Ferreira, J. B., Ribeiro, L. C., Rodrigues Fracon, B. R., & Wong, S. (2021). Vulnerability and primary health care: An integrative literature review. *Journal of Primary Care & Community Health, 12*, 21501327211049705. https://doi.org/10.1177/21501327211049705

Clark, B., & Preto, N. (2018). Exploring the concept of vulnerability in health care. *CMAJ: Canadian Medical Association Journal, 190*(11), E308. https://doi.org/10.1503/cmaj.180242

English Oxford Living Dictionaries. (2018). *Vulnerability*. https://en.oxforddictionaries.com/definition/vulnerability

Kuran, C. H. A., Morsut, C., Kruke, B. I., Krüger, M., Segnestam, L., Orru, K., Nævestad, T. O., Airola, M., Keränen, J., Gabel, F., Hansson, S., & Torpan, S. (2020). Vulnerability and vulnerable groups from an intersectionality perspective. *International Journal of Disaster Risk Reduction, 50*, 101826. https://doi.org/10.1016/j.ijdrr.2020.101826

Proag, V. (2014). The concept of vulnerability and resilience. *Procedia Economics and Finance, 18*, 369–376. https://doi.org/10.1016/S2212-5671(14)00952-6

Index

S. Castaños-Cervantes et al. (eds.), *Working with Vulnerable Populations*, https://doi.org/10.1007/978-3-031-67710-6